"I was first introduced to Dr. Marcia Sue Cohen-Liebman and her work in forensic art therapy 25 years ago when she provided a pre-conference course/workshop on the topic at the national AATA conference. I fortuitously – dare I say, accidentally – found myself in the room, listening to some of Dr. Cohen-Liebman's new [to me] and innovative ideas on how to use drawings in forensic investigations and testimonies. Immediately following, we had a brief discussion on forensic art therapy, its importance in the field and how important it was to differentiate from art therapy in forensic settings. This evolved into numerous conversations, one article, several presentations and a long-lasting mutual respect and friendship.

I have been following Dr. Cohen-Liebman's illustrious career closely with admiration and glee over the years as she has continued to hone and expand her expertise. She continues to serve as a stalwart bellwether in developing resources and training to successfully and ethically provide valid forensic art therapy.

A number of years ago, I found myself in a situation where I was asked to testify on the art completed by a man on trial for murdering one of his children and attempting to kill his other. I knew who I needed to turn to for advice and counsel – and Dr. Cohen-Liebman was readily and enthusiastically available, providing comprehensive support with patience, diligence and care regarding judicial and testimonial process and procedure. At that time, there were only a few resources available about forensic art therapy, and fewer still that deconstructed carefully and in detail systematic forensic art therapy processes and strategies; the majority of which were provided by Dr. Cohen-Liebman. It is perhaps needless for me to say that I have been waiting patiently for this book for a very long time.

Well, the wait is now over, and *Forensic Art Therapy: The Art of Investigating, Interviewing and Testifying* fulfills all expectations. This book truly is the culmination of Dr. Cohen-Liebman's life's work, and it is apparent she was not going to release it until she was ready – not until she carefully dotted each "i" and cautiously crossed each "t" to diligently and clearly communicate these very sensitive procedures and experiences. And we, the readers, are better for this.

Through detail and deconstruction, and her artful examples and vignettes, Dr. Cohen-Liebman simultaneously demystifies the practice of applying an art therapy-based process to investigative procedures while systematically demonstrating the intricate and careful knowledge needed to robustly and ethically investigate, interview and testify. As a result, she has created the ultimate resource to be used by those faced with the daunting task of forensic engagement and throughout Dr. Cohen-Liebman demonstrates why she is *the* forensic art therapist."

David E. Gussak, *PhD, ATR-BC, Florida State University, professor of art therapy and project coordinator of the FSU/FDC Art Therapy in Prisons Program*

"A book on forensic art therapy has been needed for a very long time. This socially and culturally vital domain is one where the specialized understandings of a sophisticated art therapist can make a critical difference in determining the truth. The author's vast experience in the delicate process of forensic investigation with youngsters who have been victims of or witnesses to abuse is unique and therefore extremely valuable. All who are involved in seeking justice for traumatized children will benefit from her thoughtful creation of a protocol that helps little ones tell their stories through art. This book is a wonderful and welcome gift to the professional community."

Judith A. Rubin, *PhD, ATR-BC, former president and honorary life member of the American Art Therapy Association, and author of* Child Art Therapy, The Art of Art Therapy, Introduction to Art Therapy and Artful Therapy

"The expertise and wisdom shared in this book is welcomed and long overdue for all clinicians who work with traumatized children. Children, equipped with developing cognitive and language skills, often struggle to explain the horrors of abuse through words. These trauma-informed methods to integrate verbal and art interventions are proven effective, promoting novel approaches to investigate and document childhood sexual abuse. The Common Interview Guideline (CIG), explained in great detail, provides clinicians with the structure to gain critical evidence amidst the often overwhelming context of abuse. Dr. Cohen-Liebman, a well-recognized expert in this field, has documented her findings following more than two decades of research and clinical work. Developed through practices of great insight and compassion, the CIG is a sensible and well-informed approach. Outlined recommendations are supported by extensive explanations of how trauma impacts the mind and body in childhood. Clinicians of all disciplines can benefit from this book for the courageous treatment of childhood abuse."

Marygrace Berberian, *LCAT, ATR-BC, LCSW, clinical assistant professor and director of the NYU Art Therapy in Schools Program, New York University*

Forensic Art Therapy

Forensic Art Therapy is designed as an educational and informative resource for individuals from a diverse array of disciplines that engage in investigatory undertakings, interview victims and witnesses, and provide evidentiary testimony.

The material presented serves as a primer for professionals that may potentially present in court on behalf of a client. Ethical issues inherent in the forensic arena, as well as the use of novel scientific evidence in the form of drawings, legal proceedings, testimonials, and practical tips and strategies for effective witnessing, are shared. Research regarding a forensic art therapy investigative interview process, the Common Interview Guideline, examines the facilitative factor associated with the effect of drawing. When utilized as a primary resource within investigative interviews, drawing has the potential to offer support, promote empowerment and enhance disclosure. Understanding how drawing functions in investigative interviews and what it offers for the child, the team and the process contributes to ongoing research and best practice.

The text serves as a resource and a handbook for students and professionals that investigate, interview, testify and intervene on behalf of child victims and witnesses from the domains of child protection, law enforcement, prosecution, the judiciary, creative arts therapies, social work and allied practitioners in medicine and mental health.

Marcia Sue Cohen-Liebman, PhD, ATR-BC, LPC, LPAT, is a forensic art therapist, child interview specialist, educator and child advocate who assists victims and witnesses of interpersonal violence, maltreatment and traumata.

Forensic Art Therapy

The Art of Investigating, Interviewing, and Testifying

Marcia Sue Cohen-Liebman

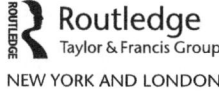
Routledge
Taylor & Francis Group

NEW YORK AND LONDON

First published 2023
by Routledge
605 Third Avenue, New York, NY 10158

and by Routledge
4 Park Square, Milton Park, Abingdon, Oxon, OX14 4RN

Routledge is an imprint of the Taylor & Francis Group, an informa business

Library of Congress Cataloging-in-Publication Data
Names: Cohen-Liebman, Marcia Sue, author.
Title: Forensic art therapy : the art of investigating, interviewing and testifying / Marcia Sue Cohen-Liebman.
Description: New York, NY : Routledge, 2023. | Includes bibliographical references and index. | Identifiers: LCCN 2022039417 (print) | LCCN 2022039418 (ebook) | ISBN 9781032125367 (hbk) | ISBN 9781032125343 (pbk) | ISBN 9781003225041 (ebk)
Subjects: LCSH: Forensic psychology. | Art therapy.
Classification: LCC RA1148 .C64 2023 (print) | LCC RA1148 (ebook) | DDC 614/.15—dc23/eng/20221122
LC record available at https://lccn.loc.gov/2022039417
LC ebook record available at https://lccn.loc.gov/2022039418

ISBN: 978-1-032-12536-7 (hbk)
ISBN: 978-1-032-12534-3 (pbk)
ISBN: 978-1-003-22504-1 (ebk)

DOI: 10.4324/9781003225041

Typeset in NewBaskerville
by Apex CoVantage, LLC

Pour mes enfants, Les amours de ma vie,
Tu es mon coeur et mon âme

It is no revelation that you are my inspiration and my motivation
You foster determination, devotion, dedication
Do not let the imprudence of procrastination rob you of aspirations
Make each moment purposeful, meaningful, joyful
May perseverance and passion guide, drive, impel and fulfill you
Follow your heart, pursue your goals, trust your judgment, and stay
    true to your ideals
Share your gifts with the world
Impart your goodness
Impact others through deeds, words, thoughts and actions
Engender compassion, kindness and forgiveness
May truth, candor, and respect resonate within your convictions
Be responsive and receptive
Genuine and authentic in your endeavors and pursuits
Possibilities and potentialities are endless; listen, learn, discover,
    explore
L'dor V'dor – from generation to generation
For your patience, understanding and love, *todah rabah*

Contents

Acknowledgements

I have always been fascinated by the narratives that shape, define or connote existence, whether through fate, faith or destiny. Perhaps individuals either erroneously or expectantly determine through trial, error or chance how life unfolds. Perhaps this interest or curiosity transposed my path to facilitating accounts of experienced events through imaginal and verbal expression. To help others uncover, decipher, process, resolve and integrate on some level that which cannot be articulated in a linear form.

Reassessing the circuitous route that we embark upon as we transverse our unknown path hopefully stimulates awareness of self and other and promotes insight and cultivates interest while contributing to expansion of mind, memory, intellect and enquiry. Indelibly, the individuals we encounter and the cumulative experiences we collect underlie how we progress, develop and improve individually and professionally.

The circuitous route, unknown and unscripted; fosters perspective; influences worldview and impacts acquisition of information, knowledge and material that may be viewed and incorporated on a conscious or unconscious level be it provocative or propitiatory or mollifying in some way. Within our collective conscious lies the filaments of the myriad of experiences and expectations that emanate from the individuals and events or happenings encountered as we journey through life.

An array of individuals has contributed and, in some manifestation, shaped my path and impacted my lived experience through direct contact or transitory influences. I credit many with challenging me to see different, hear louder, ignore boundaries and pursue my vision. I am humbled by the reciprocity of words, levity, support and succor whether covertly or overtly. Although some may be unaware of the indelible mark left by a mere comment, a singular thought or the commingling of ideas, I wish to convey my sincerity and gratitude for the time, aptitude and propensity that others have selflessly shared, whether known or unknown, deliberate or unintentional. The confluence of so many factors, facets and personalities have impacted what I have cultivated and continue to pursue. Many have provided, whether intentionally or not, guidance, support, sustenance and, yes, silence when appropriate and needed. The power in silence speaks volumes. Responsive listening underlies self-awareness.

Many garner acknowledgement and gratitude for time and talent, intellect and truth. Various realms intertwine, blurring friendship and kinship. To the varied family, friends, supporters and influencers from the realms of art therapy, investigative interviewing, child advocacy and related yet diverse disciplines, as well as students, professionals, practitioners, clients, nonoffending caretakers, thank you for entrusting me to listen, support, dialogue, teach, learn, receive and share. Your receptivity and engagement have truly inspired and enabled me to continue to grow and develop on so many levels.

Believing in oneself is not a given, one must learn to do so through the interactions and feedback that one is afforded through authenticity, veracity, generosity and reciprocity.

Spheres of gratitude commingle with recognition and acknowledgement. First and foremost, Ellen Horovitz, without you there would be no manuscript in its current vestige. Without Ellen this book would not have come to fruition, as it was Ellen who cultivated, mentored and fostered the belief that indeed this just might materialize into a viable resource for professionals, including art therapists and others that work to effect change and advocate for others within and external to the legal system. Thank you for your introductions and your encouragement. You have been onboard with this project since the beginning, and I have you to thank for your graciousness, your consummate professionalism, insight, wisdom and truthfulness. Your belief in me and your unwavering support are incredible, just like you. You have given so much of your precious time and encouraged me. I cannot thank you enough for all of your optimism when I was pessimistic and for helping me to keep moving forward. Thank you for your indelible commitment to this project and to being the most ardent champion of this material. Your recognition of the need for dissemination of it and your commitment to the potential value and impact of this text is inspiring and heartening. I thank you for sharing your participation in the forensic arena and for allowing me to work with you in this context. You are inspirational, genuine and one of the most incredible people I know. You are simply amazing on so many levels and in so many ways! You are so talented, creative and spirited. Thank you for the many gifts that you bestow through your very presence and essence; friendship, mentorship, authenticity, faith and so many more.

Dave Gussak, from the beginning you have been one of my staunchest supporters. I thank you for beginning a dialogue so long ago that truly was transformational and proved to be impactful. It continues to shape the work that each of us has come to own, define and propagate. From our initial conversation (once we dealt with my true identity) the mutual respect and the convergence of thoughts and ideas truly spawned a special working relationship. It has been a most exciting and intriguing path to witness your development and expansion within the forensic arena and the strides you continue to take and create. Thank you for the various roles you have inhabited and for challenging me to keep refining and defining the scope of this sub-specialization. Mostly, thank you for your sense of humor, friendship and unwavering support.

Nancy Gerber, you have been one of my biggest supporters through the years. I thank you for your interest and curiosity which have helped me to expand my worldview and my thought process, especially with regard to my research. I thank you for the countless hours spent in discourse. You have always encouraged me to take my work to a larger audience. I appreciate the support you have demonstrated in my nontraditional focus and application of the modality. You have travelled with me along this path and invested much time and effort to support and guide me, for which I want to thank you.

Sherry Lyons, this work began under your auspices, and for that I thank you. Funny memories of discussing thesis-related material with Peachy, the Moluccan cockatoo, on my shoulder snipping the phone lines as we spoke (yes, really dating myself now with a phone that was attached to a wall via a cord). Never will forget thinking that my defense was going in the wrong direction when we discussed the prospect of an art therapist as a hired gun in a legal proceeding. Fortunately, we got past that, but it was truly a seminal point of discussion. Forever grateful to you for entrusting me to continue the work you began with the psycho-legal practice devoted to custodial matters when you moved West.

Certain individuals permeate our existence and grace our lives. Even though they may no longer inhabit the physical sphere, their presence is no less impactful and engulfing.

Two people dear to me, Ron Hays and Laura Greenstone, both inspiring and elevating forces, in so many ways. Ron was a supporter from day one of this novel approach to the modality. He provided words of encouragement and wisdom as I navigated unchartered ventures. He never faltered in his support. He shared his perspective, and his words provided grounding and an often much needed and welcome reality check with regard to the world I found myself interacting with, which was very different and necessitated a nuanced approach.

My friend Laura Greenstone, who I miss dearly and daily. I know you are clapping. Laura, I thank you for continuing the conversation with me and for your presence in mind, body and spirit. You always had words of inspiration. I miss your wit and keen insight. I recognize the role you played in helping me to see the merit of perseverance. You exhibited such courage and such fortitude in all you committed to and all that you encountered in life, in practice and in the ethics you subscribed to always. May your memory be for a blessing and may your nature transcend existence through the work that continues in your name.

Marygrace Berberian, thank you for your extraordinary patience and steadfastness. You provided an avenue for me to share my work, and I thank you for that and for this. You were so kind and so considerate and so willing to wait for me. Thank you for sharing your thoughts at the beginning of this process. I so appreciate and value your feedback regarding the necessity for this material and the viability of the text as a resource for individuals providing support to the identified populations. I truly am grateful for your time and talent in recognizing the void that exists, and I hope that this manuscript will help eradicate some paucities and contribute to strength-based approaches to fostering resilience in children and youth. Thank you for the opportunity to contribute to your brilliant book and for your continued support.

Judy Rubin, you are indeed one of my favorite people. As I have said, you just make me smile. Your innate personality and outlook are so authentic and genuine. I appreciate you always speaking with me and taking time to chat. Thank you for befriending me so many moons ago and for always being a shining beacon within this profession and to so many people. Your keenness and alacrity with regard to interacting and engaging encapsulate who you are which is so gratifying. Thank you for believing in my work and for your unconditional encouragement and support. Your integrity and honesty are admirable. You are so down to earth, so humble, so warm and so sincere. I am grateful just to be in your orbit. Thank you for the gifts of goodness and kindness that permeate all that you do and all that you are. I am so grateful for your generosity and willingness to endorse this long-awaited project.

For my family and friends, near and far in space, time and heart, my sincerest gratitude for listening to me, loving me and supporting me unconditionally.

Mom

Dad

Kelly

Aunt Cheri

Love and appreciation cannot convey or contain my sentiments but please know how much I value and cherish each of you and all that you give and offer.

LL, thank you for your love and support in every realm and for enabling me to pursue my passions and projects.

In addition to the dedication M & S – just know my hopes for you are high, my dreams are powerful and my love for you is incomparable. Someday I hope you will appreciate how much you taught me as I sojourned along the path of motherhood.

You have been tolerant, considerate, patient, understanding, forgiving and supportive throughout and I thank you for the gifts that each of you are and for loving me without question.

Thank you to the students and professionals I have worked with, learned from and enjoyed meeting in courses, presentations, workshops and trainings. Every course and presentation afford opportunities for enlightenment and altering perspective to encompass ways of seeing not previously entertained or explored. Thank you for your participation, your presence, your interaction, response and engagement.

The children and families that I have had the honor to assist throughout my career, thank you for entrusting me with your narratives, for sharing your imagery and your bravery. I have learned so much about resilience, strength, faith, hope and forgiveness. Thank you for trusting the process and letting imagery provide a means for voice and agency. Each and every one of you have taught me so much and motivated me to work harder, endeavor to do better and think broader about cultivating self-expression. Thank you for helping me appreciate the power of drawing and imagery, as well as the purpose and premise of art therapy to empower those that have been rendered powerless irrespective of circumstances. May vulnerability, hidden truths and forced silence not impede expression, but strengthen and promote it. Strive to find the expressive vehicle that provides sustenance, justice, empowerment, integration and resolution.

My thanks and appreciation as well to those who have participated and assisted me with my research endeavors.

So many others – but truly not enough space to say all of the things I might like to. A few words of thanks to a few special people.

Angelique A. – I owe you such a tremendous amount of thanks and appreciation for always being there for me. Thank you for your unadulterated support. A good friend indeed who listens, provides perspective and is not afraid to challenge me and make me expand my worldview. Always willing to lend an ear and provide me with what I need in the moment and to help me move forward. You are without a doubt one of my biggest and most generous supporters on so many levels and in so many ways. Thank you for always, everything and any time.

The Beckers – Appreciation and gratitude for the many ways you have supported me and shared compassion and creativity.

Cathy L. – You have been there since Hahnemann, and I truly value your friendship and your point of view, always. Through the years we have been through a lot and we share much. Thank you for walking beside me and for your friendship, your insight, your kindheartedness and your openness.

Kathy C. – What can I say, except thank you for your truth, your convictions, your openness, your receptivity and reciprocity. Your positivity and outlook are inspiring as is your perseverance. You do not let life get you down, instead you find the strength and courage to keep moving forward, always. Thank you for sharing your spirit and vitality. We just pick up where we left off – so wonderful to have that kind of support, love, friendship and trust.

Lisa B. – Thank you for being you and for listening and offering support always and unconditionally. You are special in so many ways; friend, mother, believer and supporter.

Carrie L. – I love you for everything that you do and for who you are, my sister, my friend. You are the sweet, considerate, caring, compassionate person that you have always been. You instill hope, faith, love and laughter. Thank you for never doubting and always assisting.

K and A – Family through and through – you have walked this road with me, heard it all and still you root for me, love me and support me. I know I can always count on you both. K your support, presence and truth have and continue to sustain me through life's trials and exaltations. Thank you for all that we have shared and for always being there for me, yesterday, today and tomorrow.

Angelina G. – Your presence is calming. You always create order out of chaos and for that I am in your debt. You are family to me and always will be. Thank you for everything that you do and for always returning with a smile and a sense of humor. Your laugh is precious.

Christine J. – What can I say except thank you. Thank you for always being in my corner and for taking care of business along the way. You provided unbridled support through words and actions. Thank you for truly seeing and acknowledging the value of this work – thank you for saying what others did not – thank you for your goodness, your kindness and your friendship.

Angie A. – Such a kind and giving heart – your generosity knows no limits. Thank you for believing in me, for your encouragement, your uplifting, generous and gracious spirit. You continue to support and inspire via love, fellowship and determination.

Shante M. – How can I not acknowledge you? You have been part of this long and winding road through thick and thin. Memories and moments that have defined these past 20-plus years – wow. Stay true to who you are and never change. Constancy and consistency are treasures that demarcate everlasting relationships.

J.J.F.B. – Strength to you, comfort and peace – your resilience and perseverance are inspiring. I am in awe of you, your powers know no limits and your creativity and tenacity are truly incredible. Sharing, caring and believing – innate traits – thank you from the heart.

Mrs. K. – you know who you are – thank you for your friendship, your clarity, your goodness, your kind and compassionate soul. Thank you for always doing, giving and never questioning. A true mensch.

John Myers – you have been a force throughout the years. I remember one of my initial encounters watching and listening and observing your use of PowerPoint. You changed the focus of my world. Thank you for all that you have done on behalf of children and victims. All that you have contributed to the nomenclature of investigative interviewing and child advocacy. You truly deserve to be acknowledged and recognized. Your indefatigable body of work has influenced and inspired and continues to impact victims and witnesses while enhancing the scope of practice.

So many others, please accept my global thanks for the care, concern and compassion that you have imparted whether in recent years or during the long haul. I know who you are, and I extend my deepest appreciation and ask for your forgiveness for not including each of you here.

Finally, I want to express my deepest gratitude and appreciation to the editorial team at Routledge who were willing to take a risk on an idea. An idea that became a manuscript that was 20-plus years in the making. Through the attention and devotion of a dedicated team, the idea became a reality. I especially wish to acknowledge all that Amanda Savage and Katya Porter did to support this project and see it through to completion. I wish to let you both know that I truly am grateful for all that you did to make this possibility into a reality, and I apologize for any and all inconvenience that transpired along the way. Without your commitment and determination, the potential for this book to exist may not have happened. Thank you from the bottom of my heart. I have learned so much through this process. I thank you for your patience and diligence. Last but not least, I want to acknowledge and thank Balaji Karuppanan, Project Manager and his team at Apex CoVantage for all of the hard work, dedication and assistance in bringing this manuscript to fruition. Thank you all for your time, help, professionalism and support.

> *Crayons and markers, paper and clay these are the tools I use everyday*
> *With media in classrooms the students explore the innate character of materials and more*
> *Rather than spend our time with a textbook which may be irrelevant and perhaps even bore*
> *I implore the students to learn through exposure, via experientials and to pour*
> *Their thoughts and reflections into a visual journal to explore*
> *On a daily basis to cultivate interest, dynamism and more*
> *We record our thoughts and what we have discerned*
> *Through visual depictions in which introspection is born*
> *My teaching philosophy is predicated upon keeping the students engaged and informed*
> *And transferability to real world application of all we have learned*

Foreword for *Forensic Art Therapy*

There are times when being a therapist is difficult. I suppose being in any of the helping professions stirs a similar quandary in others. But there have been several cases that affected me so virulently that I cried, became angry and even questioned ethical responses in others as well as myself (Horovitz, 2005). It's not only that the work is hard but also it places a toll on you. This drain can be in the form of physical, spiritual and/or emotional duress. Those first few raps at the door are very hard and can feel much like your system has become dis-eased. Fortunately for you, the reader, this book has arrived thanks to Dr. Marcia Sue Cohen-Liebman.

In a recent conversation with my brother, Len Horovitz, MD (2022), we spoke about Marcia's book and his present-day experience as a medical expert witness; we both lamented that neither of us had been trained for court-adjudicated situations. He, too, wished there had been a book like Marcia's to prepare him for judicial situations. Unfortunately, it is trial by fire (no pun intended), since while ethical issues may be covered in medical/therapeutic training, preparation for legal issues is sadly ignored.

When looking at factors from a family systems perspective, the toxicity can affect more than the IP (identified patient), thus making the impact even greater. When transitional conflicts are handed down from generation to generation (McGoldrick et al., 1999) (such as in sexual abuse cases), the consequences can be devastating. For most, perpetuating dis-ease is clearly more comfortable than change, and thus family members are apt to continue to recycle the same belief system thus reinforcing the perpetual state of inertia (Bullock, 1998; Horovitz, 1999, 2005, 2020, 2021; Tolle, 1999). It is easier to be wedded to pathology than to embrace change. Most patients that enter therapy are long on pathology and short on change; otherwise, they might not be in our care.

A Failed Promise

In the late 1980s, I had a sexual abuse case whose legal outcome (presented to both a New York and Illinois judge) almost caused me to leave the field. I was contracted by the states of Indiana and New York to work with a young girl, aged eight, herein known as Melissa, who had been sexually abused. Her history was atrocious. From her infancy until she was adjudicated to live with her paternal grandmother and father's aunt, she had been physically neglected and sexually abused. Her abuse was at the hands of two people.

Her father was employed as a janitor at a church. Father's first wife (herein called Cindy 1) had been a prostitute. She was the biological mother of Melissa and her younger six-year-old brother Karl. When she birthed both her children, she performed heinous sexual acts on them, such as sticking dowels up Melissa's vagina and rectum and Karl's rectum, binding them with rope and leaving them in darkened closets for long periods of time. Fortunately, for Melissa and Karl, Cindy 1 left when they were approximately four and two and a half years old, respectively. Shortly after that, father married Cindy 2, who moved in with her 21-year-old brother, Ron. In time, Cindy 2 gave birth to Angela. Ron began to sexually abuse both Melissa and Karl, and I later learned that Karl was forced to have sexual intercourse with the baby in front of Ron. All three children, Melissa, Karl and Angela, were found naked in a detached garage on an old mattress when child protective services intervened after a tip from a neighbor.

Melissa and Karl were taken out of father's custody and placed to live with his mother and sister (in Rochester, New York) (a questionable decision at best), and the baby, Angela, was placed in foster care. Cindy 2 remained with the father, and the father was seeking to regain custody of all children. Karl was placed in therapy with a social worker in a family service agency (with whom I had two joint sessions with the children, paternal grandmother and aunt), both children were adjudicated to the paternal grandmother and aunt, and Melissa was placed into private individual art therapy with me. We had 12 sessions total, one conjointly with her brother, Karl; another with her brother, aunt and paternal grandmother; and our last session was with her father, brother and her brother's social worker.

At best, I was presented with a psychosocial history that so reminded me of the infamous case of *Sybil* (later made into a movie in 2007) that I knew I would be facing a huge undertaking from a legal, spiritual and personal position. Because the case was shared between two states and two different judges, it indeed complicated an already difficult situation.

Since Melissa was in my care, I gave her the following diagnostic tests in the first few sessions: the House Tree Person (HTP) test (Hammer, 1975), the Kinetic Family Drawing (KFD) test (Burns & Kaufman, 1972), the Silver Drawing Test (SDT) (Silver, 1985), the Cognitive Art Therapy Assessment – Clay and Paint (CATA subtest only) (Horovitz-Darby, 1987; Horovitz, 2022) and the Bender Gestalt test for Children (Koppitz, 1963). While she was clearly bright and functioning almost in the age-appropriate range, her responses indicated severe physical, emotional and sexual abuse issues.

During the second diagnostic session, Melissa talked the entire time about Karl's being bad and feeling responsible for him. "Karl gets to sleep with Daddy and Daddy likes him better", she stated. Then she drew the sexually explicit picture of herself and Ron, Cindy 2's brother, who was one of the perpetrators revealed in this case:

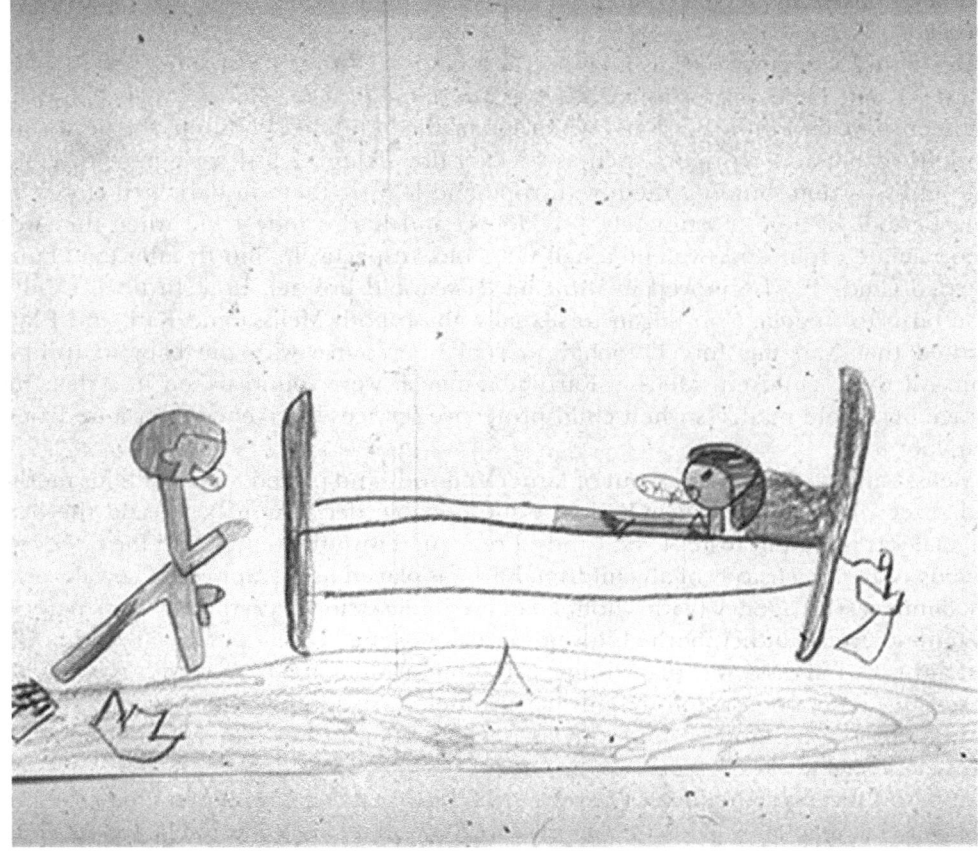

Figure 0.1 Melissa's sexually explicit picture of herself and Ron, one of the perpetrators in this case.

In this picture, Melissa told of the daily circumstances with Ron. He would lock the bedroom door, place the lock in his pants, command Melissa to undress, hang up her dress by the bed and then force her to have sex. In this sexually explicit picture, Melissa is pictured on the bed saying "NO" as Ron approaches her and says "YES". Both are naked.

In the next picture, "SEX that is wut he had" (sic), Melissa places herself again protesting and saying "NO". It is also repeated next to the title on the page. While the picture is like the first, in this rendition, Ron is illustrated penetrating Melissa's vagina. Both these pictures were created in the second meeting. While this might signal that the client is entrusting very private information, given how damaged this child was, it was not such a surprising response. Sexually abused children tend to glom onto passersby quite quickly to obtain the nurturance that they so desperately desire. The sexual abuse literature also attests to this type of behavior, as well as the ultimate confusion of sex, love and loyalty. Clearly, both Melissa and her brother Karl struggled with these issues.

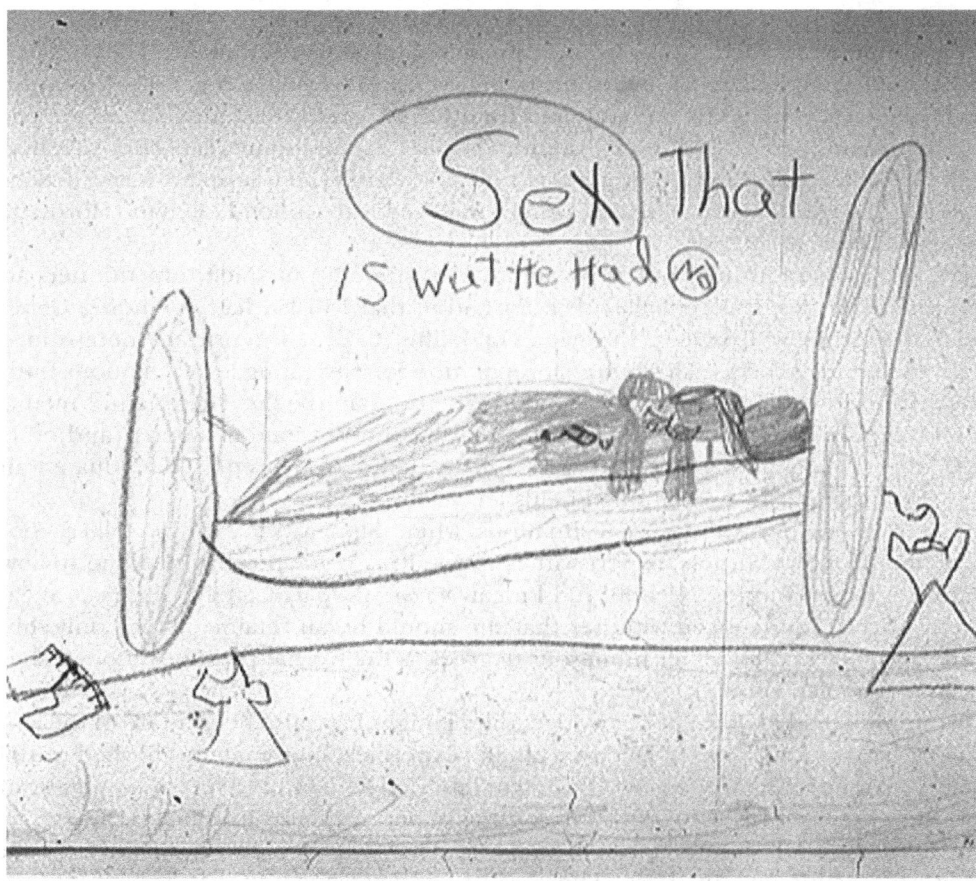

Figure 0.2 Melissa depicted herself protesting and saying "NO" when the perpetrator was sexually abusing her.

Speed ahead months later: The judges from Indiana and New York states deliberated the fate of these children, that is, whether the children should remain in the custody of the paternal grandmother and aunt (and continue therapy) or be returned to the father's charge. Both Karl's social worker and I advocated for the children to remain in New York State and recommended continued individual and family therapy. I submitted a very detailed report of my work with Melissa and Karl and included photographic representation of our sessions, including the artwork. Much to my shock, the Indiana judge disagreed with the New York State judge's recommendation, which concurred with mine. Because Indiana had jurisdiction over this shared case, both Melissa and Karl were yanked from their New York placement and sent back to live with the father.

Shock fails to describe the feelings that emerged after the sentencing of these children's fate. I was stricken to the core. I felt guilty remembering the day that Melissa begged me to take her home and my promise that I would do my best to keep her safe. I failed her, and the system failed her. While her outcome was clearly outside of my control, it didn't stop my feelings of devastation. While unable to alter the Indiana judge's decision, had I the knowledge now available in Marcia's opus, I would have been amply prepared and sought legal counsel for preparation of this case.

Years later, I attended a presentation by Marcia at an American Art Therapy Association conference. I knew I had to bring her to my university as a guest lecturer. In a word, her presentation was brilliant, and I wanted my graduate students to experience firsthand what I had missed in my training. While it is now many years after the aforementioned case had devolved, it matters not, as it wasn't the last time I was called as a witness to the court, the most recent being published with Cohen-Liebman (Horovitz & Cohen-Liebman, 2020).

The preparation in this book is paramount for students, incipient practitioners and seasoned clinicians. It is replete with information that I wish I had, including Cohen-Liebman's formative Common Interview Guideline (CIG), a forensic art therapy investigative interview process. This book is preparation for navigating legal situations future forward and should be a staple in every graduate program (be they therapeutic, medical and/or educational). In fact, I would go so far as to necessitate this book (and others that Cohen-Liebman recommends) as a staple in a stand-alone, required graduate training program in the aforementioned fields.

In fact, in one of my latest legal situations, when talking to Marcia, we talked about everything from lay witness, expert witness, voir dire, to my possibly needing my own counsel as expert witness. No one, and I mean *no one*, prepared me for what was ahead, except Marcia. I have joked with her that she should be on retainer, as the only thing she seems to lack, despite her numerous degrees, is the official JD title, although she is certainly schooled enough.

In addition, had I known of her work earlier, I might have also been aware of the landmark case that spiraled out of Dr. Myra Levck's expert testimony, later published in 1990 (Levick, Safran & Levine). To even have that knowledge to offer to future lawyers would pave the way for more art therapists to serve as expert witnesses in court.

In sum, this book should be required reading not just for graduate health fields but for every practitioner out there. There will be a day when you will be thankful that you have this encyclopedic information at your fingertips to prepare you for the legal challenges ahead. I wish I had this book years ago, but I am ever grateful that Cohen-Liebman has finally amassed this information for all. It is a necessary gift and with that repeatedly, I am in Dr. Marcia Sue Cohen-Liebman's debt. Thank you from your community, present and future.

Dr. Ellen G. Horovitz, ATR-BC, E-RYT500, C-IAYT
Canandaigua, NY
https://yogartherapy.com

References

Bullock, C. (1998). *The path to healing: Experiencing God as Love.* The Assisi Institute.

Burns, R. C., & Kaufman, S. H. (1972). *Action styles and symbols in kinetic family drawings (KFD).* Brunner/Mazel.

Hammer, E. (1975). *The clinical application of projective drawing techniques, fourth printing.* Charles C. Thomas.

Harvey, M. A. (1984, June). Family therapy with deaf persons: The utilization of an interpreter. *Family Process, 23,* 205–221.

Horovitz, E. G. (1999). *A Leap of faith: The call to art.* Charles C. Thomas.

Horovitz, E. G. (2005). *Art therapy as witness: A sacred guide.* Charles C. Thomas.

Horovitz, E. G. (Ed.). (2020). *The art therapists' primer: A clinical guide to writing assessment, diagnosis, and treatment* (3rd ed.). Charles C. Thomas.

Horovitz, E. G. (2021). *Head and HeART: Yoga therapy & art therapy interventions for mental health.* Handspring Publishers.

Horovitz, E. G., & Cohen-Liebman, M. S. (2020). A de novo case: Efficacy, telehealth, and supervision within a legal confine. In E. G. Horovitz (Ed.), *The art therapists' primer: A clinical guide to writing assessments, diagnosis and treatment.* Charles C. Thomas.

Horovitz, L. H. (2022, July 2). Personal Communication.

Horovitz-Darby, E. G. (1987, October). Diagnosis and assessment: Impact on art therapy. *Journal of Art Therapy*, 127–137.

Koppitz, E. (1963). *Bender gestalt test for young children: Research and application.* Grune & Stratton.

Levick, M. F., Safran, D., & Levine, A. (1990). Art therapists as expert witnesses: A judge delivers a precedent-setting decision. *The Arts in Psychotherapy, 17*, 49–53.

McGoldrick, M., Gerson, R., & Shellenberger, S. (1999). *Genograms, assessment and intervention.* Norton.

Silver, R. A. (1985). *The silver drawing test of cognition and emotion.* Ablin Press.

Tolle, E. (1999). *The power of now.* New World Library.

Preface

Drawing is much more than a picture, a tool or a strategy in an investigative interview. This text presents a novel approach to interviewing children about experienced events by elevating drawing from a secondary resource to a primary component within the interview process. This text will introduce and consider the advantages of an art therapy–based investigative interview process that evolved from my work as an art therapist and a child interview specialist.

The intrinsic benefit associated with imaginal expression is central to appreciating drawing as a facilitative agent in the exploration of experienced events that may be traumatic in nature. The text shifts the focus on drawing from an ancillary aid or an adjunct confirmatory tool to that of a primary resource within an investigative interview process. Open-ended prompts or invitational prompts are considered best practice for eliciting free recall and stimulating a narrative response in an investigative interview of a child victim or witness. To understand and appreciate a child's experience when exposed to a traumatic event, marks on paper in tandem with a child's associations are considered within a relational context through examination of an art therapy investigative interview format, the Common Interview Guideline or CIG. Drawing functions as an open-ended prompt within the CIG and serves in a primary capacity.

When utilized as a primary resource within investigative interviews, drawing has the potential to facilitate fact-finding, promote empowerment and enhance disclosure. Understanding how drawing functions in this context and what it offers may provide an alternative to traditional verbal interview processes and contribute to ongoing research about the use of drawing within investigative interviewing, as well as knowledge pertaining to the underlying mechanisms associated with the effect of drawing. A possible outcome of the text may be an appreciation for an art therapy–based interview process and a response to the call for "how, when, and whether drawing should be introduced in forensic contexts" (Pipe et al., 2004, p. 451), as well as to determine the relevance and appropriateness of the use of drawing in forensic interviews (Driessnack, 2005).

This book has been in a formative state for many years. The premise was to capture the essence of forensic art therapy or FAT and provide an orientation and a conversance with the dynamics that underlie the novel practice. This introductory text will provide insight as well as an overview of the origins, the foundations and the procedures associated with this nontraditional art therapy practice. This novel application of the modality is prefaced around three interrelated domains: investigation, interviewing and litigation which encompasses the art of evidentiary presentation, or investigating, interviewing and testifying. The pragmatic nature of the text will position it as a resource and a handbook for students as well as professionals interested in understanding how drawing and art therapy assist in the facilitation of recall, fact-finding and disclosure of information related to experienced events that may be traumatic in nature.

In addition to introducing FAT, the scope of information included will provide a reference and resource for professionals and students on a range of intertwined subjects, including investigative interviewing, effective witnessing, evidentiary material, reporting mandates, multidisciplinary team investigations of child sexual abuse allegations and other relevant topics. This text is long overdue as a complement for the graduate course on FAT I developed, as well as for the workshops, classes and seminars I have conducted and presented through the years.

Routinely, I receive emails or phone calls from art therapists and others seeking advice and consultation with regard to courtroom participation, effective witnessing and drawing as evidentiary material. I have toted and tripped on plastic bins and cardboard boxes of materials for many years. I have spent time and money at Kinkos and Staples collating packets of information and resources which have been inserted into green notebooks and folders. As I have told participants through the years, keep the packet – some day you might need it. To this effect, I have provided consultation and instruction to individuals potentially engaged in courtroom proceedings, something that I find is often lacking in graduate school curriculum. When one is subpoenaed to appear in a courtroom without prior exposure, training or guidance, trepidation and anxiety manifest. This book will hopefully be an aid to address this paucity and serve as an instructional and resourceful manual for multidisciplinary professionals who confront child maltreatment and serve victims through investigating, interviewing, collaborating and ultimately explicating their role and involvement through testifying in judicial proceedings.

This text will appeal to a multidisciplinary audience, including individuals who intervene at the initial stage of investigation when an allegation of child sexual abuse is suspected. Child maltreatment is not relegated to a specific profession or discipline. As such, individuals from child protection/welfare, law enforcement, prosecution, child advocacy, mental health, medicine and investigative/forensic interviewing, as well as professionals and graduate students in psychology, criminology and the social sciences, along with creative arts therapists, will benefit from exposure and familiarity with the material contained and addressed.

Additionally, this text is intended to offer a contribution to the research and study that pervade the use of drawing within the context of investigative interviewing. The concept presented here, which derived from my practice, is prefaced around art therapy teachings and is an original perspective. Although drawing has been considered and studied with regard to interviewing, it has not been addressed from an art therapy perspective. The information presented here is offered to demonstrate the potentiality of an art therapy–based process in which drawing functions as a primary resource within the investigative interview format. Given the nature of art therapy, which encompasses and integrates ideas and concepts pertaining to the creative process, imagery, a dedicated relational context, and psychodynamics, an appreciation for why drawing from an art therapy perspective as a primary means for enhancing fact-finding will hopefully emerge.

The interview guideline (to be explained) will offer a format that may be modified or adapted according to the population. The guideline is amenable to a myriad of situations and is transferable for investigations by interviewers exploring allegations of an interpersonal nature. The framework for interviewing can be adapted and utilized by professionals to explore experienced events within a construct that is developmentally sensitive, culturally aware and forensically defensible.

The guideline provides a frame for how to establish and maintain rapport, elicit facts and conclude positively while incorporating drawing as an open-ended prompt within the process rather than as a secondary support wherein drawing is introduced after a disclosure or to confirm or clarify a statement. Interviewing is a skill that not every-one is qualified to do, yet understanding the process is important for every member of the investigative team. Information derived from investigative interviews contributes to additional investigative pursuits and determination of interventions and supportive recommendations.

Graduate-level programs designed to prepare students for professional practice in psychology, social work, child protection, law enforcement and creative arts therapies will benefit, given the sections on effective witnessing and judicial and legal tenets, as well as investigative interviewing. This information and knowledge are not part of stand-ard graduate curricula, at least in the creative arts therapies (as far as I know), rendering a dearth of opportunity for comprehension and practice. Guidance directed at court-room participation and even mandated reporting is not always part of advanced train-ing, necessitating on-the-job learning once a situation has surfaced, which highlights a need for education and support.

In a survey conducted as part of my doctoral practicum, creative arts therapists in the Northeast and Mid-Atlantic regions engaged in some form of child advocacy were questioned about preparatory or introductory education. The majority of respondents reported no knowledge or background about the legal system as well as a lack of gradu-ate training directed at preparing for legal involvement. Many expressed that exposure to this material would have made an impact and been beneficial as graduate students for eventual professional interaction. Personal statements by survey respondents indi-cated that most had to acquire information, education and training on the job. Many expressed a lack of enthusiasm for such work given the paucity of programming and instruction designed to familiarize and prepare individuals for possible and often even-tual courtroom engagement as well as effective witnessing.

This text will offer material to supplement programs of study by fomenting awareness and responsiveness that judicial engagement demands. The information is intended to inculcate cognizance of basic stratums that underlie effective witnessing and judiciary acuity, which is predicated upon preparative practice and engagement as well as pre-paratory mindfulness. The manuscript also addresses the basic tenets and constructs associated with FAT, which fills the void for a viable resource and reference tool about this nontraditional application of art therapy.

Although not everyone will work in this capacity, the information pertaining to reporting, testifying, witnessing, judicial protocol and procedure, as well as presenta-tion of evidentiary material in the form of drawing, may at some time in a student's or professional's career be relevant and pertinent regardless of one's affiliation, be that art therapist, social worker, investigator, interviewer, member of a multidisciplinary team or a child advocate. The text is designed to provide information and material to minimize apprehension, combat confusion and instill understanding in an effort to vanquish vul-nerability on the witness stand. The lack of preparation is probably one of the most significant detriments when one is requested to provide testimony within a courtroom context. In the event courtroom attendance is requested or testimonial and evidentiary contributions are mandated, the material presented is offered to quell the unknown, assuage participation and lessen the angst that accompanies such interaction.

Author's Note

The text invites active participation by perusing material in a manner that is most ben-eficial to assist the reader either as a resource, a reference, a guide or an educational and informational text. The material presented in each section is not meant as an isolated entity, but rather it is offered in support of a conceptual framework and as such is related to what precedes and sets the context for what ensues. It is not meant to be presented as inert, but rather in the vein of a Prezi, an interactive and moving presentation where comprehension of information is contingent upon the parts to appreciate the whole (forensic art therapy or FAT) yielding a dynamic construct.

In organizing the material for the text, it was incumbent to present information in a logical and cohesive fashion; however, the difficulty in doing so rendered organizational liberties given temporal and spatial confines. Material is presented in a linear fashion because the configuration dictates such; however, the material is intended to be amalgamated, meaning that information overlaps and interacts, encouraging integration on multiple levels. The text is divided into parts to assist the reader with the acquisition of material applicable to investigating, interviewing, and witnessing culminating in a mock court section. The latter promotes the integration of various information providing the reader with a foundation for effective and compelling testimony. The reader is encouraged to seek out what is most prudent for the intended application whether as a novice or a seasoned professional. As such, perusing the text from cover to cover may not be the goal but rather attending to the material as a resource and supplementary guide may be appropriate. The book concludes with a section devoted to recent research on the use of drawing within the context of investigative interviewing. Significant to this section is the literature review that considers how drawing and drawings have been explored by researchers in various disciplines and how the research has been applied within the realm of investigative interviewing. Also, of note is the section devoted to school-based bullying and the parallels to child sexual abuse which appeal to the call for exploration of different types of victimization and possible associations.

I believe in providing comprehensive and informative resources. I appreciate and understand that too much information can be overwhelming or not purposefully poignant. Collating material from my treasure trove of plastic bins that have long housed my eclectic mash-up of teaching materials, including notes, outlines, hand-outs, supplemental information and PowerPoint slides, the bins continue to gather dust and crack as time moves forward (I should have bought stock in Kinkos and Rubbermaid many years ago). Respectfully, the proffered materials have resulted in provision of a pared-down compilation of supplemental resources and materials for students, professionals and participants in courses, workshops and presentations. Less hard copy and more digital provisions have contributed to select materials organized in a signature green folder or binder. Eventually, I began to succumb to technological advances with regard to collating and distributing materials (such as CDs and jump drives) to be current and environmentally aware.

Frankly, it became too difficult to bring stuffed packets with me when traveling via planes, trains and automobiles. Eventually, it was seemingly prohibitive and too expensive to ship or pack individual resource notebooks for large gatherings, although for many trips I did just that. As I write this, I cannot help but smile at a recollection. Exiting a small regional airport, waiting for me was a dear friend and colleague who was originally set to transport me into town in his teeny tiny, forgive me, "clown car" (the type where a dozen or so clowns pile in at the circus and then disembark and the audience is stunned into disbelief as it counts the number of clowns that emerge from the seemingly confined space). The look on my friend's face was sheer amusement as he surveyed the assortment of suitcases and the medley of hand luggage when I emerged. Fortunately, he and his bestie, an art therapy giant, had decided at the last minute that she would accompany him and much to everyone's relief, drive her (full size) car to the airport before we all went out to dinner. Just the image alone of trying to stuff everything into the clown car (no offense intended to clowns or tiny cars – just my association) catapulted us into hysterics the entire evening.

Through the years, I have received many gifts in the form of pictorial imagery, wherein I am depicted garbed in various hues of green, my favorite color. I like to thank the giver and assure that the artwork is valued, appreciated and will be viewed. That is the premise upon which I share my materials. I encourage students, participants/attendees, professionals and lay readers to consider the included materials as offerings to be tucked away until such time as a situation arises and clarification or edification is sought about a specific (identified) topic.

For many years, I have conducted expert witness forums for various audiences. On occasion, I encounter participants who share personal anecdotal references regarding how the green folder was stashed away in the event of a subpoena or some other court entanglement. One individual who stopped me in a corridor not too long ago, kindly introduced herself and explained that she had attended a workshop of mine years earlier. This former attendee wanted me to know that she had followed my suggestion and put the green folder aside to be retrieved in the event a request was received to appear in court and testify. Much to her chagrin, she received a subpoena to appear in court to discuss her involvement in a particular case. She shared that she thought about the workshop and unearthed the green folder. From it, she was able to cull materials and information to help her prepare and present testimony. It was nice to know that the folder served as a resource and provided some measure of calm for this individual.

As such, the intent for the material contained herein is as a resource or a reference. At the very least the material is intended to serve as a catalyst on the designated topics across the spectrum of readers: professionals, students, multidisciplinary team members or individuals interested in learning more about the featured related and intertwined subjects encompassing art therapy, forensics, investigative interviewing, child abuse and a compendium of related topics, especially the value of the use of drawing within the presented context. Finally, I hope the information serves not only as a scaffold for the courses and workshops I teach but also functions as an implement for the plethora of individuals committed to serving and supporting child victims and witnesses. The intentionality of sharing my narrative and materials extends beyond the picture frame.

Note Regarding Drawings and Imagery Included in the Text

Case examples including vignettes are a result of amalgamated and aggregated cases that represent a diverse populace encompassing child abuse, child custody, domestic violence, interpersonal violence including bullying and other specified populations. The case examples are not intended to represent a particular case, a specific child or a designated family and are fictionalized for demonstration purposes. As such, the imagery presented may not have been specifically created for the fictional vignettes but serves as a means to illustrate the essence of what is communicated and how information is shared within the context of FAT. Identifying information has been masked, altered or reconceived. Although there is much to say about each individual drawing, respectfully, the emphasis for inclusion is not necessarily the pictorial content rather, the artwork fosters contextual understanding. As such, this is not a narrative about the drawings; instead, the drawings are used to elucidate the narrative.

Description of the Text

The intention of collating this material within this context is twofold. First to serve as an orientation to forensic art therapy; second, to provide a resource for students, professionals, art therapists and multidisciplinary team members or just an interested reader who might be required to give testimony or participate in a judicial proceeding and may not have acquired introduction or experience in this realm. The information contained is not merely consigned to a text in support of the corresponding course I developed and taught for many years for second-year master's students. The material contained herein is also supplemental for the expert witness forums I conducted for art therapists and other professionals with regard to effective witnessing and evidentiary presentation. Both platforms demanded a multitude of resource materials and hand-outs. Through the years I complied and compiled accordingly. To have the opportunity to bring into existence a text that explains and contains relevant material in a tangible and manageable format epitomizes the culmination of myriad pursuits. Overall, the text is presented as a resource and guide not only for the course I developed on forensic art therapy but as informative for a wider audience engaged in addressing the compound issues surrounding child maltreatment within the various contexts of investigating, interviewing and testifying.

The first section is informational and provides insight as to how forensic art therapy evolved and emerged. Material is presented narratively with precursors identified that contributed to the development of the sub-specialization of art therapy. The focus then shifts to an investigative interview guideline that is predicated upon art therapy. The latter sections are offered to familiarize and acquaint participants with process, protocol and procedure pertinent to forensic proceedings. A mock court exercise will be discussed with regard to effective witnessing to demonstrate an experiential method of acquiring and honing skills. Practice or training exercises as well as tips accompany the material to assist individuals with the development of efficacious and proficient skills. Finally, recent study of a forensic art therapy investigative interview process will be shared, including findings and implications for future study as well as recommendations. The review of literature salient to the use of drawing within investigative interviewing and related topics is presented. Bullying is also addressed including parallels with child sexual abuse.

The incorporation of drawing into the realm of investigation, which encompasses interviewing, as well as testifying and witnessing, will be considered through anecdotes and modified vignettes to illustrate the benefit and impact drawing affords in service to these separate yet interrelated domains. The advantages associated with the use of drawing for victims and witnesses, investigators and the process of inquiry, as well as presentation of evidentiary material, will be elucidated through consideration of relevant literature and research, as well as exemplars. Each part or chapter includes references, resources and supplemental material.

Summary of Parts I–V

Part I is constructed to introduce forensic art therapy, including the various components that overtly and covertly contributed to the establishment and emergence of the nontraditional application of the modality. The section will define and explain the basic tenets of forensic art therapy, including its origins and the foundational constructs.

Additionally, the operational components that contributed to the development of forensic art therapy are presented and discussed to establish the context from which this application emerged, including multidisciplinary team investigations of child sexual abuse.

Content is presented in a systematic fashion to showcase the development of forensic art therapy, including principles and practices, component elements and relevant features that demarcate the practice. Given the integration of art therapy and judicial precepts, social science and law will be examined to provide context for the commingling of traditionally divergent systems that underlie forensic art therapy. Next, the distinctions and differences, as well as the similarities that pervade forensic art therapy (FAT) and art therapy practiced in forensic settings (FS), related but separate modes of practice, are considered. Specifically, the role of the art therapist, settings, populations, goals and objectives associated with FAT and FS are delineated. Emanating from my original premise that the manner in which I utilized the modality differed from more traditional applications of art therapy, FAT extended the boundaries of art therapy praxis into the nontraditional realm of investigation, which is explained. Different types of interviewing, forensic and clinical, are examined in an effort to clarify the distinctions that demarcate FAT and denote the novel process.

Part II is devoted to discussion of a FAT investigative interview process, the Common Interview Guideline (CIG). The use of and the integration of drawing within the interview process is examined. Drawing is used as an open-ended prompt and functions in a primary capacity in the interview process. The component phases associated with the CIG are explained in depth, and the attendant criteria that accompany each phase will be described. The integration of drawing within the designated phases is addressed and highlighted.

Part III is concerned with legal proceedings, reporting mandates, evidentiary presentation and testifying. Professionals and students, whether or not actively engaged in child protection endeavors, as well as investigatory undertakings, will be presented with information pertaining to judicial process and protocol, as well as testimonial capability and qualification. Ethical issues inherent in the forensic arena and the use of novel scientific evidence in the form of drawing will be discussed.

This section is designed to provide guidance and prudent information for anyone who may find themselves called into court either as a lay/fact or expert witness. The chapter culminates with examination of a landmark case to illustrate how the principles discussed are applied and integrated in a judicial proceeding. The case, *Wilkerson v. Pearson* (1985), established the credibility of art therapists as expert witnesses and the validity of drawings as judiciary aids. General acceptance of art therapy and its reliability within the scientific community was established in the precedent-setting case. The application of legal principles as described in the section, as well as the qualification of an art therapist as an expert witness, will be examined. Review of the case fosters an understanding of the intricacies involved in the complex realm of judicial proceedings and provides a forum for integration of concepts highlighted in the text. The judge discussed the acceptance of art therapy and its reliability in his opinion in the following manner which, when repeated on the witness stand, is impactful:

> This court is satisfied that Art Therapy has a sufficient scientific acceptance and basis. It is not a test such as a breathalyzer that establishes a result given certain facts. Rather Art Therapy is a modality of treatment that is subjective in nature but has

within its discipline fundamental criteria that if found to exist lead to certain inferences and conclusions. To this extent such evidence is reliable.

(*Wilkerson v. Pearson*, 1985, p. 338)

The preparatory work one must engage in prior to the multidimensional experience of
courtroom participation is highlighted and discussed in Part IV. Modeled upon mock
court curriculum, this section will consider litigation tactics and courtroom strategy to
enhance performance on the witness stand. Practice tips pertaining to preparation, presentation and qualification are highlighted. Tips for effective witnessing are presented,
and practice exercises are described. The section is essentially a primer for anyone who
may end up in court and be required to provide testimony and present evidentiary
material.

Information will be introduced through examination of mock court, an experiential
process that will acquaint readers with process, protocol and procedure as it pertains to
judicial proceedings. Information and guidance for individuals who may need to testify,
present evidence or supply records is addressed. The use of mock court provides a frame
for examination of foundational material relative for effective witnessing. Practical tips
for testifying, including strategies for managing direct and cross examination are shared
to assist with readiness for potential courtroom engagement and to afford the reader
with resource material for preparation and presentation in a courtroom context.

The final section, Part V, will discuss a recent study that examined the use of drawing within an art therapy investigative interview process, the CIG. The literature associated with the use of drawing in investigative interviewing, which has been described
in connotations both positive and negative is explored. The study of an art therapy
investigative interview process to consider the efficacy of the use of free drawing as an
open-ended prompt within investigative interviews of children who may be victims of or
witnesses to interpersonal violence is presented.

The study compared an art therapy–based investigative interview process that incorporated free drawing in the capacity of an open-ended prompt to a verbal investigative
interview without the use of drawing through content analysis. Concepts that factor into
the study, including investigative interviewing, forensic relevance, open-ended prompts
and the drawing effect, are reviewed and a summary of the methodology, findings,
implications, limitations and ramifications for future study are addressed. The themes
that emerged from this qualitative comparative analogue study, fact-finding, imagery
and relationality, are congruent with the CIG, which is predicated upon rapport building, attunement to a child's developmental capabilities, fact-finding and minimization
of re-traumatization. Analysis of the data identified the use of imagery as enhancing
children's abilities to communicate accurate and relevant information. Imagery, visual
(mental) or graphic (pictorial), appeared to be the facilitator, or perhaps the factor that
stimulated and triggered recall and memory.

In this section, the underlying precepts associated with art therapy, including imagery,
the creative process, the dynamic relationship between art therapist and client and the
newly framed acknowledgement of the neurobiological underpinnings of the modality (King, 2016), are considered in relation to the application of drawing as a primary
source within the process of fact-finding. The encoding and recall of trauma, which are
linked to sensorium, appear to offer a context for understanding imaginal disclosure.
Traumatic memories are thought to be stored in image form, rendering art therapy
an appropriate or effective method for uncovering traumata, given the use of imagery
(Wadeson, 2016).

The emphasis on imagery as a means to convey traumatic exposure is examined in relation to the study which considers the question: *How does drawing facilitate disclosure of experienced events of school-aged children in an art therapy–based investigative interview process when compared to a verbal investigative interview process?* Secondarily, the "drawing effect" was explored from an art therapy perspective. Relevant literature is reviewed, given that researchers who have studied the use of drawing and its effectiveness regarding personal expression have shifted focus pertaining to the expediency of drawing within interviewing. Researchers that have investigated this topic for many years put forth in 2009 that their primary concern has shifted from "the practical issue of whether drawing works to the more theoretical issue of why it might work" (Gross, Hayne, & Drury, 2009, p. 967).

An approach to investigative interviewing that is predicated upon art therapy principles and practices may be a viable response to the paradigm shift that has emerged in investigative interviewing. How drawing works, rather than if drawing works, is a current focus of research with an emphasis on identifying and understanding the underlying mechanisms of the drawing effect. In addition to responding to current research initiatives, the literature review addressed how drawing facilitates fact-finding and memory recall through consideration of the three foundational principles of the CIG: drawing as an open-ended prompt; the dialogical and relational process; and the encoding, storage and recall of (traumatic) memory in image form. Ultimately, this study may support the recognition of drawing within investigative interviews of children and the impact on enhancing children's abilities to communicate about personally meaningful experiences. Understanding how drawing in the capacity of an open-ended prompt facilitates fact-finding in an art therapy–based investigative interview process may potentially contribute to the inconclusive and debatable antinomy that surrounds the use of drawing in investigative interviews of school-aged children.

The study will potentially contribute to the discussion surrounding interviewing best practices for victims and witnesses by providing an alternative to traditional verbal interview formats. An art therapy–based investigative interview process may offer a viable resource to assist children and investigators in the exploration of allegations that may be traumatic in nature.

References

Driessnack, M. (2005). Children's drawings as facilitators of communication: A meta-analysis. *Journal of Pediatric Nursing, 20,* 415–423.

Gross, J., Hayne, H., & Drury, T. (2009). Drawing facilitates children's reports of factual and narrative information: Implications for educational contexts. *Applied Cognitive Psychology, 23,* 953–971.

King, J. (Ed.). (2016). Introduction. In *Art therapy, trauma, and neuroscience: Theoretical and practical perspectives* (pp. 1–10). Routledge and Taylor & Francis Group, LLC.

Horovitz, E. G., & Cohen-Liebman, M. S. (2020). A de novo case: Efficacy, telehealth, and supervision within a legal confine. In E. G. Horovitz (Ed.), *The art therapists' primer: A clinical guide to writing assessments, diagnosis and treatment* (pp. 280–303). Charles C. Thomas.

Pipe, M. E., Lamb, M. E., Orbach, Y., & Esplin, P. W. (2004). Recent research on children's testimony about experienced and witnessed events. *Developmental Review, 24*(4), 440–468.

Wadeson, H. (2016). An eclectic approach to art therapy revisited. In D. Gussak & M. Rosal (Eds.), *The Wiley Blackwell handbook of art therapy.* Wiley-Blackwell.

Wilkerson v. Pearson, 210 New Jersey, Super. 333, 335. Chancery Division. (1985), 122–131.

Introduction

In 1997, I presented a preconference course at the American Art Therapy Association's (AATA's) annual conference. The presentation was based upon my work and was entitled "Forensic Art Therapy". During the day-long platform, I discussed in detail the nature of my work, which was nontraditional in variant ways. The notion of forensic art therapy as a subspecialty within the field of art therapy was presented. The novel investigative art therapy approach was presented, and the mode of practice was introduced.

Specifically, I addressed the discriminating elements that demarcate the practice and characterize it as distinct from art therapy approaches that are construed as interventive or evaluative. My work is different from art therapy practiced in forensic settings, which is aligned with a more traditional clinical application. A quote that I particularly favor and one that I typically open presentations with, especially when the audience is composed of art therapists or graduate students, states:

> Art Therapists are challenged to broaden their own definition of the use of art therapy and the settings in which it might be profitably practiced. This integration has emerged due to art therapists demonstrating the value of art therapy to those in a position to assess demand.
>
> (Smart, 1986)

Throughout the day, I highlighted the particularities that characterize and distinguish forensic art therapy (Cohen-Liebman, 1997). I defined the working definition for this investigative technique in the following manner: "The application for art therapy principles and practices within a forensic context to assist with legal matters in dispute" (Cohen-Liebman, 2007).

Prior to presenting the all-day preconference course, I began to second-guess myself. Was forensic art therapy a separate entity from art therapy practiced in forensic settings? I had defined forensic art therapy as an investigative mode of art therapy practice. In my opinion, forensic art therapy extended art therapy practice beyond diagnosis and treatment into the nontraditional arena of investigation. To me, art therapy in forensic settings was a more traditional art therapy approach, albeit with specified modifications in deference to the population(s) and the various settings in which practiced.

Determined to substantiate and confirm distinctions, differences and similarities between art therapy practiced within a forensic setting and the investigative work I was doing, I thought it best to make some inquiries and conciliate my burgeoning concern that perhaps my work was an existent entity. At the time, Dave Gussak, an art therapist known for his work with offenders, had a text, *Drawing Time* (Gussak & Virshup, 1997), slated for imminent release. I contacted the publisher and requested an advance copy.

DOI: 10.4324/9781003225041-1

My intention was to peruse the text to confirm and give credence to my belief that indeed my work, which entailed an investigative method, differed and diverged from the clinical application invoked by Dave and other art therapists practicing and providing treatment in forensic settings. I wanted to firmly establish that forensic art therapy was a novel and burgeoning application that embraced the work I was engaged in and had developed and implemented rather than a new identity for an existing mode of practice.

I decided to dial (yes, I am dating myself) Dave Gussak. Although there is an anecdotal story about this auspicious telephone conversation which I love to share with my students and in my trainings, I will not print it here; suffice it to say that after overcoming his initial reticence to speak with me, Dave became increasingly intrigued by the conversation. He was genuinely supportive of the forensic art therapy dichotomy I was detailing. Of course, his fascination extended to the fact that I had secured access to his soon-to-be-released text before he himself had obtained a copy, which promoted intrigue and certainly cannot be discounted. We arranged to meet at the forthcoming AATA conference where Dave attended a portion of my presentation.

Although Dave was observed leafing through his text, he listened, watched and conferred that indeed the work I was detailing and describing differed from art therapy practiced in forensic settings or with identified forensic populations. We determined and agreed that our work and approach represented different modes of art therapy practice with discernible distinctions as well as proclivities that tended to meld. Dave subscribed to my contention that forensic art therapy and art therapy practiced in forensic settings were not the same and indeed had differences and similarities. Primarily, both approaches had an association with the judiciary or a relationship with the legal system. Art therapy as practiced in forensic settings provided treatment and addressed interventive measures as the result of a judicial decision. Forensic art therapy, in contrast, was predicated upon fact-finding and was enacted for investigative purposes to assist with a judicial or legal matter in dispute. Differences in approach, application, objectives and outcome were solidified between the two art therapy modes of practice, leading to discernment of particularities that were manifest. These were determined to exist in the role of the art therapist, the setting(s) where practiced, the population(s) served, the intentionality of the application and goals as well as objectives.

Dave and I decided to explore the differential espoused by the two practice methods by engaging with additional conference attendees, specifically art therapists, in a focus group. A dialogue with practitioners associated with forensic settings was initiated. These individuals were engaged in more traditional facets of clinical work with modifications (as previously noted) relevant to population and setting. In other words, these art therapists were using art therapy for intervention and evaluation with individuals in some type of setting that was forensically rooted. Discussion ensued with art therapists who worked with forensic populations, meaning incarcerated or remanded to locked units that had a forensic connection, as well as outpatient settings with a forensic nexus. Distinctively, these populations were utilizing art therapy as a result or in response to a judicial decision or while awaiting sentencing.

The focus group confirmed the existence of forensic art therapy as a separate method of practice and as a distinct entity. Although commonalities were identified, discriminating properties were determined that distinguish these two art therapy practices. The focus group on forensics illustrated that my work differed significantly from the work associated with the art therapists who engaged with clients in forensically oriented settings and provided art therapy services after a legal decision had been made or while a client was awaiting a decision to be handed down.

In contrast, forensic art therapy was used to procure information within an investigative or fact-finding process and contributed to the resolution of a legal matter in dispute. At the time, the scope of my work revolved around child sexual abuse and child custody cases. Forensic art therapy rendered a mode of art therapy that was concerned with fact-finding or investigative endeavors and was based upon the juxtaposition of art therapy principles and practices with forensic canons and judicial tenets.

I believe that Dave's intentions that day were true and not directed by his desire to thumb through my copy of his book. Mutual respect, a collegial partnership and an enduring friendship resulted. We embarked on a path to educate and enlighten our peers, colleagues and the profession on the differing art therapy approaches. Dave's acknowledgement as well as the colloquial verification of the integrity of forensic art therapy as a distinct and unique mode of art therapy practice was affirmed, which was important since my work had been developed and implemented prior to this propitious interaction.

Forensic art therapy was recognized as a viable and pragmatic method of practice, distinct from art therapy practiced within a forensic setting. Acronyms to differentiate the distinct modes of practice emerged: FAT for forensic art therapy and FS for art therapy in forensic settings. I was informed, however, by a very dear friend, mentor and fellow art therapist (may he rest in peace) that FAT meant family art therapy; however, never having heard the moniker utilized to reference family art therapy, I reserved and adopted the ellipsis and continue to refer to forensic art therapy as FAT and art therapy practiced in forensic settings as FS.

Excited at the prospect of working together and sharing the supposition that our respective practice of art therapy was different yet had tangible connections, Dave and I decided to co-present our distinct modes of practice the following year at the annual conference. We configured and submitted an abstract, as is procedural, which was duly accepted. We set out to organize our separate information and combined our insight and experience to develop a paper that we co-presented at AATA, which led to an article that was published in the *American Journal of Art Therapy* (Cohen-Liebman & Gussak, 1998; Gussak & Cohen-Liebman, 2001). In the article we discuss our work by outlining and defining similarities and differences, addressing goals, settings, objectives, population(s), role of the art therapist and advantages associated with each method of art therapy practice. Through our combined efforts, we ultimately communed and highlighted information to the art therapy community. These various platforms propagated the distinctions and similarities promulgated by FS, a more traditional mode of practice, and FAT, which amalgamated art therapy and forensics.

Melding art therapy within the realm of investigative interviewing resulted in an original application. Creating a space for myself within this unlikely merger meant I was straddling two very distinct realms: I was not practicing art therapy in a conventional manner since I was not providing traditional clinical services as a therapist. I did not provide treatment or therapeutic intervention. Rather, my art therapy background buttressed my role as a child interviewer or child forensic interview specialist. As a forensic interviewer, I was schooled in a bevy of subjects and knowledge-based competencies that were not art therapy-based. This nurtured an intersection of subject matter from very different arenas as investigative interviewing was developing into an autonomous discipline. A blending of therapeutic and judicial norms was forged that was not necessarily compatible, yet fostered the development of a hybrid practice in which art therapy and judicial canons were juxtaposed resulting in a forensically defensible, yet intrinsically supportive process: forensic art therapy.

The conceptualization of a subspecialty within the field of art therapy was established. Subsequently, I was invited to teach a graduate-level course at Hahnemann University (currently Drexel University in Philadelphia) that specifically targeted this newly (at the time) emerging domain. Drexel was the only university to offer a course specifically devoted to forensic art therapy. There is no textbook per se for the course that was offered as an elective for second-year master's-level students in art therapy (which I taught from 1997 to 2017). Over time, the format changed in step with the demands of the university (switching from semesters to quarters), and the material was adapted from weekly to intensive offerings (summer or weekend condensed versions) as dictated by the department. Eventually, professionals were allowed to take the course for continuing education credit.

References

Cohen-Liebman, M. S. (1997, November). *Forensic art therapy*. Preconference course presented at the annual conference of the American Art Therapy Association.

Cohen-Liebman, M. S. (2007). Parent support group: A non-traditional use of art therapy. In D. Spring (Ed.), *Art in treatment: Transatlantic dialogue* (pp. 68–85). Charles C. Thomas.

Cohen-Liebman, M. S., & Gussak, D. (1998, November). *Investigation versus intervention: Forensic art therapy versus art therapy in forensic settings*. Paper presented at The American Art Therapy Annual Conference.

Gussak, D., & Cohen-Liebman, M. S. (2001). Investigation vs. intervention: Forensic art therapy and art therapy in forensic settings. *American Journal of Art Therapy, 40*, 123–135.

Gussak. D., & Virshup, E. (Eds.). (1997). *Drawing time: Art therapy in prisons and other correctional settings*. Magnolia Street Publishers.

Smart, M. (1986). Expanded work settings for art therapy. *Art Therapy, 3*, 21–26.

Part I   The Art of Investigating
Forensic Art Therapy

Introduction

Appreciation of the underlying principles and foundational nuances that contribute to the emergence of a novel method or technique provide the context from which practice derives. The factors that contributed to the configuration of forensic art therapy, a nontraditional mode of practice, will be identified. The circumstances that subsequently shaped this psycho-legal practice, including the origins of impetus, will be explored. The climate as well as the context from which forensic art therapy emerged is also addressed. Exploration of the underlying dialectical elements that commingled will be discussed. The resulting platform that transpired conflated art therapy principles and practices, the use of drawing, investigative interviewing and forensic tenets and judicial canons.

To ground my work and identify the geneses from which forensic art therapy emanated, I begin with a paradigm shift. The foundational roots for my sub-specialization were birthed as I explored topics for my second master's thesis. I was determined to concentrate on a nontraditional use of art therapy, which resulted in the intersection of art therapy and the judiciary. My interest centered around art therapists as expert witnesses in child sexual abuse litigation. I spent many hours combing through the library of a local law school and using the legal database (LexisNexis) to seek out cases that referenced art therapy. Trying to unearth and ascertain the extent to which art therapy and art therapists were identified in the law literature, I found very few references (at the time). Art therapy, when it was identified, was noted in relation to cases on appeal, or the use of drawing as evidence was briefly mentioned. Art therapy was not a central aspect of the cases I located, nor was the use of free drawing. Probing the literature, I realized that the locus of control was not singularly relegated to the law literature. Rather, my exploration merited refinement of definition and expansion into a plethora of multidisciplinarity. A medley of sorts, a foreshadowing of my future work. The rudimentary and formative stage of development would eventually coalesce across disciplines melding social science and law while intersecting art therapy, psychology and forensics. As such, an amalgam of sorts was fostered encompassing art therapy, clinical precepts and judicial principles.

Forensic Art Therapy Origins

To define and establish the origins of forensic art therapy (FAT), a nontraditional art therapy approach formulated on investigation, it became apparent that comparing it to

DOI: 10.4324/9781003225041-2

what was already existent was necessary. I began to explore fields of practice that were relevant and related to the work I was engaged in and that I was developing as a sub-specialization. Embarking upon an odyssey of sorts, I resolved to define and articulate the basis of my work and establish a cohesive framework. This was predicated upon the actual work I was doing that emanated from my position at a not-for-profit agency that was tasked with coordinating multidisciplinary team investigations of child sexual abuse cases.

Prior to my forensic work, I was employed as part of a clinical team at an alternative high school. The position actually evolved from an internship I had secured at the school which became a full-time art therapy position. Each enrolled student was assigned a primary clinical and educational team member. The students received their education at the school due to behavioral and emotional issues and were unable to be maintained in a mainstream setting. After a year of working in the setting, I realized that I was not being challenged – at least not the way I wanted to be despite a case load of individual students, facilitator of group art therapy sessions and working conjointly with a clinical and educational staff.

At the time, art therapy positions were not in great demand in the area where I lived. Specific positions ascribed to art therapy were few, necessitating one to think outside the proverbial box and be creative. As such, it was imperative to respond to position listings that were in allied professions such as social work, psychology and counseling. Taking a leap of faith, I responded to a blind ad in the newspaper. The listing described a position that was seeking an individual to conduct mental health assessments for sexually abused children and their nonoffending caregivers. Not having previously responded to a blind ad for a job, I thought that I might not have addressed it correctly and as such I re-sent the materials. At any rate, I was selected to interview for the position. The rest, as they say, is history but suffice it to say that the ad was subtle in declaring what I was embarking upon. The agency itself was in an inchoate stage of development and was fostering a position within the multidisciplinary investigative community. Objectives were directed at bridging cultural gaps and diminishing barriers to inter-agency collaboration within the professional community that served maltreated children, specifically sexually abused. The setting was ripe for an innovative investigative approach. Promulgating interaction and securing engagement from external agencies, I began my work within a milieu that was promoting multidisciplinary cooperative investment and collaborative relationships.

The organization was designed to bring representatives from the various agencies charged with investigating allegations of child sexual abuse together and to work as a team. Throughout the hiring process I met and spoke with representatives of the multidisciplinary team that I was to work with in a newly developing concept. Art therapy was virtually unknown to these individuals, yet my background and research pertaining to the integration of art therapy within the judicial system and art therapists as expert witnesses in child sexual abuse litigation (Cohen-Liebman, 1991, 1994) coupled with the potentialities of the modality in this nontraditional realm resonated and cultivated interest.

Originally hired to conduct mental health assessments of child victims of sexual abuse, my position changed as team members, predominantly from the fields of law enforcement and child protective services, requested assistance with investigative interviews of minor children, pre-teenagers, adolescents and on occasion developmentally delayed adults. The factors that demarcated my role were recast, adapted and modified as I was routinely asked to conduct interviews on behalf of team members while fostering a collaborative and cooperative process across disciplines. My role evolved from mental health evaluator to child interview specialist coupled with clinical director.

Authenticating the work I was doing meant defining it in an inclusive manner, meaning I had to address the roles I was straddling daily: art therapist, forensic interviewer, child advocate, crisis counselor, group facilitator and mental health practitioner within a multidisciplinary setting that was not therapeutically oriented. Primarily, I was responsible for facilitating the fact-finding process and conducting investigative interviews to elicit information for different investigative entities; a process that invoked a shift in gestalt. My position promoted interaction and engagement across cultures and disciplines that traditionally did not work in tandem. What seems common and is advocated today – the need for cooperative and collaborative agreements, shared interactions and the imparting and sharing of information across disciplines – was emergent when I began this work. I was consigned to strengthen, promote and develop cross interaction among agencies and representatives that previously had explored allegations independently.

Separate yet parallel investigations had been the standard mode of investigation prior to the emergence of a shared team concept. This mentality contributed to child victims and witnesses being exposed to multiple interviews as well as multiple interviewers which was stress inducing and potentially a source of revictimization. Interagency collaboration and minimization of secondary victimization through coordinated and cooperative relationships among the agencies or systems mandated to protect and serve was progressive and timely. The concept was a burgeoning response to this societal issue and was proliferating in communities across the country.

The multidisciplinary team approach as described was applied to reports of abuse allegations advancing an integrated model for investigation. Collaborative interviews among agencies increased, as did joint interviews between law enforcement and child protective services. Representatives assigned to individual cases from the two primary investigative agencies, law enforcement (often, but not always, the special victims unit) and child protective services (CPS), were encouraged to participate in this novel venture. As such, joint or lead interviews to explore allegations became integral to the process and contributed to the expansion of services as well as the embrace of the benefice derived from a multidisciplinary response to child sexual abuse cases.

As time went on and referrals increased, partner agency representatives requested additional assistance with collaborative interviews and the concept of teaming. My role shifted from mental health evaluator to forensic interviewer or child interview specialist. In response to the identified need for a skilled lead interviewer, I began attending state-of-the-art trainings dedicated to investigative interviewing and the facilitation of team processes while also participating in professional skill building conferences sponsored by professional associations and related organizations. At the time, investigative interviewing was still in a nascent stage of development but ultimately would develop into a mainstream profession.

Exposure and study revolving around what at the time was considered best practice regarding investigative interviewing were becoming endemic. There were many areas of interest and knowledge-based competencies to explore and absorb. State-of-the-art interviewing seminars were convened in various venues around the country. These forums offered instruction and interactive engagement directed at fostering educa-tion surrounding best practices based on the literature and research that was current at the time. Topics that ranged from rapport building to question continuum to the use of media and tools within interviews were areas of focus within these platforms. Peer review was another area that garnered attention. Research and literature proliferated in response to and out of respect for the myriad of interwoven topics that contributed to the field of investigative interviewing of children. Taken together, exposure, training, education and experiential opportunities coupled with hands-on interaction translated into state-of-the-art practices that were responsive to developments within the field. Research and scholarship were cultivated and stimulated a profusion of publications addressing a range of related topics for multidisciplinary investigations of child abuse and investigative interviewing.

The use of media, tools and props within investigative interviewing is a topic that has meted ambiguity. It is an area that has been characterized as developing in response to the need to supplement the interview process. In the literature (to be discussed), it is purposed that some of these techniques and supports may lack an empirical basis for implementation as adjunctive measures within investigative interviewing. A larger discussion relating to implanting such measures including the use of drawing will follow.

It would be remiss of me not to address how I felt as an art therapist engaged in this burgeoning realm as I integrated my background and experience with a forensic lens. As an art therapist engaged in fact-finding and investigative interviewing, it was very disconcerting that drawing was typically relegated to an ancillary position. The overall lack of art therapy within the investigation as a contributory voice was disheartening. Determined to confront this void, I approached the facilitator at a week-long inter-viewing seminar. She was neither interested nor impressed with the topic. Attempts to instill awareness or even stimulate curiosity were disregarded and the status of drawing was not elevated beyond a tool, prop or aid and art therapy was dismissed. Frankly, the nonchalance was an untoward reaction. Through the years I have attempted to reconcile diffidence (my own) with courage and conviction. I have presented, taught and published aspects of my work and I am pleased to have this opportunity to detail and share Forensic Art Therapy in this form. I sincerely hope that the text will promote appreciation and understanding of this amalgam of art therapy, forensic and judicial tenets.

Underpinnings of Forensic Art Therapy

The confluence of art therapy, social science and forensics underlie FAT. As my jour-ney deepened, I realized that I was bridging fields that did not typically unite. FAT commingles distinct modes of thought – social science and law – which are unique entities not profoundly enmeshed. Understanding the dichotomy that is existent between law and the social sciences resulted in appreciating the differences that engulf these separate domains. The epistemology and ontology of these two fields are dissimilar, yet FAT fostered the need to integrate these very distinctive realms. The underpinnings of FAT encompass a host of areas not included in standard art therapy curricula, which will be articulated. These modules contributed to the devel-opment and establishment of this application and thus extend the nomenclature associated with it. This assemblage distinguishes forensic art therapy from traditional art therapy applications.

Forensic art therapy addresses

- reporting mandates, legal proceedings, testimonial capability and evidentiary material
- ethical issues inherent in the forensic arena and the corresponding impact on the art therapist
- how drawing factors into the realm of investigative interviewing
- three ways that drawing can be used within a legal context
- use of drawing as evidentiary material in a legal or forensic context
- populations impacted by interpersonal violence, including child victims and witnesses

---

Forensic Science Versus Social Science

Forensic mental health practice is identified as distinct from clinical practice. Although it has been recognized that "clinical and forensic practice are generally incompatible" (Myers, 2019, p. 37), reconciliation of these different approaches is contingent upon a melding of different philosophies and theoretical frameworks. Law is designed around the premise of resolution. Resolving disputes or legal matters through reliance upon the law, as well as deference to legal precedents, is standard in judicial matters. Law is attributed, applied and deciphered in relationship to maintaining and advocating for the protection of constitutional rights with respect to individuals and organizations. Judicial decision making, however, often relies on the translation of social science (Perry & Wrightsman, 1991).

Social science assists in legal contexts through the provision of data. Social science practitioners are sanctioned to provide information to individuals within a court of law who may not possess awareness, understanding or appreciation of how the law is applicable in understanding people or behavior. Social science practitioners educate, enlighten, clarify and correct through informing and explaining, articulating and offering information regarding traits, characteristics and behaviors associated with individuals and/or groups of people.

Experts from the social sciences organize, integrate and interpret data from empirical studies (Gould & Stahl, 2009; Perry & Wrightsman, 1991). Educating the trier of fact (judge or jury) about individual and group behavior is the jurisdiction of social science. Rather than make decisions on behalf of a judicial officer, information is presented and education is provided to empower the trier of fact (judge or jury) to render a decision regarding a particular issue (Perry & Wrightsman, 1991). Observations or information, singularly and in combination with other pieces of data, yield meaning or lend a basis for inference or interpretation that guides conclusions and recommendations (Gould & Stahl, 2009). These efforts assist the trier(s) of fact in the decision-making process and contribute to the resolution of legal matters in dispute. Upholding scientific as well as clinical standards is paramount when social scientists are invited to participate in a court proceeding or when asked to provide assistance and help with legal matters.

In summary, the role that is assigned to each discipline with respect to a legal matter differs. The focus of law is order and protection of constitutional rights, representation of specific individuals and organizations within the legal system, and the resolution of disputes by relying on legal precedents (Perry & Wrightsman, 1991). Legal issues are determined in an absolute fashion within the context of how law is applied and interpreted. In contrast, social science focuses on upholding scientific and clinical standards, offering explanation about the behavior of both individuals and groups of people, thereby offering the means for a trier of fact to render a decision resulting in the resolution of a legal matter in dispute.

Epistemology (Knowledge) and Ontology (Reality)

Law and social science are predicated upon distinct and diverse epistemologies (knowledge and understanding) and ontologies (realities). Epistemological underpinnings of the legal system contrast with those of the social sciences. The former is based in scientific objectivity, while the latter is considered more subjective (Milchman, 2011). In the most basic sense, scientific knowledge is construed as objectively valid, while subjectivity is often associated with clinical applications. In order to best meet the expectations of the legal system, there needs to be a balance between the two (Milchman, 2011). Elements delineated from both scientific and clinical epistemologies combine to strengthen expert opinion in a court of law (Gould & Stahl, 2009). Current trends in forensic mental health assessments support adherence to scientific principles and practices while also recognizing the validity of clinical methodologies.

The legal system adheres to a conceptual framework in which truth, veracity and validity are underlying principles. The epistemology of law is "a mode of inquiry with the purported goals of discovering truth and avoiding errors" (Ward, 2006, p. 350). Facts and evidence are central to legal findings. The establishment of a burden of proof is paramount to the legal system. Standards range from "beyond reasonable doubt" to "a preponderance of evidence", depending upon the nature of the judicial process. In deference to judicial protocol, the issue before the court necessitates a determination of true or false. In the social sciences the aim is to evaluate through observation, interaction and clinical procedures (Gould & Stahl, 2009). The objective is to address the needs of the client. The establishment of a burden of proof is not the goal, and absolutes are not the priority for social science.

Elements delineated from both scientific and clinical epistemologies combine to strengthen expert opinion (Gould & Stahl, 2009).

Integration of the ontological foundations of forensic and social science results in a comprehensive fact-finding approach (Gould & Stahl, 2009). FAT commingles forensic and social science epistemological and ontological dogmas, resulting in a pragmatic investigative approach. Ontologically there are very different realities between the legal system and the social sciences, resulting in a dialectical confluence which is pragmatically oriented. Investigative interviews that derive from FAT are based on a scientific framework, while subscribing to an art therapy paradigm (Cohen-Liebman, 2016). The melding of different philosophies and theoretical frameworks supports the pragmatic nature of the process (Cohen-Liebman, 2016).

Legal System (Law)	Social Science
Objective	Subjective
Conceptual framework in which truth, veracity and validity are underlying precepts	The aim is to evaluate through observation, interaction and clinical procedures (Gould & Stahl, 2009)
The epistemology of law is "a mode of inquiry with the purported goals of discovering truth and avoiding errors" (Ward, 2006, p. 350)	The objective is to address the needs of the client
Facts and evidence are central to legal findings	The establishment of a burden of proof is not the goal, and absolutes are not the priority
The establishment of a burden of proof is paramount to the legal system	Fact-finding is construed as information gathering
Standards range from "beyond reasonable doubt" to "a preponderance of evidence"	

Law	Social Science
Order and protection of constitutional rights	Focus on upholding scientific and clinical standards
Represent specific individuals and organizations within the legal system	Understand the behavior of individuals and groups involved with the legal system
Resolve disputes by relying upon legal precedents	Resolve disputes by organizing, integrating and interpreting data from empirical studies
Decide legal issues in an absolute fashion	Inform triers of fact to assist them with decision making (Perry & Wrightsman, 1991)

Forensic Counseling

It became increasingly apparent that to distinguish FAT as unique and novel, it had to be compared to what was extant. To appreciate what actuated the nontraditional mode of practice that merged art therapy with judicial tenets, the underlying sensitivities necessitated identification. This contributed to the development of a conceptual model for the construct of FAT, which was predicated upon the intersection of law and social science.

Forensic counseling seemed to best correlate with the forensic parameters that underlie FAT. The definition identified a specific set of skills and experiences that merited modification from traditional counseling methods to address and meet the distinct needs of the legal system. Forensic processes differ from mental health processes and garner a different approach given the strictures associated with a forensic context. When melded, a psycho-legal orientation emerges; hence, the descriptor for FAT was identified.

The essential features associated with forensic counseling seemed to correlate with what I thought resembled the type of skill set invoked in FAT, including the need to modify traditional (art therapy) practice to be compliant with judicial practice. The requirements for the work necessitated a specific set of skills and experience that were modified such that they met the demands dictated by the legal system. Concomitantly, traditional art therapy practice, including the requisite skills attributed to an art therapist, were integrated with judicial canons in compliance with adherence to forensic procedure. This adoption best suited the nature of the setting and the demands of the position.

- a specific set of skills and experience
- traditional counseling skills modified for the legal system
- forensic processes are different from clinical assessments
- psycho-legal process

Synthesis of Social and Forensic Science

FAT commingles social and forensic science tenets with art therapy conventions. The pragmatic use of art is congruent with the pragmatic nature of the interview process. Interviews happen in an intersubjective matrix that has a corresponding influence on the process. A meaning making experience rather than an aesthetic one is fostered. A child assists in the fact-finding process in a developmentally congruent manner through self-expression that invokes verbalizations in tandem with self-directed or free drawing. Enabling a child to communicate and express his or her experience via imagery and verbal associations is the pragmatic piece of the process (Cohen-Liebman, 2016, 2017).

FAT juxtaposes basic art therapy tenets with forensic and clinical methodologies, including clinical understanding, scientific thinking, thorough observation and judicial procedure. The convergence of behavioral science and legal standards of admissibility (Gould & Stahl, 2009) underlie FAT, which is informative yet supportive, legally compliant yet clinically responsive (Cohen-Liebman, 2016). The synthesis results in a supportive process that meets the standards of the legal system. Art therapy is not a part of the legal system in a traditional sense; however, it offers individuals a way to relate experienced events in a nonthreatening way. The process is predicated upon creative methods of expression procured within a relational context. Within the forensic interview process, the use of drawing promotes elicitation of information that may otherwise not be communicated due to the encoding and recall of traumatic material (Cohen-Liebman, 2017).

FAT originated from the integration of art therapy principles and practices with standard forensic procedure and protocol. It adheres to forensic interviewing principles yet has clinical overtones due to the intrinsic art therapy foundation. FAT is based upon the inclusion of nondirected or free drawing within the investigative interview format. In this context, drawing functions as an open-ended prompt to facilitate recall of experienced events. Often obstacles that impair or inhibit self-expression are mitigated using free drawing in the investigative interview process (Cohen-Liebman, 1999, 2017).

Definition of Forensic Art Therapy (FAT)

FAT is defined as

The juxtaposition of art therapy principles and practices with standard forensic procedure and protocol.

FAT emerged out of a dialectic fusion of two unrelated but integrated practices. The commingling of social sciences and law resulted in an amalgamation predicated upon a construct rooted in forensics and art therapy. This intersection constituted an innovative and unique mode of practice in which client-based drawing is central to the process. The development of FAT extended the parameters of the field of art therapy beyond evaluation/diagnoses and intervention/treatment into the realm of investigation, a novel application (Cohen-Liebman, 1999, 2002, 2003; Gussak & Cohen-Liebman, 2001). FAT is a fact-finding endeavor, directed at the resolution of legal matters in dispute. The processes embedded in FAT foster support for victims and witnesses in communicating experienced events that may be traumatic in nature without compromising forensic integrity (Cohen-Liebman, 2017, 2021).

> Forensic art therapy and the use of drawing as an open-ended prompt within a forensic context extended the potentialities inherent in the modality of art therapy beyond traditional applications and signified the interface of art therapy within the judicial arena and as an investigative process (Cohen-Liebman, 2003).

FAT is sensitive to the parameters of clinical interviewing, yet adheres to forensic interviewing principles in order to be acceptable in a court of law. Investigative interviews that derive from FAT are based on a scientific framework, while subscribing to an art therapy paradigm (Cohen-Liebman, 2016). Fact-finding, the primary objective of an investigative interview, improves when approached within a format that is commensurate with developmental level and interactive patterns (Cohen-Liebman, 1999; Melinder et al., 2010). FAT interviews are conducted in a developmentally sensitive, forensically defensible manner. Goals of these processes include maximizing information gathering and minimizing repetitive interviews toward eliminating secondary victimization.

FAT has the capacity to meet the respective goals of the law, while protecting the rights of victims and witnesses regardless of the allegations under investigation. In a FAT interview, free drawing is incorporated in the capacity of an open-ended prompt to facilitate fact-finding and elicit a narrative response. Information gathered from the use of drawing as a primary resource and proffered in court via the art therapist provides the trier of fact with information to assist in decision making (Cohen-Liebman, 1999). The process is designed to adhere to forensic practice while safeguarding the emotional well-being of the client.

An interview may prompt initial disclosure leading to divulgence of information relative to an experienced event. Sometimes, disclosure initiates investigation or action and subsequent intervention. Although FAT is not intrinsically a therapeutic process, healing or repairment begin with the initial response to disclosure, which may be the investigative interview. The interview initiates recovery in whatever form may be pursued. Given the hybrid orientation of FAT, recommendations extend beyond investigative needs in post-processing. As such, the FAT interviewer makes recommendations that may include investigative, interventive or therapeutic services in conjunction with the team and in response to the circumstances of the case to support the child and family.

FAT

- juxtaposition of art therapy principles and practices with standard forensic procedure and protocol
- nontraditional art therapy practice
- investigative, not interventive or evaluative
- outside the parameters of normal clinical practice
- clients may come from outside of traditional art therapy practice
- investigative in nature yet has clinical overtones

The Forensic Art Therapist

The forensic art therapist works within the judicial system. Through the application and integration of art therapy practice, the forensic art therapist assists in the resolution of legal matters in dispute. The forensic art therapist juxtaposes the requisite skills of an art therapist in tandem with knowledge and understanding of judicial tenets. This juxtaposition supports an approach that is rooted in art therapy fundamentals and judicial underpinnings. FAT employs specific skills and experience on the part of the forensic art therapist, as well as modification of standard art therapy practice. The forensic art therapist utilizes elemental skills of the profession, including but not limited to child development, human behavior, psychodynamics, psychoanalytic processes and the creative process in combination with forensic tenets (Cohen-Liebman, 1999). As such, FAT lies outside the parameters of normal art therapy practice. The forensic art therapist has training and expertise that extend beyond art therapy principles and practice, embracing a range of legal and judicial components that exceed standard art therapy curricula. The FAT art therapist works outside traditional art therapy settings and outside the parameters of conventional clinical art therapy practice.

Art therapy, the profession and the practice including fundamental aspects relevant to Forensic Art Therapy are explored in the literature review in Part V including approach, inherent advantages, meaning making, dynamic relationship, triangular composition, imagery, preverbal cognition, sensory knowledge, and encoding of trauma.

Forensic Art Therapist

- assists in the resolution of legal matters in dispute
- through application and integration of art therapy practice
- works within the judicial system and subscribes to judicial tenets
- utilizes essential skills of an art therapist in combination with legal tenets

---

Forensic Art Therapy (FAT) Clients

FAT Clients

- do not seek service, since not interventive but investigative
- often involuntary
- are referred for investigative purposes
- forensic or legal matter necessitates investigation
- are referred by a system involved in an investigative or legal matter
  - law enforcement
  - prosecution
  - defense
  - child protection agency
  - judge or judicial officer
  - at times, process may be court ordered

Forensic Art Therapy (FAT) Settings

FAT is practiced in a nontraditional setting. Typically, the setting is associated with an investigative or forensic entity or a multidisciplinary interviewing center that facilitates team investigations. The setting is outside the parameters of typical clinical or traditional art therapy practice. FAT is not based upon therapeutic interventions or specific art therapy tasks; rather, it is a process that is forensically rooted and intended for fact-finding rather than treatment or diagnostic purposes.

FAT Setting

- nontraditional
- the setting is investigative in nature
- associated with an investigative or forensic entity
- outside the parameters of clinical or traditional art therapy practice
- FAT does not consist of specific art therapy tasks or interventive measures

---

Forensic Art Therapy (FAT) Goals

FAT is a mode of practice that is rooted in forensics and art therapy. It provides a platform for investigative interviewing that incorporates the use of free drawing in the capacity of an open-ended prompt. It is a process that utilizes free or client-directed drawing in an effort to engage a child and elicit free recall about experienced events and assist with fact-finding. The process is intended to safeguard the emotional well-being of a child victim or witness while adhering to forensic standards. FAT is a process that contributes to decision making or resolution of a legal matter that is in dispute given the investigative nature of the process. Information culled from an interview may potentially impact investigation, prosecution and interventive measures. Findings may contribute to determination of supportive (including therapeutic) services, additional investigative interviews and multidisciplinary response, as well as determination of next steps with regard to investigative and prosecutorial pursuits.

FAT is more than an investigative interview process. It is a mode of practice that is predicated upon the juxtaposition of art therapy and forensics. It entails investigation and fact-finding (interviewing), judicial engagement including testimonial capability and the presentation of evidentiary material (such as drawings and/or other forms of imaginal work) within a legal context.

FAT Goals and Objectives

- fact-finding process
- assists in resolution of legal matters in dispute
- investigative
- nonthreatening
- minimization of repeated investigative interviews
- child friendly
- safeguards emotional well-being of child victims and witnesses while maintaining forensic integrity

---

Art Therapy in Forensic Settings (FS)

There are inherent differences that underlie FAT and art therapy practiced within foren-sic settings (FS). Distinctions and similarities pervade the different modes of practice. As such, a dichotomy is existent. The objective of FS is not directed at influencing decision making or resolution of a legal matter that is in dispute. FS is employed after a forensic issue has been determined or during the decision-making process. FS primarily consists of interventions. Although considered a clinical application, FS may be construed as less traditional, given constraints that may be dictated by the setting in conjunction with a legal association.

> I would be remiss if I did not acknowledge the collaborative atmosphere from which this material was identified, delineated, refined and collated. I refer to the coopera-tive alliance and working relationship that were spawned with my colleague and friend, Dave Gussak. As mentioned previously, we co-presented (Cohen-Liebman & Gussak, 1998) and co-wrote an article about the dialogue that ensued surrounding our respective modes of practice including similarities and differences (Gussak & Cohen-Liebman, 2001).

The mode of treatment within a correctional or judicially affiliated setting may be dictated by the confines of the institution, which merits adaptation accordingly. In FS, the art therapist provides treatment or intervention. FS is therapeutic in relation to the setting and the situation in which it occurs. Settings include placements wherein some-one is remanded to a particular penal institution such as prison, jail, a state hospital, a detention center, a juvenile justice center and designated out-patient settings (Gussak & Cohen-Liebman, 2001). The setting is determined in response to the resultant decision corresponding to a judicial or legal matter.

Caveat

Given today's modern society, the term traditional is one to debate, as so many elements factor into what comprises the term. Many individuals (for purposes of this discussion, art therapists) may be practicing outside of what previously may have constituted a more conventional clinical environment or treatment atmosphere in which therapeutic services or task-oriented directives were specified. The term traditional is not all encompassing and as

such is used with respect to assist in differentiating clinical and forensic milieus and is not intended in any way to depreciate the nature of work or practice affiliated with or ascribed to a particular setting. The boundaries of practice are expansive and determinant upon many factors.

Role of the Art Therapist in Forensic Settings (FS)

Within FS, the art therapist functions in a more "traditional" role and provides clinical intervention or treatment. The FS art therapist is not a fact-finder and does not assume the role of investigator. Treatment or intervention is rendered after a judicial decision has been determined or while a client is awaiting sentencing but has been remanded into custody. As such the FS therapist works in a more traditional role, albeit in correspondence with the setting and the nature of the environment as well as the population (Gussak & Cohen-Liebman, 2001). The FS therapist provides intervention or therapy as a result of a judicial decision or after a judgement regarding sentencing or placement often in response to a legal proceeding.

The therapist will modify and adapt interventions and tasks in accordance with the parameters of the setting. Some art materials and media may be construed as conflictual given the nature of the setting. Concern may be prompted that items may contribute to subversive use necessitating creative interventions that allow for personal expression in alternative forms. For example, sharps (scissors) and tape may not be readily displayed or supported (flexibility is inherent with regard to choice of media within art therapy practice regardless of setting). Knowledge regarding the inherent properties and possibilities associated with different types and forms of media is fundamental to art therapy practice and impacts interaction with a client (not just in relation to judicial settings) and manifests situationally.

Caveat

Understanding the potentialities innate to different materials is not relegated to forensic settings, as media choice and selection factor into every art therapy intervention to meet the needs of clients and provide support rather than promote stress.

Forensic Settings (FS) Clients

Clients may not be voluntary, depending upon the circumstances of incarceration. Intervention is the objective as a means of helping the client help himself or herself to manage and cope within the setting, which may have imposed limitations or boundaries. FS is employed after a forensic issue has been resolved or during the decision-making process, meaning that a client may be awaiting a decision about sentencing. The process is not intended to direct or impact a judicial decision. Instead, FS addresses the needs of a client as the result of a judicial decision (or a pending determination). The FS client may engage in art therapy as a means for personal management and as a way to deal with his or her reality within the correctional milieu and to help manage or resolve internal conflicts (Gussak & Cohen-Liebman, 2001). FS is interventive in that it provides a means for a client to manage underlying thoughts and feelings. It is therapeutically motivated, not investigatory, which distinguishes it from FAT.

Forensic Settings (FS) Goals

The goal of FS is to help a client to help himself or herself and to stay safe within the environment (Gussak & Cohen-Liebman, 2001).

Art Therapy in Forensic Settings (FS)
(Gussak & Cohen-Liebman, 2001)

FS Art Therapist
- differs from art therapist engaged in FAT
- more "traditional" role but with modification to setting
- not a fact-finder
- does not function in an investigative role
- provides therapy

FS Settings
- attention to media, choice, selection and application
- modifications and adjustments as dictated by the institution
- various settings
- prison, county and city jail, state hospitals, detention centers, juvenile justice centers/youth authority, parole/out-patient settings
- not a traditional clinical setting or model

FS Clients
- discharge of underlying feelings while controlling behavior
- dealing with reality of the situation
- helping client help themselves to manage and to stay safe
- resolution of internal conflict(s)
- interventive
- may be task oriented (depending on variables)

FS Goals and Objectives
- engagement with population is not directed at influencing forensic decision making
- it is employed after a forensic issue has been resolved or during the decision-making process (meaning client is awaiting decision but has been taken into custody)
- the needs of a client are addressed in response to a resultant judicial decision or in deference to situational matters and/or concerns

Similarities and Distinctions Between FAT and FS

Both FAT and FS provide a means for self-expression for identified clients. Both are typically conducted within a nontraditional setting that has an association with the judicial system or a legal construct. Clients of both may not seek out services yet be mandated to cooperate with either investigation or intervention. FS clients may be encouraged to participate if services are available to address residual and concomitant issues, so a suggestion rather than a mandate may be made. A FAT client may be referred by an investigative authority or entity to participate in an investigative interview process, and choice is not necessarily a factor.

Similarities and Differences FAT versus FS
(Gussak & Cohen-Liebman, 2001)

Similarities
- self-expression for clients
- practiced within nontraditional settings
- association with the judicial system
- FAT clients do not necessarily have a choice regarding compliance
- FS clients may not seek out services
- FS may be strongly encouraged to participate
- FAT and FS do not focus on uncovering

Differences

- FS therapist provides intervention or therapy albeit in accord with the setting
- FS occurs in response to a judicial decision or legal proceeding
- FS is employed after a judgment regarding sentencing or placement or during the decision-making process
- FAT is associated with an investigative or forensic entity
- FAT is not based upon therapeutic interventions or specific art therapy tasks
- FAT is directed at fact-finding rather than treatment or diagnostic purposes
- FAT may contribute to decision-making or resolution of a legal matter in dispute

Uncovering FS
- uncovering in FS may be detrimental to the treatment
- may compromise the safety of a client due to exposure of history, reason for incarceration or vulnerabilities

Uncovering FAT
- since not a therapeutic session client may not be able to process and manage disclosed information when uncovering in FAT
- interviewer may not be able to address issues that merit therapeutic intervention given the nature of the interview process, which is directed at fact-finding
- therapeutic intervention may be recommended after the interview to provide the client with the opportunity to process and manage underlying thoughts and feelings associated with the allegations as well as disclosure
- therapeutic intervention and supportive services may be identified and referred

How Artwork Is Used
- FS only as far as needed to get the client to main population and stay safe
- FS to elicit information while maintaining a proper mask to keep safe within an environment that will take advantage of weakness (Gussak & Cohen-Liebman, 2001)
- FAT to elicit free recall of information and facilitate fact-finding
- drawing may be used in FAT to address court preparation (if child is to testify in a hearing), refresh and review what was disclosed previously, segue to what happens next

After Investigation/Judicial Decision, What Happens to Client and Artwork
- with FAT client, may be referred for an extended interview, to therapy, support group or other services as determined in consultation with the team
- if a judicial proceeding is scheduled, appropriate court support and prep are provided
- if used in court, artwork becomes evidence and belongs to the court
- FAT clients do not own artwork made for investigative purposes
- FS client may go to a less restrictive environment
- FS client is a ward of the court
- art belongs to the FS client or the institution depending upon the setting

Uncovering

Uncovering of material is not essential in FAT or FS, given the nature of the work and the need not to be therapeutic (FAT) and as a means for self-protection (FS). Uncovering in FS may be detrimental. It may not be necessary for the FS therapist to know at the onset of treatment why a particular client is incarcerated (Gussak & Cohen-Liebman, 2001). This information may be examined as therapy progresses to identify and address the locus of identified issues and conflicts. As Gussak (2013) has noted, in a prison setting it is prudent to help the client manage surface symptoms in order to enable the client to function in the environment and for personal safety.

With FAT, uncovering may be construed as too therapeutic for the client and for the parameters associated with the process. Given the emphasis on fact-finding and a (typically but not always) single session interview, the goal is not to promote decompensation that may result if information and issues are exposed and no provision for addressment is provided. A referral for therapeutic intervention may follow the process in consultation with the team. Resolution of underlying and associated thoughts and feelings is not the objective within the investigative context (fact-finding), and the potential to compromise the integrity of the process exists if the interview transforms into a therapeutic session. The investigative interviewer (if another member of the team takes the lead) is not presenting in a therapeutic stance and may not have a background in clinical intervention. The emotional well-being of the child may also be jeopardized if the boundaries of the process are compromised or not respected.

The forensic art therapist, while not presenting in a clinical role, is able to utilize the skills of an art therapist in combination with investigative interviewing skills. The forensic art therapist supports the child in a manner that respects forensic integrity while safeguarding the emotional well-being of the child, through the hybrid process.

> Drawing as an open-ended prompt retains a primary purpose in the interview and is used to facilitate free recall and support a child's narrative about experienced events.

Artwork in FAT and FS

Artwork provides a function in FS, as does drawing in FAT. In FAT, drawing offers a means for self-expression about experienced events. FAT contributes to the elicitation of information via free recall and perhaps a narrative within the safety of a child-centered process. FAT incorporates drawing in a supportive capacity to assist in the elicitation of information for fact-finding purposes. Within the context of an interview, free drawing is used as an open-ended prompt to facilitate fact-finding. As such, drawing is utilized and presented in the context of an invitational prompt similarly to a verbal one. Drawing is used in a primary capacity rather than as a secondary support to confirm or clarify a verbal statement. Drawing provides the opportunity for a child to relate information and discuss an experienced event via imaginal as well as verbal articulation. Often verbal elaboration follows graphic depiction (Cohen-Liebman, 1999; Kelley, 1984). Drawing in this capacity provides an avenue for engagement, interaction, rapport building, developmental assessment, fact-finding and closure.

The child's associations are critical to understanding the child's graphic depictions. The interviewer is not interpreting visual or pictorial content, but elicits information from the child through nonleading means to garner understanding and information. The information provided by the child may offer explanation relative to the allegations being explored, as well as disclosure of previously unknown material or details associated with the experienced event. Drawing and discussion of the content may contribute to the respective investigative pursuits of the team and impact recommendations as well as potential outcomes. The art or drawing(s) provide an objective, concrete record created by the child at a given point in time. Pictorial content in conjunction with the child's verbal associations enable the child to communicate in a developmentally and ego-syntonic manner. The child's associations to the self-generated graphic material reveal what the child was expressing in relation to the child's experience.

In FAT, a child's drawing may be used to refresh a child's memory, perhaps when the next step in the process is a court proceeding. Court involvement may be delayed due to unforeseen or systemic issues. Drawing created in an interview may be used to review what a child discussed or disclosed, and the child's drawing may be helpful to prepare the child for a courtroom proceeding.

Drawing created within the interview context may be presented in court as evidentiary material and serve as a judiciary aid. A child's associations to a self-created drawing may assist with remembrance or recall of earlier disclosure and in some respects provide a child with voice if called upon to testify. Drawing as a judiciary aid may delineate information that is contributory to charge enhancements, which is salient for law enforcement and prosecution as well as protective matters.

Drawing made within the interview that pertains to fact-finding does not belong to the client or even the agency that may have requested the interview, including members of the multidisciplinary team. It may be maintained in a chart or case file for preservation and be available to team members for their respective investigative pursuits and, if necessary, court proceedings. Artwork made in investigatory processes (FAT) belongs, in theory, to the court; however, the court is not a repository for evidence. The art or drawing remains with the client's file and is housed accordingly. This is a challenging matter given that a physical storage space is not maintained at court, so an agency, perhaps one that coordinates the investigation, may house client records. As such, evidence is accessible and retrievable in the event it is needed for future courtroom proceedings or to prepare a child for court as a means to refresh or review what was disclosed/discussed during the investigative or fact-finding interview process.

Protecting the child's rights, ensuring the safety of the child and maintaining the integrity of the process (FAT) are integral elements. Children are informed at the onset of the process that they are being observed and that drawing and information will be shared with the team in an effort to avert surprise or deception. "Children are not led to believe that no one else is hearing what they say. They are made aware of the standards of practice (in a developmentally congruent manner) in an effort to avoid misperceptions and false pretenses" (Cohen-Liebman, 1999, p. 192). This is explained during the initial meeting with the caregiver as well. Drawing that is not related to fact-finding that is created within the investigative interview process may not be considered part of the investigative record. As such, this material does not merit retention and storage with a child's record. FAT clients do not own artwork made for fact-finding purposes.

Children's Drawing(s), Ownership and Confidentiality

Cohen-Liebman (1999) discussed ethical and legal considerations pertaining to ownership and confidentiality of children's drawing(s) within a forensic context, which pose unique dilemmas and concerns. The reader is referred to the article for more specific information beyond what is shared. A few points to reiterate follow.

In a forensic context, confidentiality is not congruent given the fact-finding nature of the investigative interview. It is not considered a therapeutic process and is not supported as such. Information obtained within the process is memorialized (documented and/or observed) and shared with the investigative or multidisciplinary team. Information including drawing(s) made in the service of fact-finding may be presented in court as evidentiary material. "Ultimately, confidentiality is superseded by the process which entails fact-finding and evidence gathering whereas a therapeutic alliance engenders confidentiality in interaction and exchange" (Cohen-Liebman, 1999, p. 192).

Cohen-Liebman (1999) also noted that "[o]wnership is a matter that is predicated upon purpose" (p. 192). Within a courtroom context, ownership may be scrutinized with regard to establishing identity (of the creator, for example, with regard to a pictorial rendering). Within a forensic context, the purpose is to obtain information or facts and corroboration of this material. Within a court of law, a drawing may be introduced as evidentiary material to denote what was procured in the fact-finding process and to bring the child's disclosure/experience

---

(*Continued*)

(Continued)

Children's Drawing(s), Ownership and Confidentiality

(pictorial and/or verbal into the courtroom). This may connote a shift in ownership, with the concern being guardianship (Cohen-Liebman, 1999). As evidentiary material, drawing may serve as a judiciary aid which is presented on behalf of the child by an investigator or interviewer perhaps affiliated with a multidisciplinary team.

Drawing(s) created within a forensic context or a fact-finding endeavor such as an investigative interview are not extended the same privileges as drawing(s) created within a therapeutic alliance. In a fact-finding process, the nature of the drawing is delineated as documentation that is considered part of the investigative record or file, yet it is available for the team to use within the investigative process and as evidence that may be presented in court. Ethical and legal dilemmas attributed to the use of children's drawings from a forensic stance merit continued study, discussion and examination.

FS ownership is a matter that is assigned to the institution that governs the use of artwork as well as the display and maintenance of the art. Artwork in FS is used only as far as it is needed. It may be used to move a client forward, perhaps into a less restrictive milieu, and to develop coping mechanisms to stay safe (Gussak & Cohen-Liebman, 2001). FS is more task oriented in that interventions are utilized. Depending upon the needs of the client and in deference to the surroundings, art can mask dangerous issues while at the same time afford a means for interaction while maintaining mental and physical well-being within an environment that may not be receptive or amenable to vulnerability (Gussak & Cohen-Liebman, 2001).

FS	FAT
Art Therapist • differs from art therapist engaged in FAT • more traditional role but with modification to setting • art therapist is not a fact-finder • does not function in an investigative role • provides therapy	**Art Therapist** • assists in the resolution of legal matters in dispute • through the application and integration of art therapy practice • works within the judicial system • utilizes the essential skills of an art therapist, including but not limited to child development, human behavior, psychodynamics, psychoanalytic tenets and the creative process
Settings • nontraditional use of the modality • various settings • prison, county and city jail, state hospitals, detention centers, juvenile justice centers/youth authority, parole/out-patient settings • specificity of treatment within the correctional setting • not a traditional clinical setting or model	**Settings** • nontraditional • outside the parameters of normal clinical and art therapy practice • work is investigative in nature yet has clinical overtones • process is conducted in an environment not necessarily clinically oriented, but rather provides an interview space that is child friendly and child focused
FS Clients • not necessarily voluntary in a traditional sense	**FAT Clients** • do not seek service since not interventive but investigative

FS	FAT

• may be recommended for services within the environment to assist with adjustment and other needs, including personal safety and reconciliation with reality of placement
• discharge of underlying feelings while controlling behavior
• dealing with reality of the situation
• helping client help themselves
• resolution of internal conflict
• interventive
	• often involuntary
	• referred for investigative purposes due to a forensic or legal matter
	• referred by a system involved in a legal dispute or an investigative function such as
	  ○ law enforcement
	  ○ prosecution
	  ○ defense
	  ○ child protection agency
	  ○ judge or judicial officer
	  ○ at times, may be a court-ordered process

FS Goals and Objectives • engagement with population is not directed at influencing forensic decision making • it is employed after a forensic issue has been resolved or during the decision-making process (meaning client is awaiting decision but has been taken into custody) • addresses the needs of the client because of a judicial decision	**FAT Goals and Objectives** • fact-finding process • assists in resolution of legal matters in dispute • investigative • nonthreatening • minimization of repeated investigative interviews • child friendly • safeguards emotional well-being of child victims and witnesses while maintaining forensic integrity

After Investigation (FAT)/Judicial Decision (FS)

At the conclusion of a FAT interview process, drawing may serve as a stimulus to explore additional material. It may be used to segue into what happens after the investigative process. A FAT client may be referred to treatment to address trauma or other issues as identified by the interviewer in consultation with the team and in the context of the interview. The allegations may merit additional exploration in an extended interview process. A FAT client may be referred to a support group, or therapeutic intervention may be recommended and services for the family may be advocated. After investigation, a FAT drawing may be a means to refresh what was previously disclosed during a forensic interview, as court proceedings may occur after copious amounts of time have elapsed. As such, drawing made during an interview may be revisited to help prepare a client for courtroom participation. Appropriate court support and advocacy may also be suggested. For example, some communities provide resources for children and families that may participate in courtroom proceedings, including court school for children and victim advocates or counselors to assist parental figures.

As they acclimate, FS clients may be moved to a less restrictive environment. FS may encourage someone to address underlying thoughts and feelings while maintaining a proper mask (Gussak & Cohen-Liebman, 2001), which may entail balancing self-exposure. Gussak (2020) provides further discussion of the concept of masks with this population. A person may be willing to take a risk and express information when supported to do so. Use of media in FS is encouraged in relation to the needs of the client, for example, to help a client adapt to the setting and to maintain personal safety and for self-preservation (Gussak & Cohen-Liebman, 2001). Clients are considered wards of the court, and artwork belongs to the client or the institution depending upon the orientation and the dictates of the setting.

FAT and FS SUMMARY of MAIN POINTS

Similarities	Distinctions	Uncovering	Artwork	After Investigation or Intervention
FS and FAT self-expression for clients practiced within non-traditional settings Both have an association with the judicial or legal system	FS clients may not seek out services, although they may be strongly encouraged to participate FAT clients may not have a choice with regard to participation given investigative protocols	FS may be detrimental to the treatment (may compromise the safety of a client) FAT or investigation not a therapeutic session or process FAT client may not be able to process and manage disclosed information (not a clinical process) integrity of forensic process must be maintained FAT processing of information (uncovered and/or disclosed) and addressment of issues may necessitate a referral or recommen-dation within a therapeutic milieu	FS only as far as needed to get client to main population and be safe FS to elicit information while maintaining a proper mask to keep safe within an environment that will take advantage of weakness (Gussak & Cohen-Liebman, 2001) FAT artwork is used to elicit information and facilitate fact-finding court prep, refresh memory, review, segue to what happens next	FS client may go to a less restrictive environment FS client is a ward of the court art belongs to the FS client or the institution which is contingent upon the setting FAT client may be referred for an extended interview, or to therapy, a support group and other resources as indicated if a judicial proceeding is scheduled, appropriate court support and prep may be recommended for child and family artwork may serve as evidentiary material or judiciary aid

The Art of Interviewing

Interviews are considered the foci of a child abuse investigation and as such garner attention regarding best practice and application (Faller, 2014). Interviewing, however, connotes different ideals and associations. FAT is a forensic interviewing process that amalgamates forensic and art therapy approaches. Clinical overtones are present, given the juxtaposition of art therapy principles and practices with judicial ideology. One of the underlying premises associated with FAT is directed at maintaining the emotional and overall well-being of a child victim or witness without compromising the forensic integrity of the process. As such, it is a supportive practice that is legally compliant. Attributes of interviewing that factored into the evolution of FAT as a process oriented fact-finding endeavor follow.

First, consideration will be directed at interviewing versus interrogation. A child interview process differs in scope and orientation from an interrogation of a suspect or an offender. Interrogation of child victims of interpersonal violence is not best practice and is to be avoided.

Next, a brief overview of clinical versus forensic interviewing provides contextual background relevant to the foundation of FAT. The inherent differences that distinguish these processes will be identified, as well as characteristics associated with interviewers that conduct them. For the context of understanding and appreciating how FAT evolved and developed, it is important to address the variance that exists between clinical and forensic interviewing practices. There are unique differences that distinguish clinical and forensic interviewing with regard to process, procedure and interviewer conduct.

Interviewing Versus Interrogation

Interviewing and interrogation are exploratory processes, but they are different in semantics, style, goals and objectives. Interviewing is a way to acquire information from an individual that may have been a victim or a witness to a crime, whereas an interrogation is conducted to determine the innocence or guilt of an individual. Interrogation is intended to obtain information that will contribute to determining and perhaps confirming if an individual is guilty of committing a crime, as well as someone's culpability. Interrogation is a process that, by nature, is adversarial in design, although it can achieve this nuance via different frameworks. A summary of strategies and strengths as they pertain to interviewing (mainly within the context of children and youth) and interrogation is provided to demarcate how these processes differ in approach, objectives and strategy.

An interview is a process by which information is obtained within a conversational context such as a meeting. The process is planned in advance and hopefully conducted in a comfortable, warm and welcoming setting (which is not always attainable). Information is obtained in a non-accusatory manner, meaning that the tone is conversational and not antagonistic. The interviewer documents the conversation by taking notes and perhaps may record the process (depending upon the dictates of the jurisdiction where the process is conducted). Interviews have an implied timeline. The investigator conducting the interview is tasked with uncovering information that will be verified, supported or disproved within the investigation.

Interviews are considered different than a conversation given the emphasis on three things: "a definite purpose, a question-answer format, and a well-defined goal" (Saywitz et al., 2018, p. 313). Interviews have been characterized as existing on a continuum from unstructured to semi-structured to highly structured. The latter involve adhering to a script "where exact wording of questions is scripted", whereas a semi-structured process follows a prescribed guideline that addresses topics (Saywitz et al., 2018, p. 313). An unstructured interview subscribes to the premise wherein the interviewer follows the child's lead. There are pros and cons to the use of each type of interview strategy.

Interrogation is premised on a different model than an interview. The format is structured and conducted in a manner designed to elicit information to confirm innocence or guilt. The process originates with an assumptive stance of guilt, which pervades. The interrogator controls and leads the direction of the conversation; thus, the subject being interrogated is not the focus. Typically note taking is not a primary concern, as procedurally notes are not standard. Interrogations continue essentially without interruptions or disturbances, and privacy is supported. There is not a set time limit to an interrogation, as the end goal is the acquisition of a confession. Interrogations may continue until an admission is obtained, with desired facts and supporting material hopefully provided.

Interrogations may be accusatory in nature and design. These processes are conducted usually as a one-on-one interaction, although audiences devoted to crime shows may associate good cop/bad cop dyads with interrogation. Although on television this scenario is invoked, that may not necessarily exist in real-world situations, given resources and the dynamics of a particular case. Observation, however, is highly regarded as part of the process. Although interrogations are meant to be private, an observer is warranted, whether from outside the room of engagement in which observation is via a one-way mirror or another platform. Another possibility is to have an additional investigator (the observer) stationed within the space where the process is conducted but not interact as an engaged combatant or otherwise.

Interviewing	*Interrogation*
• information is obtained during a meeting • non-accusatory • conversational • notes are taken • time limited • looking for information that will be verified or disproved during investigation	• accusatory in nature and design • interrogator dominates the conversation • guilt is suspected • note taking is not typical • one-on-one interaction • privacy and no interruptions/distractions • may continue as long as needed in an effort to get a confession • should be observed by additional personnel

Comparison of Forensic and Clinical Interview Methods

Forensic and clinical interviews have distinct elements that differentiate them from one another. Inherent differences manifest in procedure, role of the interviewer, intent of the process, contextual nature, collection of information or data and memorialization as well as style. The relationship between the child and interviewer differs, as does the type of questioning. Forensic interviews require the acquisition of accurate information, while mental health processes promote expression of thoughts and feelings regardless of accuracy (Carnes, 2000). The task of the forensic interviewer is to identify "the most effective means of getting an accurate, complete report" (Everson & Boat, 2002, p. 383). The task for the clinical interviewer is to "match the interview with the individual client in order to maximize the child's ability to convey significant information" (Salmon et al., 2003, p. 65). A forensic process addresses legal issues and obtains information to assist with legal determinations (Haralambie, 1999; Mannarino & Cohen, 1992), including the ascertainment of abuse (Reed, 1996). Finally, these processes are devoted to procuring information in a manner that is objective, developmentally sensitive, comprehensive and forensically defensible (Cohen-Liebman, 1999; Davies et al., 1996) as well as culturally attuned.

Clinical Versus Forensic Interviewing

Inherent Differences
Within the scope of interviewing, there are unique differences that distinguish clinical and forensic processes. These differences manifest in the following arenas:

Clinical Versus Forensic Interviewing

Procedure
Role of Interviewer
Intent
Context
Collection of Data/Information
Style

CLINICAL	FORENSIC
• interventive	• investigative
• assumption child is telling truth	• fact-finding – no assumptions
• advocate for child	• advocate for facts/truth
• subjective reality	• alternative explanations explored
• nonspecific account	• corroboration of information
• data collection not important	• strict rules and procedures
• validation of feelings	• assess credibility and competency

OBJECTIVITY/NEUTRALITY/IMPARTIALITY	
• not neutral	• neutrality enhances the quality of the evaluation, as well as the credibility of the evaluator
	• subjective biases can compromise impartiality

CONFIDENTIALITY	
• exists, although exceptions subsist	• nonexistent

Clinical Interviewing

The clinical interview addresses the safety and well-being of the child, including protective, medical and emotional needs (American Academy of Child and Adolescent Psychiatry, 1990). A clinical process is a means to assess the needs of an individual and determine corresponding interventions and support. Typically, these processes are directed at diagnostic and treatment considerations stemming from the evaluation of a child's psychological functioning.

Clinical interviewing is subjective in nature such that the clinician is an advocate for the child, who is encouraged to express thoughts and associated feelings. What the child communicates is accepted and addressed within the context of the process. Accuracy is not integral to a therapeutic process. Veracity of disclosure and establishing credibility are not within the scope of the clinical interview. The way information is gleaned is not central to the clinical process. Maintaining confidentiality within a clinical process is a mainstay, although exceptions do exist. The clinical interviewer is not an investigator and is not obligated to decipher the information a child may disclose in relation to abuse. If abuse is disclosed or suspected, it is incumbent upon the clinician to act accordingly and report as mandated in deference to local and state guidelines. The clinical interviewer is not an investigator and as such should not conduct an investigation; rather, the duty is to file a report as required and allow the appropriate agencies to conduct an investigation in accordance with jurisdictional directives.

A clinical interview is not intended to be a neutral process. The assumption is that the child is telling the truth, and the interviewer is an advocate for the child since subjective reality is acceptable and nonspecific accounts are welcomed. The clinician or therapist demonstrates empathy and provides acceptance as well as emotional support, which may entail validation of feelings. Data collection is not pertinent to the process. A general idea of abuse is sufficient, whereas in a forensic process details are imperative (Raskin & Esplin, 1991).

Clinical Interviewing

- a clinical interview is a supportive process
- a clinical process is a means to assess the needs of an individual and to address the need for intervention
- the interviewer is an advocate for the child
- expression of thoughts and associated feelings is acceptable
- subjective interpretations and nonspecific accounts are sufficient
- collection of information is not integral to the process
- validation of feelings is supported

Forensic Interviewing

Forensic interviews are designed to adhere to scientific thinking and method. "A scientifically crafted forensic work product uses the methods and procedures of the scientific method in the gathering, analysis and interpretation of data" (Gould & Stahl, 2009, p. 398). The systematic collection of data grounds the process in scientific thinking (Gould & Stahl, 2009). Scientific methods and procedures enhance reliability and validity since the scientific method is forensically sound and legally defensible (Gould & Stahl, 2009).

Assessment of competency and credibility are factors that distinguish a forensic interview from a clinical interview. Competency is defined as a child's ability to testify in court in a reliable, meaningful manner, whereas credibility refers to truthfulness and accuracy (American Academy of Child and Adolescent Psychiatry, 1997). Credibility specifically refers to trustworthiness, while competency pertains to witness capability and whether or not a victim or witness is able to viably present information. To determine credibility of information, additional material, including details (core, peripheral and idiosyncratic), corroboration (of material disclosed) and alternative explanations (of the allegations), is explored. The exploration of an alternative or ulterior explanation is an essential aspect of the process. Alternative hypotheses are considered to demonstrate reliability and validity within a reasonable degree of scientific certainty in order to meet standards of admissibility (Gould & Stahl, 2009).

Forensic interviews are conducted for fact-finding purposes. The goal of the forensic interview in child sexual abuse cases is to find out if abuse occurred by obtaining information for a legal context. Forensic interviews adhere to rules of evidence in accordance with judicial standards. These processes are directed at facilitating a child's recall of experienced events. Additional objectives are protection and safety of children, the conviction of perpetrators (Cronch et al., 2006) and avoidance of wrongful convictions (Salmon et al., 2012). Truth is the essential criteria being sought, while fact-finding is the objective. The way information is obtained in a clinical process is not an integral factor; however, in a forensic process memorialization of information is paramount. These processes are conducted with adherence to forensic practice, which means that everything within the process is governed and must be defendable in a court of law.

A forensic process may be recorded in conjunction with the practice subscribed to by the team, which varies according to jurisdiction and mandates. Some communities record via videotape while others audio-tape. Note-taking or stenographic records may be approved mechanisms as well to memorialize and preserve the process. Team members observing the interview document material relative to their investigative dictates. As such, a forensic interview necessitates memorialization of the process, which is governed by forensic principles. Everything that is introduced and included in an investigative interview has a purpose and may need to be explained or defended in court. This extends to the interviewer, including behavior and presentation as well as the format and content of the interview proper, including use of interviewing techniques and tools. Memorialization may be subject to scrutiny in court, meaning documentation, reports and testimony may be requested.

In a forensic process there are no assumptions since it is a fact-finding endeavor and the interviewer is an advocate for the facts. Alternative explanations are explored to corroborate information, and the process adheres to strict rules and procedures. The premise is not to educate children, but rather to learn the terminology they ascribe within the context of an experienced event.

Forensic Interviewing

- objective process
- interviewer is an advocate for the facts
- truth is the essential criteria being sought, while fact-finding is the objective
- details, corroboration, alternative explanations are explored
- practice is governed and memorialized (documented)
- credibility and competency are assessed
- interviewers in a forensic process adhere to forensic practice
- preservation of data is key
- a forensic interviewer is a truth seeker
- a forensic interview is a process by which information or fact-finding is obtained for legal purposes
- the primary task in a forensic interview is to gather information and data
- assessing the probability of abuse and the child's credibility are forensic tasks
- corroboration of information is sought
- the process adheres to strict rules and procedures

Distinctions Between Clinical and Forensic Interviews

- a clinical process is subjective in nature, while a forensic process is objective
- a clinical process is not directed at establishing the credibility of a child or the veracity of a child's statements
- while the expression of thoughts and feelings is acceptable within the scope of a clinical process, in a forensic process, facts are sought

---

Characteristics Attributed to Interviewers

Certain characteristics and key factors are associated with forensic interviewers. Three concepts that are integral to interviewing and are engulfed within these processes are objectivity, neutrality and confidentiality. Forensic interviewers maintain objectivity and neutrality to elicit reliable and accurate information. Forensic interviewers draw upon knowledge from a host of competencies to facilitate the process. Professional judgment that is incontrovertible while providing nonjudgmental support is advocated. The goal is to obtain information in an objective manner. Subjective biases can compromise the impartial collection of data in an interview. As such, interviewers must be aware of their own biases which merit attention in the pre-interview meeting (to be addressed).

It is important that the interviewer not determine ahead of the process what may or may not have occurred based on background information shared in advance of the interview. Background information may contribute to how an interviewer structures a process or formulates questions. This material should not influence or contribute to the development of preconceived ideas that may infiltrate or impact how the interviewer interacts or engages. Interviewers must maintain objectivity and not enter a process with a predetermined conclusion which may alter information gathering and preclude exploration that may potentially impact the investigation. The purpose is not intended as a confirmation of an allegation but rather the elicitation of information or fact-finding.

The interviewer interacts with neutrality, which invariably enhances the quality of the process as well as the credibility of the interviewer. The interviewer may convey in a developmentally appropriate way that whatever is expressed by a child will not be judged and will be accepted as offered. Forensic interviewers need to conduct as impartial a process as possible. In this way, the process is acceptable in a judicial proceeding, and the interviewer will hopefully sustain defense of the techniques, tools and skills invoked as well as the fundamental elements associated with the interview format.

An interviewer is responsive to what is said by a child as well as what is not expressed and maintains an impartial affect along with keen listening skills. Responsive listening is important and supports how the interviewer follows the child's lead yet retains control of the process (regardless of the nature of the interview or the amount of structure that underlies it). Additionally, cognizance of nonverbal behaviors or reinforcement behaviors is essential to the integrity of the process. Seemingly innocuous interviewer behaviors of which an interviewer may not be aware of committing or exhibiting may compromise the interview, let alone jeopardize it. This may manifest as involuntarily nodding affirmatively when a child speaks or answers a question.

Forensic Interviewers

- in forensic processes, subjective biases can compromise the impartial collection of data
- neutrality enhances the quality of the evaluation as well as the credibility of the evaluator
- need to conduct as impartial a process as possible

Exemplar

For example, in observing a process in which a police officer took the lead with a child, every time he asked the child a question, he nodded his head affirmatively. The child merely responded by nodding yes to each question the officer asked her. The child did not provide verbal information or clarity as to what she was nodding yes to or why, nor was she asked to explain her responsive behavior by the officer.

Upon conclusion of the officer's brief meeting, the interview was paused, the lead interviewer was switched and the interview continued in accordance with the process. Although not ideal, it is not uncommon to change interviewers in a joint interview if criteria emerge that merit a change in the lead interviewer. In this case, the second interviewer gathered substantive material pertaining to the allegations, and in post-processing, the interviewers discussed the need for attentiveness to nonverbal reinforcement behaviors exhibited by interviewers. During the post-interview meeting, the initial interviewer admitted a lack of awareness of nonverbal behavior that appeared to stifle the child's interaction and verbalization. It was a teaching moment for the interviewers and investigators as well as the multidisciplinary team.

Confidentiality is critical for various purposes within a therapeutic relationship; however, limits or exceptions do exist. Conversely, confidentiality is not applicable in a forensic process. Information elicited in the fact-finding process is intended to be shared across disciplines involved in the investigation. Clarification is offered at the onset of the forensic interview to the child and nonoffending caregiver to avoid misnomers and misunderstanding about the sharing of information with members of the investigative team.

Exemplar

The sharing of information with members of an investigative team that is engaged in observant behavior (meaning either watching from behind a one-way mirror or perhaps via closed-circuit television) is disclosed to the child in an effort to avoid potential conflict and to mitigate the element of surprise if discovery of additional personnel is identified, perhaps coming out of the observation booth or observed standing in the hallway upon exiting the interview space. (If a child does not understand that what they say is being shared with other members of the team, discovery of such may promote an unanticipated response that may undermine the process or negate additional interviews if warranted.)

Typically, once the issue is addressed in a developmentally congruent manner during discussion pertaining to the expectations associated with the interview, the presence (understanding that observation is taking place) of additional observers is not a factor that impacts the process. If a child is concerned about an officer or the child protection worker hearing a disclosure, the child may find an alternative way to provide information within the interview context that is still observed and heard by the individuals watching. The child is aware that the entire process is being observed and documented in accordance with the dictates of the interview setting. Explanation is offered in a manner that is congruent with the child's level of functioning and discussed to avert a negative response should the child express concern.

Personally, I have had children draw and not verbalize, believing that by not speaking out loud about what they are drawing, they are not compromising a promise to not tell. A child may believe that a threat by a perpetrator will not manifest if they do not speak. For example, a preadolescent female drew stick figure dyads to indicate abuse that occurred between male relatives and herself. She clearly labeled the individuals in the drawing. She said that the perpetrators had threatened to harm her family and her pets if she told anyone what happened.

Through her drawing she was able to depict what she experienced in conjunction with limited verbalization. Her fear of disclosure was palpable, and she positioned the paper so that team members had difficulty observing through the one-way mirror. She repeated that she was told not to say anything to anyone, yet she provided salient information that identified the nature of the abuse, the identity of the perpetrator(s), the setting in which the events took place and details related to the abusive situations on paper and through her limited and somewhat convoluted associations. The latter invoked to mask her anxiety and fear.

She was able to disclose her experience in a manner that was conducive to her need to separate telling and showing with respect to the threats she had endured and the fear she was experiencing in relating the abuse. She provided a limited narrative detailing her experiences with extended family members in conjunction with her graphic depictions. Her anxiety and fear, which included fear of betrayal (that by disclosing information she would bring evil upon her family), were expressed by drawing and telling through her imagery.

The process provided a means for the child to disclose information that was purposeful for the investigation and resulted in evidentiary gathering. Drawing provided a cathartic means of disclosure as she mastered her fear(s). Drawing also empowered her to express information pertaining to multiple abusive experiences with a myriad of perpetrators while managing underlying thoughts and feelings.

Interviewer Competencies

Forensic interviewers remain neutral and objective and draw upon their knowledge of a host of competencies or knowledge-based modules (as I refer to these topics). Awareness and background in a myriad of related topics are essential for investigative interviewers in order to maximize the fact-finding process. The knowledge assists in structuring the process and fostering the elicitation of information. If a child discloses certain aspects or details of an experienced event, the interviewer, given education, knowledge and training, will follow up accordingly or be triggered to explore an allegation further to rule out or rule in certain material.

For example, if a child discloses that they were afraid something might happen to their dog if they told, the investigator should explore whether or not the child was threatened, coerced or forced to do something. Sometimes information is divulged because the interviewer connects something the child has said with something fundamental to exploring allegations of sexual abuse such as offender profiles or the process of disclosure. Maybe the child says something that seems out of context from what they are discussing but is related to a dynamic of sexual abuse such as the progression of less intimate to more intimate behaviors. The interviewer will pursue the topic for clarification in an effort to uncover additional facts and for corroborative purposes.

The interviewer will draw upon background and training to ensure a comprehensive process. Being well oriented and well versed in the dynamics and mechanics of child sexual abuse and related topics will assist the interviewer to be receptive and responsive to the information generated through the interactive process. In addition to fundamental education pertaining to forensic interviewing, child sexual abuse and the use of nonleading questions, open-ended prompts and other identified topics and subjects, skilled interviewers draw upon engrained knowledge regarding child development to uncover information while adhering to the interview process whether it is structured or semi-structured, a protocol, a policy or a guideline.

It is incumbent upon the trained interviewer to be mindful and aware of what a child is not disclosing as well as what is being communicated. If a child provides selective material, the interviewer must be attuned to what the child is trying to express through investigative means and by applying the information acquired to related topics that are pertinent to investigating allegations of child sexual abuse. A comprehensive knowledge base will contribute to eliciting additional information by following up on what the child may be trying to convey but may not cognitively or developmentally possess the language to clearly articulate. For example, if a child is discussing physical harm or being cajoled into not telling in order to maintain secrecy, an interviewer must be prepared to explore deeper through proper forensic investigative measures what information the child may be trying to provide in concert with the developmental capabilities of the child.

The dynamics of child sexual abuse are such that maintaining the element of secrecy is embedded. A child may demonstrate conflict with divulging secrets and may be fearful of the consequences (as previously discussed in the vignette earlier). It is the duty of the interviewer to develop trust with the child (which is not a simple task) within the context of the interview to allay the child's fear and reticence to discuss experienced events. Education, experience and training that are correspondent with the demands of the role will provide the foundation for how the interviewer conducts the process and supports the child.

Depending upon the information disclosed, the interviewer will draw upon background, knowledge, skill and training to explore additional fact-finding and gather more details that may be salient for further investigation either by individual or multiple agencies. For example, if a child discloses that they were made to watch television with an alleged perpetrator, the interviewer will pursue the content of what the child was exposed to when watching programming and how the viewing may have contributed to what followed or what happened next. This information may prove salient with regard to law enforcement's investigation and may yield the procurement of significant evidence that may factor into determination of charges against an individual as well as lead to potential identification of additional victims or even witnesses. The ramifications may extend to the uncovering or new discovery of evidentiary material as well as information that may direct and potentially impact investigation, prosecution and interventive decisions.

If a child describes watching television with an alleged perpetrator, the forensic interviewer versed in dynamics and mechanics of child sexual abuse and offender profiles will know to explore the context of the television show that was watched to find out whether or not a child was exposed to pornography or age-inappropriate sexual content as well as activity that may have been perpetrated by the offender prior, during or after viewing such material.

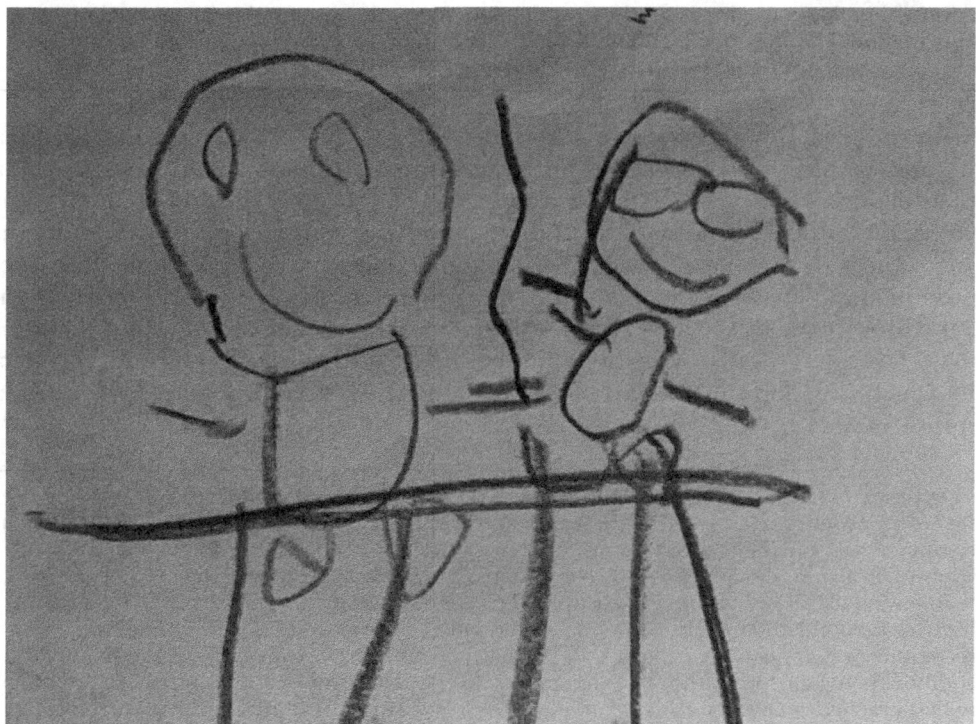

Figure 1.1 Drawing made by a six-year-old depicting several elements/facts related to alleged abuse including, setting/location, alleged perpetrator and nature of the abuse.

Drawing made by a six-year-old male molested by a teenage male stepsibling. The child depicted how he watched television with the teenager while they were sitting at the table after eating dinner. The child described that the alleged perpetrator touched him on his privates with his hand under the table while they were watching a kids' show. The child explained that no one else at the table could see what the older boy was doing to him during the television program. The child reported that if he tried to swat the teenager's hand away, the teenager would stick his nails into his leg, which he said hurt. The child said that he was afraid that the older boy would hurt him big time if he did not let him touch him down there. He said that he was afraid of his stepbrother, who had told him before that if he ever stopped him from doing what he wanted to him, he would be sorry. The child said that although he made himself and his stepbrother smiling in the drawing, he was really sad and mad. He explained that he had to try very hard not to cry because he knew if anyone found out his stepbrother would get in

(*Continued*)

trouble and come after him; however, as the child related information about not being able to cry, he indicated that he was unable to stop a few tears from coming out of his eye. He said that was the line he included next to his (right) eye. He also said that he drew a squiggly line between him and his stepbrother because he did not want to look at him because he was mean and stupid. He explained that at school there are dividers on the desks so that the kids pay attention to the teacher instead of talking to each other. The child said that he wished he had a divider that went on top and underneath the table so that his stepbrother would stop touching him when they watched TV.

The child provided a detailed narrative of the experienced event in conjunction with his drawing, which he described as he added details including idiosyncratic ones such as the squiggly line and the tear. The drawing, in conjunction with the child's associations, provided information that addressed where the abuse took place, who the alleged perpetrator was, the context in which the abuse occurred and the type of abuse perpetrated. He provided information that was relevant to the investigation, impacting eventual child protection and intervention. His drawing helped to facilitate his ability to disclose personal and meaningful information that situated the experience and offered contextual material.

With the forensic interview process there are many moving parts in that information must be processed and follow-up inquiries made to pursue and assess information as the process evolves. A strategy sometimes employed at the end of an interview involves the interviewer asking the child if there is anything the interviewer did not ask or if there is anything else the child might like to discuss or share. Sometimes such a prompt may contribute to a disclosure emerging. On occasion, a child may admonish the interviewer by saying, "Well you didn't ask about . . ." and new information is imparted, leading to discovery of additional material that is critical to the investigation, which may impact protective and interventive issues and potentially contribute to prosecution.

Competencies that factor into forensic interviewing (**knowledge-based modules**)

Knowledge, experience and skill in these arenas will enhance the interview process as well as the competency of the interviewer. It must be stated that knowing laws and criminal codes that apply to local and state jurisdiction is important, as these may vary from state to state.

The following list, although not exhaustive, identifies areas that a forensic interviewer should have background and experience with, additionally, ongoing training and supervision are recommended. If possible, exposure to and participation in peer review is suggested. In addition, being current with relative literature and research, including information pertaining to best practice, is advocated, as is familiarity with guidelines from professional organizations.

- forensic interviewing practices
- child sexual abuse
  - ◦ dynamics and mechanics
  - ◦ process of disclosure
  - ◦ delay in reporting
  - ◦ recantation
  - ◦ credibility assessment
  - ◦ competency assessment
- child development and maturational spheres
  - ◦ language/linguistic
  - ◦ cognitive/cognition
  - ◦ psychosocial
  - ◦ psychosexual
  - ◦ artistic (relevant for art therapists)
- children's memory, suggestibility, concept formation
- sexual development
  - ◦ normal

- question continuum or typology (reverse pyramid)
  - open-ended, leading, focused/directed, follow-up questions
- legal issues
- judicial proceedings
- state criminal codes
- interviewing aids, tools, props
- children as witnesses
- domestic violence
- offender profiles
- current research and literature
  - in the field of investigative interviewing
  - best practices for interviewing
- credibility assessment
- special populations
- cultural awareness
- trauma and impact
- guidelines from professional organizations
- effective witnessing strategies and techniques
- documentation, preparation and presentation of reports
- knowledge of responsibilities and mandates associated with partner agencies
- established burdens of proof
  - law enforcement
  - child protection
  - civil court
  - criminal court

The forensic interviewer is tasked with eliciting information pertaining to allegations of abuse. The process is premised around fact-finding, and the interviewer is devoted to maximizing the elicitation of information to ascertain if a crime (i.e., abuse) has been committed and procuring information regarding the circumstances and details surrounding what the child experienced. Assessing the probability of abuse and/or assessing the child's credibility are forensic tasks. Although the primary task is to gather information that will be useful within the legal system, the safety and well-being of the child are critical factors as well to prevent a child from being returned to an environment that is not safe or a caretaker that is not supportive.

Peer Review

Effective training techniques designed for interviewer skill development include the use of videotape and peer review. By participating in trainings where peer review sessions involve conducting mock interviews on tape with actors assuming roles of victims/witnesses, an interviewer can see and experience how they present as an interviewer. Viewing oneself on tape is informative and educational and often the first time may yield a wealth of information and even some surprises. Nonverbal head movements and gestures, even if subtlety executed, can have a profound impact on an interview and the information gathered or not procured. Interviewer presentation and behavior are matters of concern given the potential impact on disclosure, fact-finding and ultimately the direction of investigation and prosecution.

Peer review affords feedback in a format that is predicated upon constructive assistance directed at enhancing interviewer behavior in a safe and supportive environment. Open-mindedness and receptivity to peer review will assist in a positive and beneficial experience that is educational, informative and helpful. Often, interviewers, regardless of experience and training, are unaware of nonverbal behaviors they may exhibit. To have the opportunity to participate in an experience in which one is able to see themselves on tape (within a supervised and experiential process that affords feedback and support) can be a very rich and rewarding educational opportunity.

Clinical Provider Versus Forensic Mental Health Evaluator

Mental health professionals provide different roles according to their engagement with a child when allegations of sexual abuse are suspected. They may be called upon to provide assistance either for clinical or legal/forensic purposes. In an effort to clarify the differing roles that a mental health provider may assume, whether clinical or forensic and the distinction and applicability of such, professional organizations have provided guidelines addressing such matters, including the need to maintain separate relationships (American Academy of Child and Adolescent Psychiatry, 1990). A forensic mental health evaluation of allegations of sexual abuse is needed "when sexual abuse is suspected but has not been substantiated clearly by the formal legal or child protection agencies mandated to investigate and intervene in these cases" (Lippmann, 2002, p. 199) and "[i]t is hoped that a more extensive and comprehensive evaluation will illuminate and clarify what did or did not happen to the child, and that the appropriate legal, protective and therapeutic intervention may follow from such an assessment" (Lippmann, 2002, p. 199).

The concept of diagnosis confers divergence between forensic and clinical processes. In a forensic process information is used not to make a diagnosis, but to formulate an opinion regarding the likelihood of abuse. The treating clinician formulates a treatment plan and specific treatment goals based on a diagnosis to help the client address and ameliorate symptoms. The therapeutic relationship is not neutral and is predicated upon an empathetic response in support of the child. The treating therapist's role is to provide support, treatment and appropriate interventions to assist the child and the family, typically after the investigative process has been completed and perhaps while awaiting a judicial or litigation process. The therapeutic focus is directed at helping a child deal with associated thoughts and feelings. Safety and even prevention may also be addressed within this realm. As a clinician, an individual is a provider of treatment, not a fact-finder. Confidentiality exists with exceptions depending upon circumstances. The provider is supportive of the client and concerned with holistic welfare.

Treating Clinician in Court Versus a Forensic Mental Health Evaluator

Distinctions regarding the role of a treating clinician in court versus a forensic mental health evaluator are important because this impacts how one presents and testifies. In court, differences prevail depending upon forensic and clinical orientation. The treating clinical is typically sworn in as a lay witness if speaking to the particulars of a case. The mental health provider or therapist is not able to argue the case; rather, the role is to testify as a lay witness, which entails providing personal knowledge or firsthand information.

The issue of forensic versus clinical is relevant to the function of a mental health provider serving in the capacity of an expert witness. Within a forensic role, one purpose is to form an opinion about the matter before the court. As a forensic evaluator, confidentiality is not extended since the forensic evaluator is working for the court, not necessarily the client. Whether or not a treatment provider can be an objective evaluator is not an easy question. Typically, clinical and forensic evaluator roles are separate and thus should not be clouded. A treating mental health provider most likely should not conduct a forensic mental health evaluation or assume a dual role when working with a client.

The forensic evaluator's task is to gather information for investigative purposes. In a forensic process, the report is likely to be used for a court proceeding, and the evaluator must be prepared to submit and speak to documentation of the process. A forensic interviewer/evaluator will be expected to present his or her findings within the guise of an expert witness (of course, one must be qualified as such – this will be addressed later). The role of this individual is to provide information and essentially educate the judge and jury about the semantics that are foundational to the case at hand such as child abuse, custodial matters or interpersonal violence. The person may be asked to speak about abused children as a whole or provide information specific to the particular case. The individual, if stipulated as an expert witness, may be asked to comment about the likelihood of whether the child involved in the case is a victim of abuse; however, speaking to the issue before the court is a matter for the trier of fact to determine through the use of the expert's testimony. A forensic mental health interviewer/evaluator has a different stance from a treatment provider, which impacts the associated report. Confidentiality factors as well as privileged communications impact forensic mental health witnesses.

Treatment providers are not expected to testify; however, if requested to do so, they are considered a fact witness and will speak to the information about which they have knowledge. If testifying in the guise of a lay or fact witness, one is not expected to comment on forensic issues, the credibility of a child's statements or the likelihood of abuse. It is not appropriate for this individual to comment directly on the issue before the court, which in child abuse is the likelihood that a particular child is a victim of abuse. A mental health provider is typically not expected to testify, but there are exceptions even though the confidential alliance is ethically protected by privileged communication laws, although exceptions and limits do exist (Myers, 2011c, 2019).

Forensic or mental health forensic evaluators need to be aware that their reports, as well as they themselves, may be subpoenaed to appear in court. The likelihood that a forensic evaluator's report will be used in a legal proceeding is very real, as is the possibility of testifying. Expert witness status is most likely conferred once qualified. In this capacity, the role of the forensic evaluator is to educate about the issue before the court and discuss findings as well as the content of the report. It is the purview of the judge and jury to determine the issue before the court.

Child Custody Evaluations

Civil proceedings such as custodial matters may require the skills of forensic evaluators commissioned by the court to conduct a neutral and objective evaluation. The process may involve the parents/guardians and the child(ren) who are the subject of the dispute. The objective of a court-ordered process is to assist the court in decision making by providing objective information and informed opinions (American Academy of Child and Adolescent Psychiatry, 1990). The expert is essentially charged with the task of explaining behavioral and psychological findings in language that is applicable to the court and useful in the decision-making process. Specialized competence is required, as is familiarity with state laws (American Psychological Association, 1994).

Child custody evaluators as such require specialized knowledge and training. The role of the individual is as an expert, which means not advocate or adversary. This process goes beyond diagnosis and treatment. Although guided by the best interest of the child, the evaluator has no duty to the child or the parents. The premise is to provide information and an informed opinion to help the court determine a decision. Factors that are important in these processes include competence and ethics. The aim is to provide objective information and informed opinions to help the court render a custodial decision that is in the best interest of the child(ren). If possible, a court-ordered process in which both parents are evaluated by the same evaluator is recommended, which is consistent with the objectives of these processes.

The forensic evaluator reports to the court as such rather than to the parties being evaluated. This person cannot serve as a treatment provider and as an evaluator. Roles are distinct and separate. If the evaluator was previously engaged by the parties in a clinical capacity, the individual should not conduct the court-ordered evaluation. Previous involvement with the family may compromise professionalism as well as integrity and mar the established therapeutic relationship even if time has passed. A dual role may convolute the process since objectivity, neutrality and even confidentiality may be compromised given that the family or the parental units or the child may have formed a relationship with the potential evaluator. Within the capacity of a forensic evaluator, self-referral following completion of the process is a conflict and should not happen.

For reference about art therapists and child custody evaluations, Lyons (1993) wrote an article that discusses a psycho-legal practice that conducted court-ordered custody evaluations. She details the role of the art therapist within this construct.

Child custody evaluators require specialized knowledge and techniques. Factors that are important in these processes include competence and ethics. The aim is to provide objective information and informed opinions to help the trier of fact render a decision. Skills associated with this type of practice include:

- interviewing skills
- family and interpersonal dynamics
- child and adult development
- family law
- legal processes
- judiciary proceedings
- aim is to provide objective information and informed opinions to help the court render a decision
- testify as an expert witness
- need specialized knowledge and skill
- need to be aware of legal and ethical considerations
- familiarity with relevant case law specific to child custodial matters
- ability to communicate behavioral and psychological findings to the legal system
- ultimately provide the court with an opinion, not a custodial decision, which is the domain of the judge, who will refer to the information/report provided by the evaluator
- report contains the basis for the evaluator's opinion
- documentation will go to the court, not the parties being evaluated

Factors that will influence the outcome or the judge's decision include what is in the best interest of the child(ren) as well as the recommendations provided by the court-ordered forensic evaluator, who will assess identified areas commonly considered in these cases, which revolve around attachments, the child(ren)'s expressed preference and other factors.

Adapted from guidelines established by the American Academy of Child and Adolescent Psychiatry (1990) on Child Custody Evaluations

Exemplar

Having worked with a psycho-legal practice specifically on custody cases, the fact of the matter was the practice was contracted for its expertise, not opinion. It did not matter which party paid for the retainer up-front (mother or father) – all parties signed that the expertise provided would be accepted regardless of monetary arrangements. The totality of findings was not always in favor of the party that paid for the process. That was stipulated and agreed to prior to initiation of the multi-evaluator process. If both parties were not in agreement, then the evaluation was not able to commence. The practice was committed to an ethical, impartial, neutral and objective process.

It bears repeating that the premise was to consent to expertise, not opinion, which invariably at times might conflict with the desired outcome of the party that paid for the process when a custodial decision was made in favor of the nonpaying parental figure.

Child Maltreatment

Child maltreatment is a general term that encompasses various forms of child abuse and neglect, including physical abuse, sexual abuse, emotional abuse and psychological abuse (Miller-Perrin & Perrin, 2012). These entities are not defined unilaterally. Krugman (2018) expands upon this definition by referring to child maltreatment as "a very heterogeneous problem", and he attributes to this domain "medical care and educational neglect, child sex trafficking, pornography and child labor" (p. 10). Definitions of the different types of abuse vary by state and are often social constructs (Miller-Perrin & Perrin, 2012). State definitions are used to guide child welfare agencies in responding to reports of abuse (Drake & Jonson-Reid, 2018). "It is also important to note that definitions used in research or clinical practice may not correspond to those used by child protection because of state or local definitional differences" (Drake & Jonson-Reid, 2018, p. 15).

Definitions also vary with regard to disciplines, yet general agreement exists with regard to certain terminology. Accordingly, "child maltreatment" is used as a precise synonym for "child abuse and neglect" and "child abuse" always includes "sexual abuse" and "physical abuse," and sometimes includes "emotional abuse" (Drake& Jonson-Reid, 2018, p.14). Child maltreatment has also been considered according to acts of commission and omission. The Centers for Disease Control and Prevention (CDC) have characterized acts of commission as physical, sexual and psychological abuse and identified acts of omission as forms of neglect (Drake & Jonson-Reid, 2018). "Definitions of acts are partly a matter of public policy, including laws but also professional understanding of the nature of the acts themselves" (Conte & Vaughan-Eden, 2018, p. 96).

Differing disciplinary worldviews contribute to the challenges of defining and categorizing child abuse as either a health problem or a public safety issue (Krugman, 1999). Child maltreatment is not a singular entity such as heart disease or cancer or a health problem; rather, it falls within a myriad of domains, including "health, education, welfare or justice" (Sadler, 1999, p. 956), each with a vested interest. A multidisciplinary response is common with a coordinated response involving social sciences, health and law enforcement (Chadwick, 1999).

Child maltreatment is described as an interdisciplinary field which is comprised of a myriad of professions that must work together. This multidisciplinary interface creates challenges in the assessment and development of curriculum due to a lack of standardization in definition, education and credentialing across disciplines, professions and organizations (Vieth, 2006), signaling a lack of unification or consensus within the vicissitudes of child maltreatment. The lack of standardization for education and credentialing is an impact issue due to the diversity implicit in the convergence of different disciplines. These discrepancies impact how epidemiological questions are addressed (Friedenberg et al., 2013).

A coordinated national effort to develop policies, procedures, theory and education was initiated in 1999 (Sadler, 1999) at a summit that brought together respected leaders from the various disciplines that engage in child advocacy. At that meeting, an action plan and a movement to expunge child maltreatment was agreed upon through the advancement and support of a nationally coordinated prevention and intervention agenda (Elders, 1999; Sadler, 1999). The field of child abuse was acknowledged as "fragmented, disjointed and largely ineffective at the national level", necessitating a need for all relevant disciplines "to develop a common agenda and speak with one voice" (Sadler et al., 1999, p. 1016). The development of a "comprehensive, systemic and epidemiological framework" was endorsed by Dr. Elders (Sadler et al., 1999, p. 1015).

The World Report on Children and Violence commissioned a study to review the literature on child abuse to summarize what (at the time) was known about the epidemiology and consequences of violence against children. The study assessed the burden and encumbrance of the problem around the world (Runyan et al., 2009). The report was compiled for the United Nations secretary-general and the UN General Assembly (Runyan et al., 2009). The status of governmental programs and policies was studied. The report, which assessed the burden of violence upon children, was complicated by "variations in measurement, data sources, samples and definitions across countries and between investigators" (Runyan et al., 2009, p. 842). Difficulties in recognizing a common definition of child abuse was apparent not only on a national level but globally as well. The need for coordinated advocacy, given the variety of disciplines that respond and are impacted by child abuse, meant that an "effective catalyst to galvanize a nationally coordinated action agenda" was deemed warranted (Sadler, 1999, p. 956).

Child Advocacy

Child advocacy is an overarching term that refers to individuals, professionals and organizations that advocate for children's rights. Child advocacy engages the resources and skills of multiple disciplines, each of which contributes particular expertise to promote optimal well-being of children (Goodyear-Brown, 2012). Forms of abuse, including sexual and physical as well as neglect, require intervention as well as the skills and expertise of individuals from a host of disciplines, including law enforcement, social services, prosecution, mental health, victim advocacy and the medical community (Van Eys & Beneke, 2012). This interface creates challenges due to a lack of consensus and consistency associated with the various forms of maltreatment as well as definitions. Disciplines have to work together, share their knowledge, understand the roles and responsibilities of other agencies and forge a common language. The ability to consider alternative ideas and perspectives is fundamental to ensuring the effectiveness of multidisciplinary teams that investigate and intervene in child advocacy matters. Despite discipline diversity, protecting and maintaining the welfare of children is the primary goal in child maltreatment and hence child advocacy (Goodyear-Brown, 2012).

Child Abuse

Child abuse was not officially recognized in the mental health profession until the middle of the 20th century. In 1961, Dr. Henry Kempe, along with colleagues representing a multidisciplinary collaboration, discussed the battered child syndrome (which Kempe coined) at a symposium sponsored by the American Academy of Pediatrics. The diagnosis stemmed from physicians, including pediatric radiologists, who observed cases of infants with bone fractures and internal wounds that were determined to be nonaccidental. The multidisciplinary nature of the presentation was, according to Krugman (2018), "unique for the Academy of Pediatrics at the time" (p. 4). The response to the topic presented at the collaborative seminar, of the approximate 1,000 attendees, was disbelief and even anger (Krugman, 2018); however, a news story on the presentation cultivated response and interest in the issue that subsequently swept across the nation.

In 1962, Dr. Kempe and his colleagues, including Dr. Brandt Steele, a psychiatrist, published a seminal article in the *Journal of the American Medical Association* entitled "The Battered-Child Syndrome" which spurred child protection initiatives (Krugman, 2018) and heralded the beginning of research and literature on child abuse. Steele was memorialized as someone who "believed in the efficacy of mental health treatment and multidisciplinary approaches to recognition and treatment" (Krugman, 2005, p. 207). The work of these physicians, along with their colleagues, contributed to child abuse being recognized as a public policy issue (Krugman, 2018) and contributed to the American Humane Association and the American Medical Association developing model statutes pertaining to reporting of abuse and neglect to social service agencies by designated professionals. The initial response to the mandatory reporting laws was an influx in cases surrounding abuse.

The work of these pioneers also inculcated and advocated for a multidisciplinary approach to address the scope of the problem (Kempe & Helfer, 1968). In both their first and second edition of *The Battered Child* co-authored by Kempe and Helfer (1968, 1972), multidisciplinary response and teaming were supported and advocated. The role of the various disciplines engaged in responding to reports of abuse was recognized and outlined. This constellation of responders encompassed doctors, psychologists, law enforcement and the justice system, specifically (as noted by Krugman, 2018) "physicians, social workers, psychologists, psychiatrists, law enforcement, and civil and criminal district attorneys" (p. 6).

Reporting Laws

The first legislation that mandated reporting of child abuse was proposed in 1963 and derived from meetings convened by the U.S. Children's Bureau. This resulted in the Model Children's Protection Act, which led to the adoption of reporting mandates in every state (Myers, 2011c). Within five years every state had adopted child abuse reporting laws, which required certain professionals who worked with children to report suspected cases to child protection agencies. The laws required that professionals report suspected child abuse and/or neglect to designated authorities. The reporting requirements take precedence over confidentiality and privilege associated with the client relationship and override the ethical duty to protect confidential client information. The impetus for the laws revolved around the fact that protection and services could only be instigated when cases of maltreatment were identified or known. Reporting laws became the incentive for such identification. The laws included provisions to remove barriers from reporting by providing immunity for good-faith reporting.

According to Myers, although the level of suspicion in reporting laws may differ with regard to "triggering level of suspicion" (Myers, 2011c, p. 361), the laws essentially state "a report is required when a professional has information that would lead a competent professional to believe maltreatment is likely" (Myers, 2011c, p. 361). Myers (2011c) states that the facts of the case as "interpreted through the lens of experience and judgment" will factor into whether that threshold has been met. "Reporting is triggered by suspicion not certainty" (Myers, 2011c, p. 362). "When maltreatment is suspected, reporting is mandatory and not discretionary" (Myers, 2011c, p. 362). With regard to mandated reporting, "the child abuse reporting law supersedes confidentiality" (Myers, 2011c, p. 362); as such, only information required to meet the reporting law is necessary, meaning that not all information possessed by the mandated reporter necessitates reporting. If information is not required to be reported by the law, then that information is protected (Myers, 2011c). Although reporting statutes initially were concentrated around physical abuse and neglect, sexual abuse garnered attention in the 1970s and 1980s. The phenomenon of sexual abuse was described by Kempe as a "hidden problem" (Myers, 2011a, p. 12).

> In the early 1970's sexual abuse was still largely invisible, but that was about to change. Two related factors launched sexual abuse onto the national stage. First, the child protection system – including reporting laws – expanded significantly in the 1970s. Second, new research shed light on the prevalence and harmful effects of sexual abuse. (Myers, 2011a, p. 12)

The Child Abuse Prevention and Treatment Act of 1974 (CAPTA) is considered to be the legislation that most closely addresses child abuse (Goodyear-Brown et al., 2012). It is considered to be the fundamental legislation addressing child maltreatment in the United States (Drake & Jonson-Reid, 2018). It was also the first legislation to include sexual abuse as a distinct entity. CAPTA defines the term child maltreatment as "[a]ny recent act or failure to act on the part of a parent or caretaker, which results in death, serious physical or emotional harm, sexual abuse, or exploitation, or an act or failure to act which presents an imminent risk of serious harm" (Child Welfare Information Gateway, 2014).

The women's movement in the United States, along with other contemporary issues, influenced and impacted a deepening of awareness of sexual crimes, which sparked an elevation in interest. The enhanced recognition combined with public awareness that child abuse existed contributed to an increase in reports of child sexual abuse (Krugman, 2018, p. 6). Sexual abuse was classified as a criminal offense and fell under the auspices of law enforcement, whereas physical abuse and neglect were not necessarily considered in the same light and were consigned to the child welfare system for investigation (Krugman, 2018).

Child maltreatment is a term associated with the child welfare system, not necessarily law enforcement. Clarification regarding who constitutes an offender in child maltreatment is specific in that an individual must be a parent or serving in a caretaking role. Not all forms of child maltreatment are considered a criminal offense (Myers, 2011b). An individual outside of that capacity (caretaking) who assaults a child, whether or not a stranger, is a matter for law enforcement given that, as noted earlier, sexual abuse is a crime. Nonoffending caretakers, if aware of the abuse or if they in some way are found to have contributed to the abuse, may be considered to be a perpetrator (Myers, 2011b) or a perpetrator by omission.

Definitions that guide response from child protection agencies are established by each state. Consensus exists regarding the age when a child is no longer considered under the age of majority (adulthood) – typically 18. States determine how long after an act of abuse a report may be filed or what will trigger a report. Subsequent legal action for past maltreatment by an adult is not the onus of child protection, but rather may be addressed in the criminal or civil systems (Drake & Jonson-Reid, 2018).

With the influx of reports stemming from child sexual abuse cases and the involvement of both child welfare and law enforcement, "there had to be coordination between agencies that had never coordinated before" (Krugman, 2018, p. 7). The principles espoused by Kempe and his colleagues – specifically the need for a "multidisciplinary approach to recognition, treatment and prevention" (Krugman, 2018, p. 7) – were instrumental in the manner in which cases began to be managed. Although some in the field have recognized that the multidisciplinary team concept was initiated by the work of Kempe and colleagues, these efforts have not received the acknowledgement for this forward-thinking initiative, which in turn spurred a movement reflected in the approach to sexual abuse that emerged in the 1980s (Krugman, 2018).

Mandated Reporting

It is imperative to educate oneself about the reporting laws in the state in which one practices in order to understand what is required of a mandated reporter and the corresponding obligations associated with reporting. Reporting laws vary from state to state and may be impacted by county and other jurisdictional entities. In some states, reports are to be made to identified child protective agencies, while in others reports may go through designated hotlines either state run or associated with governmental bodies (Kemp, 2017). In some states, a reporter who is a professional may have to identify themselves and provide written documentation. Willful failure to report may result in prosecution; however, if a reporter acts in good faith, prosecution, either criminally or civilly, should not or may not be a factor. A report of suspected abuse should be made as soon as a reporter has reason to suspect. An investigation will be conducted by the appropriate child welfare agency after a report is received.

Mental health practitioners fall within the category of individuals identified as mandated reporters. Mandated reporters are required to file a report when abuse of any form is suspected. If a mandated reporter suspects questionable behaviors identified as a crime, the individual should make a report immediately. The responsibility of a mandated reporter is only to report suspicions of abuse. When in doubt, if the mandated reporter suspects abuse, a report should be made. Child abuse encompasses sexual abuse, neglect, mental or emotional abuse and physical abuse. It is not the obligation of the mandated reporter to determine if a crime has occurred. The mandated reporter, regardless of profession, is not to assume the role of investigator and is not obliged to determine if a crime was committed. That is the responsibility of the child welfare agency to determine and/or law enforcement.

For a specific example, in Pennsylvania, the Child Protective Services Law requires psychologists and other mental health care professionals to report when they "have reason to suspect that a child is a victim of child abuse" (23 Pa. C. S. A. §6311 (b)). "Reasonable suspicion is more than a hunch or a passing thought. Reasonable suspicion arises as a result of the totality of circumstances, direct observations, or background information" (Pennsylvania Psychological Association, [PPA], 2015). The Pennsylvania Child Protective Services Law states that "a report of suspected abuse is required any time the mandated reporter has reason to suspect that the crime occurred regardless of whether the mandated reporter saw the abused child in their professional capacity" (PPA, 2015). In some instances, individuals may be required to report only when they have direct contact with a child. Although any person may make a report when sexual abuse is suspected, only mandated reporters are required to do so. It is incumbent upon mandated reporters to know what is expected and how to file a report when abuse is suspected. In response to difficult cases, amendments to statutes have resulted in mandated reporters having to report suspected abuse when "a specific disclosure [is made] by any person to the mandated reporter that an identifiable child is the victim of child abuse" (PPA, 2015). It is the responsibility of the mandated reporter to make the report rather than delegate to someone else such as an assistant. In Pennsylvania, reports are to be made to a statewide hotline and a written report is to follow within two days as per Pennsylvania Child Protective Services Law (23 Pa. C. S. A. §6311 (b)) and (23 Pa. C. S. A. §6340 (a) (12)).

Once the report is made by the reporter, the child protection agency conducts an investigation and makes a determination. The purpose of the investigation by child protection is to ascertain if a report of suspected abuse is valid. How the matter is resolved and whether or not intervention is enacted are predicated upon the findings of the investigation. The determination will be consistent with the designations affiliated with the jurisdiction. Terminology varies in accordance with the statutes implemented. In Pennsylvania, for example, there is a children and youth agency in every county. Each is responsible for investigating reports of child abuse and providing services when reports of abuse are substantiated.

Substantiation and founded or lack thereof are terms that are related to maltreatment and occurrence (Drake & Jonson-Reid, 2018). Some child welfare systems use the terms substantiated or unsubstantiated, while others may subscribe to founded or unfounded or indicated (Shapiro & Maras, 2016), depending upon state regulations as applied to case findings or outcome determinants. For a case to be substantiated, state law (as indicated according to a respective state's nomenclature) requires either a preponderance of evidence (51%) or clear and convincing evidence (75%) that maltreatment was confirmed, meaning credible evidence exists or a conclusion is reached that a child has been abused. Reports of suspected maltreatment or abuse can be classified as unsubstantiated for a variety of reasons, including a lack of credible information, the allegations do not rise to the level of abuse or maltreatment (as defined by the state or jurisdiction) or an allegation may be deemed not credible due to other reasons.

Child protection and welfare agencies also receive reports that are unrelated to abuse. These cases are reported to a hotline as general protective services (GPS); however, these cases do not rise to the level of child abuse or merit corresponding investigation with regard to abuse. These types of reports may include issues pertaining to housing and living situations, level of care, truancy and injuries that are not considered child abuse yet are matters that require protective services (PPA, 2015).

Mandated Reporting Is Mandatory and Not an Option

- in some jurisdictions, some professionals may need direct observation rather than information that a child has been abused, such as daycare workers
- mandated reporting underscores the importance of being well versed and well informed about local and jurisdictional reporting mandates in the state where one sees clients or works with children
- professionals who work with children are required to report suspected abuse or neglect to child protection or law enforcement

Mandated Reporting Is Mandatory and Not an Option

- reporting laws exist in every state
- reporting laws do not require certainty; rather, the professional reports when he or she has reason to believe or suspect abuse/maltreatment
- the ultimate decision as to whether something happened rests with the investigating agency, not the mandated reporter
- the law requires good faith and reasonable professional judgement
- reporting laws provide immunity from civil and criminal liability for professionals who report in good faith (typically)
- reporting laws override the ethical duty to protect confidential information
- if a mandated reporter fails to report suspicions, he or she can be liable civilly or criminally, especially if a child continues to be abused or sustains a life-threatening or life-ending injury
- if a mandated reporter suspects abuse but fails to report suspicions, and investigation by child protection does not occur and something adverse happens to a child, the possibility exists that a mandated reporter may be brought up on charges
- it is best to err on the side of caution to protect children and youth

Protections are embedded into mandated reporting. Mandated reporters receive immunity for good faith in making reports of suspected abuse, cooperating with investigations, testifying in proceedings arising out of suspected abuse or engaging in some other actions (as put forth in PPA, 2015). Penalties also exist and are specific to felony or misdemeanor charges. A felony (more serious offense) may be charged if a mandated reporter "willfully failed to report child abuse when they had direct contact with an abused child" (as put forth in PPA, 2015). A misdemeanor (lesser offense) may be charged if mandated reporters otherwise fail to report abuse. The best means of avoiding criminal scrutiny is by obtaining "a working understanding of the child abuse reporting statute" in the jurisdiction where one practices (as put forth in PPA, 2015). Consultation with an attorney or securing legal advice is always an option to ensure that one understands the reporting mandates of the state in which they practice and what one needs to do to comply. Mandated reporters need to exercise sound clinical judgment and maintain comprehensive records (PPA, 2015). Reporters, in providing information when making a report of suspected child abuse, "should give as much detail about why abuse is suspected as possible so that the report will not simply be screened out" (Van Eys & Beneke, 2012, p. 73). Additionally, the child's contact information and the nature of the concerns that prompted reporting are to be provided.

Failure to report may engender a penalty ranging from a misdemeanor to a felony. Criminal prosecutions of such matters are reported to be rare. Reasons professionals do not report include the following:

- may fear threat with regard to the client relationship
- feel will not result in any benefit for child or family
- do not consider something reportable
- feel can better serve the child/family through the professional relationship

In Summary

- a report of suspected abuse or neglect merits investigation
- the investigating child protection agency will make a determination
- which may be aligned with one of the following (although designations may be different depending upon the jurisdiction)

(*Continued*)

- o substantiated – means credible evidence exists or a sufficient reason to conclude that a child has been abused; state law requires either a preponderance of evidence (51%) or clear and convincing evidence (75%) that maltreatment was confirmed
- o unsubstantiated or unfounded – may be related to a myriad of reasons
- reasons for failure to substantiate
  - o insufficient information
  - o inappropriate referral
  - o problem does not constitute child maltreatment
  - o a child is no longer at risk
  - o false allegations

Exemplar

Issues that arose out of a treating therapist's resistance to file a report.

The treating therapist did not want to file a report of abuse and did not until threatened by law enforcement that she was going to face charges. Her explanation: She was working with a family that was in the termination stage of therapy. During the second-to-last session, one of the minor children reported being sexually molested by an older sibling who was now past the age of majority (18). The therapist was conflicted and did not wish to alter the path to termination. She made the decision that she would handle the matter as she worked with the family to terminate therapy.

A report was made to child protection and law enforcement by a secondary source. The therapist was contacted by the law enforcement agent assigned to the case. The therapist was not willing to accept or admit responsibility with regard to her behavior and the consequences of her actions. The therapist was antagonistic and defensive with the assigned officer and steadfast in her refusal to believe that her handling of the case was inappropriate or counterproductive. She insisted that it was a family matter and that the family should continue with the termination and deal with the situation with her in the therapeutic process, thus compromising the safety of the child and jeopardizing an investigation of a crime.

The usually mild-mannered and low-key detective went through a metamorphosis as he patiently and calmly (despite I believe his desire to reach through the phone) explained to the therapist that if she did not disengage and cooperate with the investigation, she was going to be brought up on charges. Much to the therapist's indignation and true incapacity to hear what the officer was saying and explaining, the therapist relinquished her role only when she was admonished that she was going to be in legal trouble, serious legal trouble, of her own making.

The officer vividly told her that he had never encountered a therapist who exhibited such inane and sanctimonious behavior (my words, not his). Fortunately for the therapist, despite her presentation, the officer approached the situation from an educational standpoint, believing that the therapist was not willfully being noncompliant and truly thought she could do more for the family than an investigation. I think on some level the officer felt that the therapist was not being malicious, but rather the therapist either felt responsible on some level for failing the family because she had not uncovered the sibling abuse despite an extended therapeutic relationship, or she was adamant because of her relationship with the family and the community they were associated with, that she felt she was in the best position to address the situation. Needless to say, none of that mattered with regard to the investigation. The report had been made timely and appropriately by another person. The older sibling no longer interacted with the family of origin however, that did not mitigate the circumstances. The allegations, were not for the therapist to investigate or manage. The reasons for not reporting were, in the mind of the therapist, perhaps legitimate. Regardless, reporting laws still have to be respected. They exist for a reason and have a designated purpose.

The level of resistance and obtuse behavior exhibited by the therapist regardless of her seemingly supportive and compassionate stance almost resulted in the officer arresting (for the first time) an individual identified as a mandated reporter for not complying with the law.

The obligations and responsibilities that accompany reporting mandates override the therapeutic alliance and the reasons that may contribute to an individual choosing not to make a report. The therapist's devotion and determination, while perhaps admirable, were in conflict with the reporting statutes. When a situation arises, one must put personal needs, goals, agendas, etc., aside and do what is in the best interest of the client as well as comply with reporting mandates. Potential damage to the investment of the relationship (not to minimize) is moot at this point. The entire experience described was educational, informative and instructive, if not troublesome and disconcerting.

By 1986 almost every state had expanded the definition of a mandated reporter to include professionals other than medical personnel. The definition of what could be reported increased as well to include sexual and emotional abuse in addition to neglect.

Myers (2011c) provides the following pertinent information regarding reporting mandates which merit repetition.

"The duty to report suspected maltreatment is triggered when a professional possesses the level of suspicion specified in the reporting law. Reporting laws differ slightly in the words used to describe the triggering level of suspicion" (p. 361).

"Although the words differ, the basic thrust of reporting laws is the same across the United States: A report is required when a professional has information that would lead a competent professional to believe maltreatment is likely" and "Whether the triggering level of suspicion exists depends on the facts of the case interpreted through the lens of experience and judgment" (p. 361–362).

"Reporting is triggered by suspicion and not certainty" (p. 362).

"When maltreatment is suspected, reporting is mandatory and not discretionary" even if the reporter does not think it is in the best interest to report for whatever reason (p. 362).

"In-depth investigation and decision making about maltreatment is reserved for child protective services (CPS) or law enforcement – not the reporter" (p. 362).

Child abuse reporting laws supersede confidentiality; however, they do not completely abrogate it.

Disclosure is limited to the information required by the reporting law; otherwise, confidential information not required by the law is protected and not mandated to be disclosed (p. 362).

"Child abuse reporting laws override both confidentiality and privilege" (p. 368).

"Reporting laws override the ethical duty to protect confidential client information. Additionally, the reporting requirement overrides privilege" (p. 368).

Professionals "limit the information they report to the information required by law" (p. 368).

Intentional failure to report is against the law and considered to be a crime, and as Myers points out, if a reporter fails to report and a child suffers further abuse or is fatally injured, a professional may be sued for malpractice – Myers cites the case of Landeros v. Flood, 1976 (p. 362).

Myers references Seth Kalichman's text on Mandated Reporting as a good resource to clarify and provide understanding on related issues (Kalichman, 1993, 1999).

REPORTING LAWS

- reporting laws request that reporters be reasonably vigilant – no more is required
- reporters are not required or expected to investigate suspected allegations
- the purpose of reporting is to bring potential abuse to the attention of child protection and to instigate a response
- all reports of child abuse and neglect are to be investigated – this is federally mandated
- a screening function exists and is implicit in all reporting laws
- reporting responsibility is required for children younger than 18
- relationship of the perpetrator to the child figures into the definition of maltreatment
- for child protection investigations, the alleged perpetrator must be a caretaker, although it is still a criminal offense
- if the perpetrator lives outside of the home, investigation is a police matter and reported to law enforcement, not child protection
- possibility exists for dual investigations

Child Sexual Abuse

Public interest and professional concern coalesced and an increase in interest in child abuse evolved. In the 1970s programs aimed at addressing child sexual abuse emerged. Due to the nature of child sexual abuse, including the inherent inability to measure the incidence and obtain accurate accounting, an estimate of prevalence, given the barriers to measuring occurrence, resulted. Programs were created to deal specifically with the issue of child sexual abuse, which was identified as an alarming communal problem. Preponderance of professional literature before 1970 concentrated on whether the child making the allegation was telling the truth rather than focusing on the implications of the trauma upon the child. Early detection and prosecution were focal points. State legislation pertaining to the welfare of children and victims emerged in response to the deepening awareness of the pervasive nature of child abuse and the larger scope of child maltreatment, which was influenced by the CAPTA of 1974.

Child sexual abuse has been identified as a common problem that is potentially damaging to the long-term physical and psychological health effects of children and adolescents (Jenny, Crawford-Jakubiak, & Committee on Child Abuse and Neglect, 2013). This phenomenon has been described as "extraordinary in its characteristics, dynamics, causes and consequences" (Miller-Perrin & Perrin, 2012, p. 96). Sexual abuse is considered a complex event that children are ill prepared to describe (Everson & Boat, 2002). The investigation of allegations has been identified as trauma-inducing, rendering the need for reform. As such, an integrated response by the innumerable agencies and disciplines that intervene was advocated and cultivated. Contemporary trends favor multidisciplinary investigations with the core component, the investigative interview process. Resultant to these developments were research efforts to benefit children through applicability, generalizability and relevance (Poole & Lamb, 2003) on fundamental aspects related to investigative interviewing.

As noted earlier, child sexual abuse, like other forms of abuse and neglect, lacks a conceptual model and a common definition (Mathews & Collin-Vezina, 2017). This deficit has contributed to the lack of an objective scientific standard (Allen & Tussey, 2012; Brooks & Milchman, 1991). Efforts have been directed toward consensus of a common definition for this worldwide public health phenomenon and the development and validity of reliable methods for identifying victims as well as reporting (Sapp & Vandeven, 2005). Sexual abuse and sexual exploitation have been defined distinctly as "direct sexual maltreatment" (sexual abuse) and "indirect sexual maltreatment" such as pornography (Drake & Jonson-Reid, 2018, p. 14).

Investigation is often centered upon information elicited in an investigative interview. Sexual abuse is often determined from a child's statements (Faller, 2003, 2014). An investigative interview is the primary method used to acquire factual and detailed information from child victims and witnesses. Information pertaining to allegations is sought in an investigative or forensic interview. Investigative interviewing has been identified as evolving out of a need "to help avoid false accusations and ensure justice in these cases to strengthen law enforcement's ability to elicit accurate information from children" (Harris, 2010, p. 12).

Child sexual abuse allegations are difficult to investigate given that corroborating evidence is typically unavailable rendering investigators and forensic interviewers reliant upon information imparted by children (Faller, 2014; Lamb & Brown, 2006; Lamb et al., 2008; Macleod et al., 2013; Myers, 1998; Orbach et al., 2000; Poole & Lamb, 2009). A lack of physical or viable evidence and a paucity of eyewitnesses characterize child sexual abuse. A child may be the only witness or victim of such a crime (Macleod et al., 2013).

According to the American Professional Society on the Abuse of Children (APSAC), the purpose of a forensic (investigative) interview is to "elicit as complete and accurate a report from the alleged child or adolescent victim as possible in order to determine whether the child or adolescent has been abused (or is in imminent risk of abuse) and, if so, by whom" (APSAC, 2002, p. 2). Forensic investigative interviews conducted with children are typically verbal processes which focus on the acquisition of accurate and reliable information (Carnes, 2000) about experienced or witnessed events. These processes are directed at facilitating a child's recall for fact-finding purposes following alleged victimization or witnessing of a crime. Emphasis is directed at attainment of a verbal description for legal and protective purposes. Interviews are conducted to "ensure the protection of innocent individuals and the conviction of perpetrators" (Cronch et al., 2006, p. 195).

Child Sexual Abuse and Investigation

Initially, the task of investigative interviewing was assigned to child welfare professionals. With increased recognition of child sexual abuse, expansion of investigative measures was indicated. Previously child abuse and neglect were relegated to the province of child protection and civil courts. Since child sexual abuse is not only a child welfare issue but also a crime, investigation was eventually assigned to both law enforcement and child welfare and involved criminal court proceedings (Krugman, 1997). Emphasis within child protection increasingly focused on investigation with a corresponding impact on resources for other areas of importance, specifically treatment and prevention (Krugman, 1997). In response to a myriad of crises that encompassed child welfare and other social problems, in 1988, Congress passed an amendment to CAPTA by creating the U.S. Advisory Board on Child Abuse and Neglect. So many issues melded that in 1990 a national emergency was declared by this board (Krugman, 1997, p. 641). This crisis was resultant of the board's determination that there was an abject failure to "treat and prevent child abuse and neglect" in spite of the money being spent to address the issue and to rehabilitate the system. The issue was considered a cyclical spending circuit that was not working (Krugman, 1997). A plan of action was crafted in which 31 recommendations were drafted from the advisory board's report. Entitled, *Child Abuse and Neglect: Critical First Steps in Response to a National Emergency*, the steps were outlined and condensed into "Eight General Steps Required to Address the National Emergency" (Krugman, 1997, p. 630), which were identified (from the U.S. Advisory Board on Child Abuse and Neglect, 1990) as:

1. Recognize that the emergency exists
2. Acknowledge the emergency in public statements
3. Coordinate existing efforts
4. Generate knowledge (research and evaluation)
5. Diffuse knowledge through all professionals and the public
6. Increase human resources (human and fiscal)
7. Improve programs that are already in existence
8. Plan for the future

Most notably, the first indicated the need for recognition and acknowledgement (Krugman, 1997, p. 630) of the problem by public, professional and elected domains. The impact identified the need for "coordination of efforts" (Krugman, 1997, p. 630) from all levels of government, given that, "[f]or several decades, professionals working in the field have recognized that the best, most effective approach to recognizing, treating and preventing child abuse and neglect is multidisciplinary, drawing from the perspectives and methods of many areas, psychology, social work, medicine, the law and so on" (Krugman, 1997, p. 630).

Moreover, Krugman (1997) allowed, "Nonetheless, few efforts at the federal or state level have routinely been practiced this way" (p. 630). The recommendations further addressed the need for "generation of knowledge and diffusion" (Krugman, 1997, p. 630). By increasing human resources, the inception of "a new profession child protective services caseworker" materialized (Krugman, 1997, p. 630). The identification of the need for training, support and salary and the stipulation that professional schools provide the appropriate training and education through specialized curricula were advocated. This specified and referred to law, medicine, social work and additional allied professionals. Krugman vehemently stated that child abuse and neglect were relevant and merited inclusion as such. Krugman (1997) discussed the response to the report and lessons learned. He credited Dr. Kempe's public acknowledgement with catapulting awareness such that an instigated response resulted and cultivated action (Krugman, 1997). Kempe and his associates are also credited with the establishment of the National Center on Child Abuse and Neglect (Kemp, 2017).

Precursory Methods to Multidisciplinary Investigations

To address the needs of both law enforcement and child protection, joint investigation was advocated. It was determined that children might be better served through a coordinated and cooperative approach in which law enforcement and CPS combined their respective skills and expertise (Miller-Perrin & Perrin, 2012). Joint processes became the standard approach to investigation in the 1980s by most states (Faller, 2014). A need for "integrated systems to follow children through the process" was identified (Kempe, 2007, p. 165), including the need to change social and cultural moirés (Kempe, 2007). Multidisciplinary interaction was identified as prudent by various individuals across the spectrum of disciplines, including medicine.

Early identification of the need for collaborative and cooperative relationships between responding agencies, spurred by recognition of efforts to do better, was identified in various allied professions, including medicine (Dr. Suzanne Sgroi) and mental health (Dr. John Yuille). Sgroi, a pediatrician, advocated for a joint interview process. Her opportune work on the subject fostered progress toward an interface predicated upon law enforcement and child protection co-interviewing. Sgroi's (1982) handbook on the mechanics and dynamics of child sexual abuse is considered a seminal text and is recommended reading for anyone working with this population and engaged in multidisciplinary investigations. Dr. Yuille is credited with developing early on the Step-Wise protocol or guidelines for interviewing children (1991, 2002), which inculcated standards associated with these processes.

Eventually, child protection laws in the United States were amended to include collaborative investigations, given that professionals from various disciplines are mandated to respond to reports of child sexual abuse. As such, multidisciplinary collaboration was determined to be a viable approach for identification of victims by agencies and professionals that were mandated to report, protect, investigate and intervene.

A multidisciplinary team is composed of individuals that represent a host of backgrounds, experience and expertise. Representatives from diverse fields and disciplines, including law enforcement, mental health, medicine, prosecution and social services, work together and blend their respective skills (Cohen-Liebman, 1999). It is the combination and integration of these diverse resources that contribute to comprehensive investigations. The disciplines that comprise a multidisciplinary team have distinct and specific investigative needs. Additionally, law enforcement and child protection have specific burdens of proof to substantiate findings of sexual abuse (child protection) or a criminal offense (law enforcement) in accordance with agency mandates.

Early modes of investigation were directed at attempts to identify victims through multiple interviews conducted by a myriad of interviewers representing a host of disciplines (depending upon the nature of the report and the allegations). These processes might incorporate leading questions and other suggestive techniques (Ceci & Bruck, 1995) that are no longer considered state-of-the-art practice. At the time, any means necessary were used to gather information regarding child maltreatment and sexual abuse allegations (Faller, 2014). Such processes were found to be counterproductive with regard to investigation and detrimental to the emotional well-being of victims and often impacted recovery.

Information required by a particular discipline was found to be correspondent with the investigative needs of other entities engaged in fact-finding. Prior to agreements and a dedicated commitment to collaboration and a shared approach to the exploration of allegations, a lack of cooperative measures and sharing of information were the norm, and victims were subjected to repetitive processes.

Investigative Interviewing	
Origins	*Description*
Forensic investigative interviewing developed as a means of gathering information from children who may have been victims or witnesses to crimes, including sexual abuse (Faller, 2014).	Investigative interviews are directed at facilitating a child's recall for fact-finding purposes. Emphasis is directed at attainment of a verbal description for legal and protective purposes that is accurate and detailed (Faller, 2014; Katz et al., 2014; Malloy et al., 2011; Patterson & Hayne, 2011).

Origins of Investigative Interviewing

The proliferation of multivictim sexual abuse cases in the late 20th century and corresponding media attention (Cheit, 2014; Faller, 2014; O'Donohue & Fanetti, 2016) began to spur public awareness and contributed to reconceptualization of investigation, including interviewing. Research and data regarding interview practices were galvanized. Research initiatives directed at exploring various aspects of investigative interviewing burgeoned and influenced the development of interview guidelines and protocols (Faller, 2014; Lamb et al., 2008; Poole & Lamb, 2009), which proliferated in the 1990s (Poole & Lamb, 2009) and contributed to recognition of forensic interviewing as a dynamic and evolving profession (Everson & Boat, 2002; Faller, 2014; Olafson, 2012; Poole & Lamb, 2009). Collating research on topics identified as central to the process of investigative interviewing, Reed (1996) provided "a set of general guidelines" based upon research and what at the time was considered best practice and is still referenced today "for increasing accuracy" within the interview process (Kemp, 2017, p. 220).

Investigators and forensic interviewers are reliant upon the information imparted in forensic interviews by children (Lamb et al., 2008). Elicitation of factual and detailed information from child victims and witnesses in investigative interviews is the primary objective sought by investigators in these processes (Faller, 2014; Katz et al., 2014; Malloy et al., 2011; Patterson & Hayne, 2011).

Efforts to obtain credible and reliable accounts from children began to focus on interview practices and techniques (Faller, 2014). Interest also focused on interviewer behavior. Specialized training and skills to determine the best method for eliciting credible and reliable information from children were advocated, leading to research and reform of investigative interviewing. Strategies and techniques to support the interview process and facilitate elicitation of accurate information proliferated (Harris, 2010), as did study directed at the development of interventions that enhance children's self-report and subsequent testimony (Katz et al., 2014).

An investigative interview is the primary method used to acquire factual and detailed information from child victims, making a child's statements a determinant in assessing allegations of sexual abuse (Faller, 2003). There is consensus about the value of the investigative interview; however, the role it serves in investigation of allegations of child sexual abuse is mixed. While the investigative interview has been referred to as "the centerpiece of the investigation" (Faller, 2014), these processes are also considered to comprise one part of the investigative process (Poole, 2016).

Investigators are reliant upon the information imparted by children in forensic interviews, given that self-reporting by victims and witnesses is often the primary source of information when sexual abuse is suspected because corroborate evidence is often unavailable (Faller, 2014; Lamb & Brown, 2006; Lamb et al., 2008; Macleod et al., 2013; Myers, 1998; Orbach et al., 2000; Poole & Lamb, 2009).

Multidisciplinary Approach to the Investigation of Child Sexual Abuse

The focus on revitalizing process and procedure to ensure the safety and well-being of child victims culminated in streamlining the number of times a child had to speak about experienced events. The development of a multidisciplinary response predicated upon cooperative and collaborative measures was designed to improve investigation and enhance prosecutorial outcomes. The backdrop against which a movement toward coordinated team response was spawned emanated from a need to eradicate revictimization and resulted in the emergence of a concept that continues to dominate these processes. The idea placed victims and witnesses at the forefront of investigation rather than the intervening systems. Prior to reconceptualization, investigative efforts were conducted in a manner that was (later) considered to be contributory to revictimization and, as such, merited reconfiguration to minimize negative impact by the lack of a harmonized systemic response.

Child sexual abuse is not relegated to one profession. No single agency, individual or discipline has the necessary knowledge, skills or resources to provide and fulfill the succor and enquiry necessitated. Rather, as a phenomenon, child sexual abuse invokes a response and investigation by many professionals in different fields.

Current focus encompasses representatives from agencies that intervene in the initial stages of investigation working together within a conjoint or team manifestation. This produces a diverse and comprehensive base of knowledge resulting in a more complete understanding of case issues given the commingling of multiple perspectives and worldviews. By contributing ideas and speaking with counterparts across agencies, pragmatic and practical ideas emerge, encouraging discussion and promulgating joint decision making. Multidisciplinary checks and balances ensure that a system as such is procured so that actions are coordinated. Multiple points of view contribute to a holistic approach that is comprehensive and inclusive. This approach helps to minimize secondary trauma induced by systemic intervention propagated by multiple interviewers and repetitive interviews that predate a coordinated multidisciplinary response.

Through cooperative and collaborative investigative protocols and interagency agreements, professionals gain a better understanding of and develop respect for each other's roles and expertise within the process. By blending skills as well as knowledge, an effective and integrated response for intervention, investigation and prosecution is achieved. A multidisciplinary approach to child sexual abuse investigation is predicated upon combining the experience and expertise of the various team representatives. Amalgamating different and complementary knowledge and skills contributes to a more comprehensive approach and process. Lines of communication are established and strengthened, allowing members to appreciate the respective duties assigned to other professions/agencies and associated expectations that accompany each discipline.

The idea of cooperative working relationships produces results that strengthen the investigative process overall. Information is available and readily provided, resulting in the workload being a collective process. No single agency shelters the responsibility of investigation in isolation. Communication among agencies and front-line investigators contributes to transparency and timely exchange of material. This contributes to investigative and interventive strategies which are clearly defined and delineated.

Prior to cooperative and collaborative endeavors, discrepancy often resulted in children being interviewed multiple times by a myriad of investigators from varying systems. This complex interplay of investigation contributed to recantation, denial and withdrawal by children. Voicing experience might merit repeated and multiple interviews as well as engagement with a host of individuals. This contributed to fear and a lack of not feeling supported, as well as instilling in children that disclosure was not accepted or believed, resulting in revictimization by the agencies/disciplines designed to protect (California Child Victim Witness Judiciary Advisory Committee, October 1988).

Multidisciplinary Interview Centers: California Initiative

Problems inherent in the investigation of child abuse and neglect were spotlighted in the 1980s by adverse publicity garnered by several multivictim, multisuspect sexual abuse investigations, many in California (Cheit, 2014; Faller, 2014; O'Donohue & Fanetti, 2016). Two models for investigation seemingly began to develop simultaneously in different parts of the country in recognition of a need to strengthen and revise efforts to explore allegations and to enhance prosecution. In California (1987), Multidisciplinary Interview Centers (MDIC) and in Alabama (1985) the National Children's Advocacy Center (NCAC) were in nascent stages of development. Both were committed to combating and improving, as well as streamlining the process for child victims/

witnesses, nonoffending caretaker(s) and enhancing prosecution of offenders. In the MDIC and NCAC models, the emphasis was directed at interviews that fostered "objective, developmentally sensitive and legally defensible" processes wherein interviewers obtained information on behalf of a team (Davies et al., 1996, p. 189). Both models were designed to undermine the negative impact associated with multiple, repetitive and excessive interviews (Pence & Wilson, 1994a).

In California, under the auspices of the attorney general's office, the Child Victim Witness Judicial Advisory Committee was established in 1986 through the enactment of the California Child Victim Witness Protection Act. The legislation was initiated in response to a recommendation of Attorney General John K. Van de Kamp's Commission on the Enforcement of Child Abuse Laws (California Attorney General's Office, 1988). A committee was appointed, with members selected for their experience, expertise and breadth of knowledge in working with child victims of sexual abuse. The 20 members represented professionals from the multidisciplinary and multijurisdictional fabric of child sexual abuse, including the judiciary, criminal prosecutors, county counsels, the defense bar, family law specialists, law enforcement, child welfare services, probation, developmental psychologists and child abuse prevention experts (California Attorney General's Office, 1988).

An invitational conference on child sexual abuse with these representatives revealed issues and concerns regarding the investigation and prosecution of child sexual abuse, as well as systemic problems for which reform was advocated. Consensus formed around the need to reconfigure the process of investigation and identification of victims. A team concept was advanced. Examination of investigative and judicial practices and procedures as they pertained to child victims and witnesses resulted in recommendations for minimizing or reducing unnecessary repetitive interviews and court appearances of children. Proposals for streamlining and improving investigative and judicial practices and procedures were formulated. Identifying the need for systemic change to minimize secondary trauma contributed to the development of a pilot study (California Attorney General's Office, 1994).

The pilot study was enacted in California to determine how to enhance and increase prosecution of these cases. The principles invoked and proposed for streamlining and improving investigation were correspondent with the NCAC model, which was established in 1985. This model was conceived as "a one stop shop" wherein services for families and children were provided in a central location, preventing the need for multiple interactions across agencies. The NCAC subsequently became the model for Children's Advocacy Centers (CAC). Today, there are more than 700 accredited CACs around the country (Van Eys & Beneke, 2012). According to the Office of Juvenile Justice and Delinquency Prevention or OJJDP which supports "the work and expansion" of advocacy centers, in 2021, approximately 939 centers served and assisted almost 390,000 children thorough investigation, prosecution and treatment (OJJDP, 2022).

The California committee reached agreement on several issues. Child sexual abuse is not an entity to be investigated singularly by an isolated profession. A multidisciplinary approach was determined to be an effective solution for streamlining the process for child victims and witnesses and nonoffending caretakers. Remedial measures directed at improving prosecution were identified. The group recognized the value of reconfiguring investigation, as well as the benefit of a team process given that child sexual abuse is not an entity investigated singularly by an isolated profession. The belief that any agency or discipline could take the lead regarding investigative interviewing was a seminal construct. The American Professional Society on the Abuse of Children (APSAC), a multidisciplinary membership organization, was created in 1986 to support professionals who serve children and families impacted by child maltreatment and violence (American Professional Society on the Abuse of Children (n.d.), www.apsac.org/mission-and-vision).

In response to the primary mandate to make findings and recommendations for minimizing or reducing unnecessary repetitive interviews, the committee found that children are often emotionally and psychologically traumatized by the investigative process. It was determined that children were likely to be traumatized by exposure to multiple interviews conducted by unfamiliar people rather than from multiple interviews conducted by the same person. Additionally, it was determined that trauma is compounded when the interviewers are untrained in child development and forensic interview techniques (California Attorney General's Office, 1988).

Recommendations and study led to the development of multidisciplinary interview centers, which were conceived as community-based resources where teams come together and work in tandem to assess sexual abuse allegations through a collaborative interview process. The recommendations, although configured for the state of California, were transferable and intended to be replicated in other communities and jurisdictions.

Accordingly, the committee established three policy goals for reducing the psychological and emotional impact to child victims in the investigative process: reduce the number of interviewers, minimize the number of interviews and ensure that comprehensive interviews are conducted by qualified interviewers. The committee believed that implementation of these proposals would improve the fact-finding process, protect children and reduce revictimization of victims. To achieve these goals, the committee proposed the creation of special centers for interviewing child victims and witnesses and identified key components to be adopted including; the development of interagency agreements and protocols for interviewing child victims and witnesses, certified child interview specialists (to conduct comprehensive interviews), documentation of the interviews (memorialization of the process), and case review by the multidisciplinary team (California Attorney General's Office, 1988).

The committee stressed that these components and the process proposed for integrating them (as outlined in the report) provide "the foundation for achieving the Legislature's objectives of improving and streamlining the investigative processes on behalf of child victims and witnesses and minimizing unnecessary repetitive interviews". Further, these recommendations "lend themselves to application in any jurisdiction willing to undertake a cooperative approach to investigating child abuse" (California Attorney General's Office, 1988).

The California committee recognized that not every jurisdiction would be able to establish separate centers to interview child victims due to various determinants, including economics and practicality. The model pioneered in Huntsville, Alabama, under the auspices of District Attorney Bud Kramer (later congressman) was identified as the most promising approach to achieving the objectives proposed by the California study and pilot project. The Huntsville model advocated for centralization of professionals and coordinated interviews and investigative procedures. As such, the California committee sought to identify the underlying process and components of the Huntsville model to enable and promote implementation in any geographical or organizational environment.

The California Child Victim Witness Judiciary Advisory Committee (California Attorney General's Office, 1988) identified these essential elements and proposed them as amenable to adaptation in other communities:

- the creation of special centers for interviewing child victims and witnesses
- the development of interagency agreements and protocols for interviewing child victims and witnesses so that the number of interviews is reduced
- require comprehensive interviews be conducted by certified child interview specialists
- memorialize the information gathered by a child interview specialist, including the facts of the alleged abuse and the child's statements
- require that the information gathered during the comprehensive interview be used in lieu of additional interviews whenever possible
- establish multidisciplinary teams to review cases after the comprehensive interview and make recommendations on the case and the needs of the child victim/witness
- adopt procedures to ensure that initial medical evidentiary examinations are conducted by physicians with expertise in diagnosing child abuse
- provide child victims with mental health services

The National Children's Advocacy Center

The NCAC was established in 1985 and has served as a model for other communities since its inception (Van Eys & Beneke, 2012). The center grew out of a community child sexual abuse task force formed in 1983 under the guidance of then District Attorney Robert E. "Bud" Cramer Jr. and was originally proposed to the Huntsville/Madison County Community Task Force on Child Sexual Abuse in 1984. The center was a direct response to the district attorney's awareness of the critical need to redesign a system that was thought to revictimize children. Prior to its inception, as noted by the committee in California, children were subjected to multiple investigative interviews by multiple professionals with minimal or no coordination.

Critical features of the model centered on the conceptualization of a multidisciplinary team, investigative protocols and cooperative working relationships among the intervening agencies. "The CACs evolved their own multidisciplinary teams for the purposes of making prosecution of offenders more likely while trying to minimize the potential trauma of the investigation and court process for the child victim" (Krugman, 2018, p. 7). Shapiro and Maras (2016) acknowledge advantages of multidisciplinary teams, including "the proper and expedient collection of evidence", "shortened response time and length of time devoted by investigators", "reduction in the duplication of services by agencies" and "accountability as each individual conducts his or her investigation under the view of others" (p. 298).

The Huntsville task force brought together representatives from CPS, law enforcement, prosecution, mental health and the medical community (Shapiro & Maras, 2016). The task force defined professional roles in investigation and intervention to improve the system's response to child abuse, including sexual abuse (Van Eys & Beneke, 2012). Efforts resulted in strong working relationships with clear investigative guidelines for an intervention system designed with the child victim as the primary focus. The initial function of the NCAC was to provide a safe place for children where the multidisciplinary investigative team could meet and where children would receive comprehensive services in a centralized setting resulting in "a one stop shop" concept.

The underlying premise surrounded centralization of the professionals who intervene in the initial stages of investigation. The belief was that many of the obstacles that hindered investigation and prosecution would be circumvented if cooperative agreements between agencies existed. The concept, although novel at the time, developed into standard practice and has been adopted and adapted by communities throughout the country and around the world (Shapiro & Maras, 2016).

The National Children's Alliance (NCA), the membership organization for CACs, was established in the late 1980's. The NCA, the national association for the network of Children's Advocacy Centers developed an accreditation process for CACs as well as ten standards of practice (Van Eys & Beneke, 2012). These standards ensure "effective, efficient and consistent delivery of services" by CACs (Van Eys & Beneke, 2012, p. 72). The standards are directed at forensic interviewing, multidisciplinary response and community outreach and education and also address victim advocacy as well as other standards of practice (National Children's Alliance, 2010; Van Eys & Beneke, 2012).

Regional centers followed in the early 1990s to provide training and technical assistance as well as networking opportunities to communities to assist in the establishment of CACs. The four regional CACs "coordinate with state and local CACs" (Cheung, 2012, p. xxi). The regional centers were developed to assist communities seeking to establish or enhance CACs by providing "consultation, training and technical assistance to facilitate and support coordination among agencies" (Cheung, 2012, p. xxi) throughout the developmental phases of a CAC, from conception to implementation, and by providing ongoing support. As such, services include assistance to multidisciplinary teams and professionals seeking to establish or improve a community's response to child abuse (National Children's Alliance, n.d.).

In 1988 the NCAC in Huntsville expanded its services to include on-site mental health therapy for children and their families; extended assessments; crisis counseling; and individual and group therapy for victims/witnesses, siblings and nonoffending parents or caregivers. Unique to the investigative format was the inclusion of clinical staff who provided consultation to the multidisciplinary team at weekly case review sessions regarding therapeutic, age-appropriate interviewing and intervention issues to ensure expertise and adherence to professional standards and guidelines by the team. Case consultation and in-service training were also provided to community agencies and personnel as part of the NCAC model. Extended assessments for children that the team felt might benefit from more than a single-session interview process integrated a clinical aspect. Groups were designed for victims and families to provide information about the court process and to provide educational support in relation to the criminal justice system (Cohen-Liebman, 2007).

Art Therapy and CACs

Art therapy was offered in both group and individual sessions at the NCAC as a communication tool to help sexually abused children work through issues associated with abuse. Art therapy was incorporated to provide therapeutic intervention as a means to facilitate the expression of thoughts and feelings not easily verbalized. The CAC model embraced the intrinsic value and inherent therapeutic contribution of art therapy within the healing process (Cohen-Liebman, 1996). Art therapy as an interventive measure was incorporated within established CACs as part of the therapeutic program in Huntsville, Alabama, and Dallas, Texas (Cohen-Liebman, 1996, 1997b).

The use of art therapy within the CAC concept fostered a duality given the nontraditional use by Cohen-Liebman in Philadelphia, Pennsylvania: investigative technique versus treatment modality (Cohen-Liebman, 1996, 1997b, 1997c, 1999). My use of the modality was developed for investigative purposes, a novel approach rather than as a therapeutic intervention, given my role as a child interview specialist. At the time, the center where I worked was oriented toward investigation and did not provide therapeutic services. If deemed appropriate and purposeful (in consultation with the team at the conclusion of an investigative interview process), referrals for therapeutic and/or support services might be recommended or suggested, as well as resources in conjunction with interventive and investigative recommendations.

CAC programs that incorporate art therapy as part of the initial stage of investigation, as well as programs that utilize art therapy as a treatment modality, were discussed at the 1996 American Art Therapy Association (AATA) conference (Cohen-Liebman, 1996). The implementation of art therapy within nontraditional settings and as a forensic investigative method was explained. The viability and pragmatic use of art therapy within the CAC model, as well as the duality art therapy afforded within the model, were presented with consideration of programs offering investigation and intervention or therapuertic services at the time. CACs embraced the intrinsic value and inherent contributions of art therapy within the investigative and healing processes (Cohen-Liebman, 1996). The utilization of art therapy within the context of multidisciplinary team investigations of child sexual abuse was explored. The investigative interview process was outlined and explained, including the advantages associated with the use of drawing within the investigative interview process. Benefits identified for the child, the team and the process were elucidated.

The original CAC model inculcated fundamental components that include specific criteria and procedures in relation to the philosophy and mission. One of the primary goals of CACs is to improve the process of forensic interviewing and minimize the number of times that a child is interviewed, while another aim is "to coordinate child abuse investigations involving CPS, law enforcement, medical and other agencies, by making a single interviewer responsible for providing information to all of the members of the multidisciplinary team" (Shapiro & Maras, 2016, p. 298). Each CAC is configured and designed by professionals and volunteers in response to a community's needs and specifics, given the resources allocated for the establishment of a CAC. The delivery of services is coordinated, specific and amenable to serving designated clientele.

CACs embrace various orientations in conjunction with the founding principles that initiate the need for a CAC in a particular community. CACs can be not-for-profit freestanding entities, state based, prosecution based or hospital based. No single model for an ideal concept exists, because each community develops a center in response to identified needs and in accordance with the feasibility of a given community's resources. The conceptual frame is organized within the mandates of the investigative partners and agencies and supported by written agreements that underscore cooperative and coordinated working relationships. While each agency maintains its mandated role for handling cases of abuse, mutually agreed upon procedures are adhered to, providing a structure for practice and interaction. This collaborative team initiative promotes coordination among agencies that respond to allegations of child sexual abuse and has propagated across the country.

Team Concept

A team concept has many advantages, beginning with joint decision making by the agencies that intervene at the initial stage of investigation. Interagency collaboration fosters understanding and appreciation of the respective roles and investigatory mandates of each specialty/agency, including discipline-specific roles, protocols, mandates and burdens of proof. Shared decision making is conferred upon multiple perspectives, contributing to a more thorough examination of the facts. Written signed agreements among agencies provide a framework for coexisting and communal interaction, which fundamentally ensures that victims and families receive comprehensive services.

A successful multidisciplinary approach respects and builds upon the different and complementary knowledge and skills of the professionals involved. The commingling of expertise and experience contributes to a cooperative and coordinated response that is detailed in signed agreements. Agencies develop procedures for responding collaboratively in a timely and efficient manner. A team approach advocates for a coordinated response among all agencies, which encourages collective decision making that is supported by the sharing of information and receptivity to integrating multiple perspectives.

Contemporary processes were predated by the confluence of myriad investigators pursuing independent investigations, which contributed to case management issues as well as discrepancies in findings. The potential for contaminated prosecutorial pathways was not uncommon when different entities presented discrepant or divergent findings. As a result, a streamlined collaborative and coordinated approach was advocated to mitigate potential conflicts, response and adjudication. A team is comprised of individuals that are charged to work together and blend their respective skills and abilities in promulgating an effective course of action that minimizes secondary trauma induced by the investigative process (Cohen-Liebman, 1999). The multidisciplinary approach results in an integrated response through the interplay of experience, discipline-specific expertise, knowledge and skills. This confluence is predicated upon a "shared burden" as well as respect for independent agency roles and mandates (MacFarlane, 1995; Pence & Wilson, 1994b; The National Network of Children's Advocacy Centers, 1994). "When MDT members clarify their roles and communicate effectively among disciplines, the quality of aid to affected families increases" (Van Eys & Beneke, 2012, p. 96).

> Effective teamwork depends upon the individual and collective ability and willingness of the group to work together in an interdependent environment in which team members and disciplines must depend upon each other to do their part toward a common set of goals. Likewise, the individual capacity and willingness to trust the others to fulfill their role with competence and treat one another with respect are all necessary components of success. In the end, the key to effective multidisciplinary work is all about integrating the knowledge, skills, resources, and authority distributed among the team to a common end: the protection and healing of the child (Wilson & Pence, 2018, p. 400).

Some programs have advocated for lead interviewers who are specially trained to conduct interviews on behalf of all team representatives such that independent discipline interviews are not a necessity. Other models rely upon trained members from each agency so that the lead interviewer role is responsive to the needs of the case and is assigned accordingly. The emphasis is on a shared and cooperative team approach, where the responsibility and weight are collective endeavors. "Ultimately the primary goal of most multidisciplinary teams related to child maltreatment is to improve the response of all involved disciplines through coordination, cooperation, and communication" (Wilson & Pence, 2018, p. 388).

In some communities, joint interviews are the standard whereby law enforcement and social services may interview a child together, while in other locales the interview is conducted on behalf of the team by a designated lead interviewer. Joint investigative protocols promote cooperative working relationships. Typically, interviews are intended to be single-session processes unless the team determines at the conclusion of an interview process that additional information is needed or if circumstances dictate that the child might benefit from a more in-depth interview – then an extended process might be proposed.

Investigative Interviewing Practices

A joint or common interview guideline or protocol reflects a shared, agreed-upon standard of practice. Depending upon the community, a process may be developed in accordance with the innate practices or a process that is recognized may be adopted or used. Various protocols for investigative interviewing exist. Currently, there is not a single format that is considered to be a homogenized protocol; rather, the interview process applied within a community is contingent upon various factors.

Some states or regions in the United States have adopted and subscribe to a preferred format and advocate that team members attend and participate in prescribed training programs affiliated with a specified interview protocol (Vieth, 2006). Other communities have developed or incorporate practices based upon existing practice. Component parts or phases associated with an interview protocol or guideline may vary with regard to title or format; however, the objective or intention is comparable (Cohen-Liebman, 1999). Guidelines are employed internationally as well (Cheung, 1997), and certain countries have created designated structures for interviewing such as Great Britain (Home Office, 2007).

A team process with a dedicated interview format promotes best practice for various reasons. Whichever format is utilized (protocol, guideline, policy) is dependent upon local jurisdiction. Typically, team members are introduced to the process and mandated to attend training. The construct of interagency guidelines is supported. The team understands the process and is comfortable observing, knowing that specific information pertinent to an agency's needs is included in the design of the investigative interview structure. Additionally, a consistent, agreed-upon investigative interview method is warranted because it affords certain advantages; the process is accepted in court (specifically the jurisdiction where interviews are conducted), team members understand the process and procedure, a common language is existent which contributes to collective processing and comprehension and the weight and responsibilities are shared. The burden of investigation is not relegated to a single interviewer or agency.

There are distinctions between a protocol and a guideline. A protocol is a predetermined process that may have a scripted element to it and follows prescribed phases in a certain order. A guideline is a composite of the information needed by all of the various investigative bodies that are involved. Guidelines provide fluidity in that a prescribed process that adheres to a specific format is not the goal. Rather, a guideline incorporates different phases that may be engaged as the process dictates rather than followed in a predetermined fashion. A guideline is a composite of the discipline-specific information that is required by the respective agencies melded into a single process, although identified component phases do exist; however, they do not merit strict adherence to an ordered process.

Protocol	Policy	Guideline
• step by step process	• standardized way of conducting	• fluid
• order is followed	• implies predetermined process	• flexible
• strict or rigid order	• noncompliance may be problematic	•not structured per se
		• not rigid or predetermined
		• move in and out of phases/ stages in conjunction with child's presentation

A protocol may be considered a step-wise process, meaning steps or phases are adhered to in a predetermined manner, whereas a guideline is not. A protocol may also invoke a scripted process. Protocols and guidelines are composed of phases; however, a guideline allows for flexibility and fluidity in movement (of or between the phases), whereas a protocol typically follows a customary succession or process. Both decrease the need for additional individual discipline-specific interviews since the information mandated by each investigative agency is procured within the scope of the process and explored within the interview format.

A common interview limits the number of interviewers a child is exposed to and reduces the number of times the child needs to be interviewed. The interview is designed to capture as much information as possible to assist each investigator in making a determination as to whether or not an agency's burden of proof is met, if a child is safe and next steps with regard to investigation, intervention and possible prosecution.

Interviews can take one of three formats:

- A joint interview consists of a collaborative process between law enforcement and child protection.
- A lead interview is conducted by a trained interview specialist, who conducts the interview on behalf of the participating agencies who observe the process. These interviews are not conducted in isolation. They are considered a team process, and the expectation is that representatives for each agency/discipline will be present to observe and document the process as per agency dictates and support the interviewer.
- A team interview connotes an endeavor by which any member of the team from any of the participating agencies who has been trained and is qualified may conduct the interview on behalf of the team. A decision as to who will take the lead is decided among the team members and considered in relation to the case dynamics in concert with the presentation of the child.

Representatives from agencies that intervene in the initial stages of investigation work together as a team and blend their respective skills to minimize secondary trauma induced by systemic intervention (Cohen-Liebman, 1999).

Philadelphia CAC

The Children's Advocacy Center in Philadelphia (PCAC, currently the Philadelphia Children's Alliance) was established in 1990 as a collaborative effort between the district attorney's office, the police department and the Department of Human Services that evolved out of the Law Enforcement Child Abuse Project (LECAP). LECAP was a consortium that was initiated in the 1970s to address issues pertaining to child abuse investigations, which corresponded with developments emerging across the country. Then district attorney, Ed Rendell, assembled a varied group of professionals from the fields of law enforcement, the judiciary, mental health, child welfare and medicine to explore measures for enhancing collaborative approaches to child sexual abuse investigations. LECAP encompassed representatives from 30 public and private agencies that served children in the city. The eclectic group of professionals was cultivated from a plenitude of disciplines and agencies directly and indirectly engaged with child welfare (Cohen-Liebman, 2007). This diverse group of individuals shared a commitment to system reform and improved service delivery to child victims including the promulgation of a coordinated response at the initial stage of investigation (Cohen-Liebman, 2007).

In the 1980s LECAP began to explore how other areas in the country were addressing the issues associated with investigation of these cases. The group identified the NCAC model in Huntsville, Alabama, as a plausible and adaptable model for implementation in the city of Philadelphia, given the focus on multidisciplinary investigations. In 1986 an initiative to improve and streamline child sexual abuse investigations in the city commenced. This undertaking resulted in the development of the PCAC that stemmed from a three-year grant provided by the state of Pennsylvania (Cohen-Liebman, 2007). The PCAC was designed in accord with the rudiments prescribed by the NCAC model that was propagating throughout the country.

The nonprofit was configured as an entity to coordinate and facilitate multidisciplinary child sexual abuse investigations. PCAC was initially conceived as a free-standing, independent facility that provided space for front-line investigators who responded to allegations of child sexual abuse. Meeting space was allocated for external agencies (specifically law enforcement/special victims unit and the Department of Human Services [DHS]) to send assigned representatives when cases were referred for coordinated investigative interviews. Additional personnel from invested agencies were invited in accordance with the dynamics relative to a case and might include representatives from one of the children's hospitals, the district attorney's office and others depending upon the professionals who were involved. Therapeutic and medical services were not offered at the PCAC at that time. For many years these services were obtained off-site or referrals to external resources were provided on a case-by-case basis.

This was the environment that I was hired to work in, a relatively new concept. The premise was not fully formed and would undergo various permutations as the center strived to meet the mission and purpose it was intended to serve. Promoting the idea of coordinated and cooperative multidisciplinary team investigations of child sexual abuse cases was in a formative stage of development at that time in the city.

A need for a centralized interviewing center was recognized, and a push for co-location of all major systems soon followed; however, the reality of co-location was many years to come. Prior to that happening, the agency where the interviews were conducted adhered to the CAC model, where children and nonoffending caregivers received an integrated response. The concept was simple: a nondescript location that blended innocuously into the community and did not call attention to itself or the mission in an effort to maintain safety, comfort and anonymity for all involved in a particular case, secure in the sense that only the victim or witness, nonoffending caretakers and professionals were permitted inside. Anyone identified as the perpetrator was not invited to attend or participate.

Role and Responsibilities

Teaming was a new concept, as was joint investigative interviews wherein representatives from law enforcement and child protection worked conjointly. Agency representatives were schooled in their respective disciplines such that prior to the development of joint protocols, collaboration between the investigative systems was not common. Understanding "one child, one narrative" meant that a dedicated process would eliminate the need for repetitive interviews by multiple investigators, yet this was a relatively new theme at the time. The concept meant that a child could be interviewed such that the information mandated by each investigating agency was addressed in a single or conjoint practice. The process designated the gathering of information for the investigative systems in relation to respective agency mandates.

The job required diplomacy at times, given the diversity inherent in the participating disciplines that applied to worldview, burdens of proof, agency mandates and investigative roles. Team members, depending upon what agency they represented, contributed varying perspectives that were discipline specific. Working together as a team and sharing information necessitated the ability to take another perspective or to be receptive to a belief system that differed from one's professional orientation to strengthen the process and best support victims and families.

An implicit aspect of my role was tactfully instructing or providing guidance and support to team members about best practice. For example, educating team members about "dos and don'ts" associated with interviewing, such as discouraging touching of any sort during an interview process, given that a child was present because of some type of interpersonal event. Semantics dictated that we abstain from even a gentle hand on the back out of respect and with safety and precaution in mind for the child as well as the interviewer. In one instance, a female officer picked up a child and sat the youngster on her lap during an interview. After the interview concluded, discussion ensued as to why this was not best practice. The officer, clearly offended, explained that she wanted the child to understand that police officers are friendly and they help children. It was a teachable moment that led to a lively discussion given the array of viewpoints from child protection, law enforcement, mental health, prosecution and advocacy.

Additionally, the development and implementation of educational and informational groups was designated for nonoffending caretakers, as well as groups for siblings (Cohen-Liebman, 2007). These groups were not designed for therapeutic purposes, but rather the intent for nonoffending caretakers was premised upon the provision of education and information pertaining to the investigative process. The sibling groups were oriented as educational and supportive endeavors for family members of victims or witnesses of interpersonal violence.

Most importantly, my role, as previously mentioned, transformed from mental health evaluator to child interview specialist. In response, I developed a framework for investigative interviewing premised upon guidelines and best practices populating at the time (Cohen-Liebman, 1996, 1997a, 1997b, 1997c). Integrating my background and experience in art therapy with the investigative interview process I utilized, a common interview guideline was formulated. Additionally, I created an accompanying training curriculum for front-line investigators.

The multidisciplinary investigation of child sexual abuse allegations was a burgeoning concept at the time. The PCAC stemmed from and adhered to the CAC model which was developing around the country. Centers were being established to centralize services for victims and their families and conformed to a national movement dedicated to streamlining investigation and enhancing prosecution. The center was established to facilitate the multidisciplinary investigation of child sexual abuse cases. It was designed as a free-standing entity so that the various agencies that intervene at the initial stage of investigation were not co-located, but rather sent representatives when cases were referred and interviews scheduled. As an external resource, space was allocated to house representatives from the responding agencies when their presence was needed inside the building. The facility was designed to be family friendly and child centered. The only way to gain entry was via a buzzer system.

The center, which had at some point in time been a residence, was situated on an animated and lively street. Pedestrians frequented the restaurants, mini-marts, drugstores and street vendors and contributed to the busy scene along with the noise from vehicles on the street. On a rather unremarkable day, someone pushed the buzzer outside the nondescript door on the ground floor of the townhouse. The center blended into the surrounding neighborhood, which was consistent with the foundational principles as a measure not to call attention to the nature of the work, which was a veiled effort to maintain safety and security for victims, staff, agency representatives and nonoffending caretakers. Not expecting any clients that afternoon, the office manager answered the intercom and inquired as to who was buzzing and why. The response was a loud "FBI". Everyone within earshot (staff and a police officer who happened to be finishing up a case) looked at each other. The office manager said that we only let individuals with scheduled appointments into the building. To be expected, the voice on the other end of the intercom was not too happy and again stated "FBI" and something to the effect of "we need to come inside". The center was intended to provide a safe and welcoming environment for child victims and their nonoffending caregivers and to provide sanctuary for those inside. As such, entry into the building was not taken lightly regardless of the voice demanding to be let inside.

The police officer in the building went down to speak with the unknown individuals, and much to our surprise, they were indeed FBI agents. The incident reinforced the need to be alert and actively screen. We did not want to admit an offender who may have learned when an investigative interview was taking place and wanted to gain access to a victim or a nonoffending caregiver. The buzzer enabled a measure of control regarding who was able to come in and not allow someone masquerading as someone they were not into the building and potentially threaten or compromise victims, families, staff or investigative processes. We were not moved by the FBI's declaration that they needed to be let into the building, and we staunchly defended our position that was intended as a protective measure. Fortunately, the officer spoke with the two agents and explained our reticence, as we were not interested in being arrested for doing our job. The agents merely wanted to ask a few questions about a car that had been parked on the street for an extended amount of time, and frankly, no one had any awareness regarding the vehicle or information to provide.

Child Interview Specialists

A child interview specialist (CIS) gathers the information necessary for each individual discipline to minimize the need for repetitive interviews. The role was conceived to improve the fact-finding process by synthesizing the material required to meet the respective purview associated with each investigating agency. The use of a trained CIS is designed to improve the fact-finding process and eliminate secondary victimization induced by systemic intervention. The CIS contributes to the team process before, during and after the interview. The CIS facilitates the pre- and post-interview discussions and contributes to recommendations regarding additional investigative measures and possible therapeutic and supportive interventions not only for the child but for the family if warranted. If an extended process is needed, perhaps due to a child's reticence to engage or interact, or if the team is concerned about new or additional information that was disclosed or not explored fully, an extended interview may be considered. The hope is that the same interviewer is selected to continue the process. The CIS follows the child's lead while at the same time maintaining control of the interview, including the direction and focus (Cohen-Liebman, 1999).

CISs are trained in various areas or competencies to support the ability to conduct comprehensive, developmentally sensitive and culturally aware interviews. The CIS assists the agencies in pursuing their respective burdens of proof while at the same time maintaining a safe and protected environment for the exploration of allegations. Training in child development is essential for the CIS, who will use the knowledge to assess a child's skill level and expressive-receptive capabilities or communication and interactive patterns and behaviors. The CIS translates this information by modifying and adapting language and communicative patterns, so engagement is congruent with the child's presentation. The process is focused on meeting the child where the child presents developmentally, which encompasses cognitively, linguistically, socially and emotionally as well as artistically (with regard to an art therapy-based process; artistic skills correlate with other developmental spheres and provide information and insight about a person's level of functioning).

Child Interview Specialists

- conduct comprehensive, developmentally sensitive, culturally aware, forensically defensible interviews
- role is to gather information for each discipline
- minimize the need for repetitive interviews
- limit number of interviewers
- the objective is to improve the fact-finding process and eliminate secondary traumatization
- process is a composite of investigative information needed by the various systems
- follow child's lead while maintaining control of the interview

---

Knowledge-Based Competencies Associated With CIS

Knowledge-based competencies that CISs should be educated in and have experience with are critical to conducting forensic or fact-finding interviews. Understanding and familiarity with areas of knowledge will assist CISs in conducting thorough processes by following the information elicited. The CIS follows the child's lead and facilitates the fact-finding process. The CIS needs to be aware of what a child is communicating to follow up and garner information relative to a child's experience. Knowledge of competency-based content will support the CIS in this endeavor by providing background and information regarding what a child might be trying to express in relation to an experienced event.

The knowledge will contribute to how the interviewer follows up and facilitates the process, especially when a child may lack the skills to articulate what happened, perhaps due to developmental incongruency or the lack of vocabulary. The lack of understanding of an event/act may preclude a child's capability to express what their experience was or to express it clearly. Conversely, children with limited communication skills or very young children may still be able to convey what was experienced with the communicative or expressive abilities they possess. In situations where a lead interviewer is responsible for facilitating and conducting interviews, some researchers and professionals have advocated for education in the realms of developmental and clinical psychology "to ensure that they understand both normative and nonnormative growth and development" (Shapiro & Maras, 2016, p. 373).

Areas that factor into forensic interviewing contribute to the development of skills and knowledge-based competencies. Experience and education in these arenas enhance the interview process as well as the competency of the interviewer. Identified topics include child development, which encompasses the maturational spheres of language, cognition, memory and suggestibility. The last two are important concepts that factor into evaluating the credibility of a child's statements. Additional areas that are central to conducting interviews include knowledge about child sexual abuse, including the mechanics and dynamics, as well as disclosure, which is construed as a process, not an event. Additional topics related to child sexual abuse that a CIS is trained in include why a child might delay in reporting abuse, denial of abuse and recantation. Knowledge of sexual development is also warranted. To understand a child's experience and comprehend if information disclosed might be incompatible with a child's developmental level, exploration is merited to assess how the child acquired the information. Listed below are competency or knowledge based criteria for the CIS however, the list is not exclusive and not all encompassing as knowledge is cumulative and criteria evolve.

Competency or Knowledge Base Curriculum for a CIS
Caveat – the topics are not exclusive as knowledge is cumulative and competencies continue to evolve

Familiarity with current research and literature is essential for each competency

Child Development	Sexual Abuse	Interviewing	Forensic Practices	Interviewers
normal/abnormal	dynamics	skills and techniques	credibility assessment	refrain from bias
psychological	mechanics	strategies	forensic protocols	awareness of nonverbal behavior
sexual development	process of disclosure	best practices	judicial process	awareness of reinforcement cues
linguistics/language communication patterns/ expressive/receptive	recantation	current research and literature	state criminal codes	neutrality to enhance credibility
cognition/cognitive	other forms of maltreatment including physical abuse, neglect and emotional abuse	special populations	children as witnesses	objectivity
behavioral	effects/impact		forensic interviewing	impartiality
psychosexual	offender profiles	cultural competencies	legal proceedings	nonjudgmental support
memory	trauma/impact/ response	use of aids, tools and props	competency assessment	cultural acuity awareness and sensitivity
suggestibility			current research	responsive listening
children as witnesses		question continuum	question continuum	minimization of interviewer influence

In addition to understanding child sexual abuse, several other areas merit education, training, understanding and ongoing supervision. A CIS should be familiar with offender profiles. This information will provide the CIS with comprehension of information that may merit exploration in a forensic interview. For example, if a child were to disclose that a neighbor had molested her sister when the girl was nine and then the child being interviewed stated the same happened to her by the same offender, the interviewer should explore the pattern of abuse. Understanding the type of behavioral patterns and interactions that are associated with a regressed versus a fixated offender will clue the CIS about potential areas that need to be examined in the interview context to support the acquisition of facts that may lead to additional investigation and/or impact prosecution such as determination of charges.

Each competency is relative to facilitating a process that is all encompassing. This is prudent not only for the child but for the team as well. A process that omits exploration of information that may be salient for investigation and prosecutorial needs may be detrimental. In addition, omissions in the interview may impact the safety of a child if information is not pursued, given that the safety and protection of the child may be compromised. If, for instance, the alleged perpetrator has access to the home or if the nonoffending caretaker is maintaining an alliance with the alleged perpetrator for whatever reason, regardless of the circumstances, it may not be in the child's best interest to return home until the environment is determined to be safe and the nonoffending caretaker understands the dilemma of maintaining a relationship in whatever capacity with the alleged perpetrator be it financial, emotional or some other reason.

Additional areas that a CIS should be educated about include question continuum (types of questions and how to use them), interviewing aids and tools, legal issues affecting child abuse investigations, state criminal codes and children as witnesses. Knowledge of laws and criminal codes that apply to local and state jurisdiction is important, as these vary from state to state. The host of topics that a CIS should be versed in assist the interviewer with conducting developmentally sensitive, culturally aware and comprehensive interviews. The above list is not exhaustive but provides a foundation for the CIS.

Cultural Acuity and Competency

Understanding the nuances that may accompany a child's presentation or behavior during an interview may be understood within the context of culture. Education may alleviate misunderstanding and miscommunication. For example, a behavioral trait may be identified as a negative within the interview context when, in fact, the issue may be attributed to something other than what it seems. For instance, in some cultures it is inappropriate to make eye contact under certain circumstances.

If cultural awareness is lacking, it may be necessary for external resources to be brought in to educate the CIS as well as the team in order to conduct a culturally competent process. Understanding expectations and behavior associated with cultural nuances, practices and beliefs that one is not acquainted with may enhance interviewer proficiency and interactive patterns. Sometimes requesting assistance about a particular subject from a member of the team who may have experience or knowledge about a practice that is not customary may prove to be enlightening with regard to case dynamics. Bringing someone skilled and informed in to teach the team about a subject or topic that is not common knowledge may be prudent and beneficial for the child, the team and the process.

- forensic interviewing practices
- interview protocols, guidelines, policies
- child sexual abuse – mechanics and dynamics
- process of disclosure
- types of disclosure
- child developmental and maturational spheres, including expressive-receptive language, cognitive skills, psychosocial and psychosexual
- sexual development
- question continuum
- legal issues
- state criminal codes
- use of interviewing aids, tools and props
- children as witnesses
- offender profiles
- interviewing techniques
- current research and literature on related topics
- credibility and competency assessment
- special populations
- children's memory, suggestibility, concept formation
- cultural acuity and competency
- knowledge of laws and criminal codes that apply to local and state jurisdiction is important, as these vary from state to state

Interviewer Response

Fact-finding in response to what a child is disclosing may impact additional agency-specific or coordinated investigation. The information disclosed may signal the need for continued exploration and result in additional material being uncovered that may result in pursuance of additional witnesses, victims or details leading to previously unknown evidence. This information may ultimately impact investigation, intervention and/or prosecution. It might contribute to the acquisition of a search warrant. It may shed light on how a child understands and comprehends an experienced event, which may foster interventive recommendations. Most of all, it may be the first time a child is telling someone what their experience was. How the interviewer responds has the potential to impact additional disclosure by the child including related details and specifics of an event.

Interviewers have to be aware of their own response when conducting an interview. It is important to master one's emotions. Regardless of how many interviews one conducts, one will never encounter every scenario imaginable. Sometimes as an interviewer, it can be difficult to bear witness via a child's telling what they have been exposed to, endured or observed. Yet the interviewer has to remain nonjudgmental, supportive and maintain a fact-finding role.

Interviewers must be cognizant of emotional displays, exchanges or utterances that may impact or restrict a child's participation, including disclosure of information. A lack of awareness with regard to emotionality is a criterion for evaluation of one's ability to function as a CIS. An individual may not be able to manage a response during a process, which may be attributed to a variety of conscious as well as unconscious variables, including disclosure of information that was unexpected. Every process is distinct, and interviewers have to be open-minded, receptive and neutral. Acceptance of whatever is uncovered or divulged must be handled with diplomacy and tactfully, yet one should not discount nonjudgmental support. Humanity cannot be erased from the process; however, one must be prepared to receive the unknown and maintain a professional response.

The interviewer will have the opportunity to address and identify issues during post-processing with the team as well as decompress, although a child victim or witness may never have this opportunity to relinquish or let go of what they have been exposed to or experienced. This knowledge is humbling and contributes to interviewers' sensibility and sensitivity in facilitating these processes and being able to professionally elicit information, yet convey munificence, as noted, in a nonjudgmental yet supportive manner.

Interviewers must be honest and accept realistic expectations that accompany the role. Interviewers will find themselves in situations where difficulty managing emotions is real. Experience and exposure as well as education and training will foster the development of skills to help one manage a response and maintain an interviewer stance. The inability to master one's emotions can negatively impact a process. Supervision and peer review are assets to developing the skill set that a CIS must invoke and maintain. It is a developmental process, like any other profession, in which growth and insight coupled with awareness are requisite.

Use of Interpreters

In the event there is a language barrier and the interviewer does not speak the native language of a child referred for an interview, an interpreter may be necessary. It must be noted that the interpreter must be prepared about the nature of the interview, including the potentiality for the use of language that may be considered inappropriate or offensive. Suffice it to say that the interviewer should not be kept in the dark about the content to be explored. The interpreter may have difficulty translating if uncomfortable with the subject matter, which may compromise the process, especially if the interpreter stops translating (as I have experienced). It is necessary to prepare the individual for the possibility of what may be disclosed and the relevance of translating verbatim.

Exemplar

To offer an example of a case in which the inclusion of an interpreter was more disruptive than helpful, a child was interviewed in the presence of a Spanish-speaking interpreter and a social worker with limited Spanish-speaking ability from CPS. The interpreter was prepped about the nature of the content to be discussed. She alleged comfort with the subject matter and expressed a lack of difficulty translating whatever the child might say. She and the social worker began speaking to each other in Spanish during the interview (given the circumstances, the social worker elected to stay in the interviewing room with the child). The process was compromised because the CIS interviewer had no idea what was being said between the two professionals, who were engaged in speaking Spanish or the potential impact that the sidebar conversation may have had on the process or the child. Eventually, the interpreter refused to translate what the child was communicating given the sensitive nature of the interview. The social worker attempted to compensate for the interpreter's refusal to assist as had been outlined prior to commencement of the interview by asking the child questions and interpreting for the child in a mix of Spanish and English. The abdication by the interpreter of her role was understandable but irregular given that it happened in the middle of an interview and contributed to a disjointed and tainted process which was not in the best interest of the child, the team or the investigation. The social worker was trying to assist once the interpreter shut down; however, she merely contributed to the disintegration of the process.

In post-processing, the team discussed that outside of the process, which is routine and part of the job, often the language and subject matter are not common conversation, and as such sensitivity must be considered when interpreters are brought in to provide assistance. When someone additional is included for whatever purpose, agreements have to be reached with regard to the limits of one's ability to participate in order not to hinder a process that may not lend itself to a repeat occurrence. Once an interpreter is briefed and educated about the scope of the process, it must be emphasized that the interpreter has agreed to participate fully and as such must do the job as assigned without interruption or withdrawal once the process commences.

The Role of the Art Therapist as CIS

Education in the various competencies, including staying current with relevant literature and research concerning best practices, coupled with extensive interview training and participation in professional development training and conferences contributed to my role as a CIS. In conjunction with my background and training as an art therapist, this fusion of disparate orientations resulted in the development of a forensic/art psychotherapeutic hybrid. The foundation of this art therapy subspecialization was realized as this merger of distinct disciplines led to the development of a fact-finding and investigative process that was grounded in forensic and art therapy praxis.

By combining my respective skills, information gathering was pragmatically oriented. As a CIS with a foundation as an art therapist, I was able to conduct the interview process, support the emotional well-being of a child, facilitate fact-finding and meet the expectations of the team in gathering information relevant to individual agency mandates while adhering to forensic practice. Drawing provided the scaffolding for a child to convey salient information about experienced events. Non-verbal engagement via art materials often stimulated verbal interaction. Information was communicated pictorially in conjunction with verbal associations. The process was child friendly, child centered and maintained forensic integrity within the interview and in the courtroom.

The interview process in combination with drawing helped me provide the team with insight into a child's coping skills, level of trauma, emotional reaction to the abuse and in many cases abuse-specific information (Cohen-Liebman, 1999). Drawing as evidentiary material authenticated for the court the lived experience of a victim or witness and complemented verbalization (Cohen-Liebman, 1999). A child's narrative was graphically and verbally conveyed in a developmentally congruent manner that was objective and concretized the experienced event.

Drawing has typically been examined within the context of a tool, aid or support within the process of investigative interviewing. Even as recent research has focused on the use of drawing as a forensic tool, it has not focused on the function of drawing as a facilitator for expression of evidentiary material when used in the capacity of an open-ended prompt (similar to an open-ended verbal prompt). The capability of drawing to serve as an open-ended prompt and the effect of drawing are the subject of recent research by this author (Cohen-Liebman, 2017, 2021). The use of drawing as an open-ended prompt in a primary capacity rather than as a secondary or confirmatory accoutrement will be discussed in Part V.

My approach to art therapy is process oriented, meaning that everything is considered within the context from which art is created, including the relational milieu: the child's behavior, what the child says (associations or verbalizations), how the child manages materials and what the child depicts. All of the requisite traits associated with an art therapist are intrinsic to understanding and comprehending the dynamics of the child and the process. The essential skills and body of knowledge associated with "arts therapists" which extends beyond art therapists and encompasses other forms of creative and expressive therapies is described in the following manner.

> The arts therapist focuses upon the creative process involved in human expression and communication, the synthesizing of percepts, cognition and behavior. Recognizing and encouraging expression of these creative processes are skills for which he is uniquely trained. These skills and the body of knowledge behind them, the

ethical and moral considerations inherent in the practice of psychotherapy, are, ideally, what all arts therapists share in common. (Naitove, 1980, p. 254)

Significantly, as an art therapist, the use of drawing within the interview context assists in the assessment of information in a quick and nonthreatening manner. Information obtained is utilized to determine the structure of the interview and direct the process. Acquisition of information pertaining to a child's expressive-receptive communication skills, cognitive capabilities and maturational spheres including cognitive, social, emotional and linguistic, as well as artistic developmental level, is shared with the team to provide insight and understanding. This material is translated for the team to provide guidance regarding next steps, including recommendations, and to promote comprehension of a child's dynamics, behavior and presentation. Factors that contribute to forensic relevance such as suggestibility and credibility assessment that manifest in concert with the child's narrative or verbal expressions are communicated and explained. This in turn helps with the determination of additional investigative measures and supportive interventions.

As a CIS with a background in art therapy, incorporating the use of drawing assists the child, the team and the process. Drawing provides a way to gather information from the child, which is shared with the team, since drawing is integral to the process. A drawing may help the team understand a child's psychological, emotional and even physical presentation. Information is gathered via a free drawing and translated in conjunction with the child's associations in a manner that helps facilitate the process and provide understanding of a child's experience. The significance attributed to a child's associations or what he or she expresses about a drawing is shared and clarified in post-processing. The use of drawing within the process enables information to be elicited and communicated in a nonthreatening way. Information is discussed with the team after the interview to provide education, explanation, clarification and illumination as to what a child has expressed through the use of drawing in tandem with the child's verbal associations or narrative.

Drawing	*Cohen-Liebman, 1999*
Within the Interview	*For Children*
• develop rapport	• provide distance
• establish trust	• picture is less threatening means for disclosing/communicating
• facilitate disclosure	• drawing is an external object – it is easier to talk about a picture
• elicitation of details/	of someone than about one's self directly
facts	• disclosure in a child-centered process
• corroboration of facts	• children can gain mastery over an experience
• may elaborate	• place self in control of a situation
verbally once depict	• shift locus of control (from perpetrator)
pictorially/imaginally	• offers a safe space/way for disclosing or relating one's experience
• credibility assessment	• the process enables one to express a narrative in an ego-syntonic
• developmental	way
assessment	• express what wish would have happened
• stimulus for fact-	• depict how might have defended self or intervened (or someone
finding	else may have)
	• a means to explore and own reaction/feelings
	• relate experience indirectly or directly

(*Continued*)

Drawing	*Cohen-Liebman, 1999*
Within the Interview	*For Children*
	• catalyst for making sense of an experience as related pictorially and expressed verbally
	• depict emotional reaction/level of trauma
	• draw solutions
	• adds credence to child's associations
	• depict developmentally incongruent knowledge, which is indicative of experience
	• can depict sequence – what happened next – progression of activity
	• self-generated cues rather than reliance upon interviewer
	• respond to facilitative utterances from interviewer

Interview Protocols and Guidelines

Interview protocols and guidelines exist to provide guidance and assistance for facilitating the fact-finding process and eliciting information about experienced events. To date a singular protocol or process for interviewing child victims of sexual abuse has not been established. Investigative interviews often are conducted according to guidelines, although different communities subscribe to distinct interview guidelines or protocols in accordance with investigative entities or designations (Bourg et al., 1999; Carnes et al., 1999; Davies et al., 1996; Myers, 1998; Poole & Lamb, 1998; Reed, 1996; Sorenson et al., 1997; Yuille et al., 1993). Component parts may be identified differently, yet the content is similar not only in this country but abroad as well (Cheung, 1997; Cohen-Liebman, 1999; Davies et al., 1996; Monteleone, 1996; Poole & Lamb, 1998). Phases (or in some cases stages or steps) associated with various protocols may vary; however, shared objectives are fundamental (as previously mentioned). Although the specific phases affiliated with a particular process may differ with regard to name or quantity (of phases or steps), the integral components emphasize and coalesce around the same essential elements and seek to explore similar content.

Forensic interviews have been characterized as protocols with distinct phases through which an interviewer is expected to move in a "sequential and organized manner" through the process (Davies et al., 1996). A phased approach incorporates standard exploration through an initial preparatory phase, a secondary phase for information gathering and a third devoted to closure (Saywitz et al., 2018, p. 313). Phases have been broken down further and determined to focus on "introductions, rapport building, narrative practice, guidelines/rules, a strategy for transitioning to the substantive topic, narrative description, follow-up questioning, clarification and closure" (Steele, 2012, p. 105). Protocols and guidelines may differ in configuration and naming of phases; however, they have a common purpose and goal: information gathering, or acquisition of material related to a child's experience. "A phased approach is universally recommended which may be labelled as an interview structure, guideline, or protocol" (Steele, 2012, p. 105).

Protocols or phase-specific guidelines have advantages as well as disadvantages associated with them. Advantages of adopting standardized protocols "include greater consistency across interviewers and the establishment of minimal professional standards" and the disadvantages include "creating a de facto obligation on the part of practitioners to conduct all interviews in a particular way, not ideally suited to every situation" (Kemp,

2017, p. 219). Some researchers contend that "although most protocols rely on a simple phased format, more research is necessary to validate this near-universal approach, including the subcomponents of the phases" (Saywitz et al., 2018, p. 314).

Earlier protocols included stages that were to be followed in a systematic way and were considered to be a step-wise process predicated upon progressive advancement through each step. The Step-Wise Interview attributed to John Yuille (1991, 2002) "attempts to minimize inaccurate reporting by gradually increasing specificity in questions, starting with free recall and progressing to directive questions for clarification and elaboration of already mentioned information" and "without inquiring about anything that was not indicated directly by the child" (Shapiro & Maras, 2016, p. 206).

"The need for best practice guidelines and protocols that increase the likelihood of accurate disclosures" (Conte & Vaughan-Eden, 2018, p. 101) as well as the elicitation of information from free-recall memory contribute to research in the field. "Children access free recall memory when describing an event in their own way and with their own words, and this information is likely to be more accurate" (Steele, 2012, p. 103). One of the most recognizable protocols is the National Institute of Child Health and Human Development (NICHD) protocol. The NICHD is a highly structured verbal (linear) process (Katz et al., 2014; Katz & Hershkowitz, 2010). It has been and continues to be researched and studied (Katz, 2014; Katz & Hamama, 2013; Katz & Hershkowitz, 2010; Lamb et al., 2007, 2008; Orbach et al., 2000). As such, a body of literature surrounding exploration of the protocol exists. The NICHD includes "a preparatory phase focusing on narrative practice and interview instructions, a series of questions for transitioning to the substantive topic that becomes increasingly more focused, and rigorous use of open-ended questions" (Steele, 2012, p. 103). Research associated with the NICHD protocol has been considered significant for interview protocols, including highlighting the "benefits of eliciting as much information as possible from free recall memory" (Steele, 2012, p. 103).

More recent study of the NICHD has been directed at the use of prompts and techniques (Lamb et al., 2008; Orbach et al., 2000; Brown et al., 2013) as well as the use of drawing as a means to obtain "rich testimony" (Katz & Hamama, 2013). Although previously researchers did not support the use of media within this protocol (Aldridge et al., 2004), a study (which is examined in the literature review in Part V) in which children were instructed to draw a picture of the abuse within the context of the protocol revealed an increase in disclosure (Faller, 2016; Katz & Hershkowitz, 2010). Recent study of the NICHD protocol has been directed at the use of drawing within the investigative interview format and its influence upon children's testimonies (Katz & Hershkowitz, 2010). In addition, the manner in which drawing may offer provisional emotional support within the NICHD is a current trend under examination (Katz et al., 2014).

An Art Therapy–Based Investigative Interview Process

As mentioned previously, my initial role transformed as my position morphed from mental health evaluator into forensic interviewer/child interview specialist and clinical director. In response to the increased awareness of the utility in accord with the expansion of services, the use of a lead interviewer and facilitator was engendered to meet the growing demand for assistance and to accommodate the rise in referrals. The interview process and corresponding guideline that were used evolved out of the practices I implemented, as discussed previously. It was reflective of my integration of art therapy principles and practices with investigative interviewing and forensic standards that centered upon the incorporation of free drawing as a primary resource (to stimulate free recall).

The process was predicated upon the juxtaposition of art therapy with forensic investigative interviewing techniques and judicial tenets. The use of free drawing was integral to the process.

As an art therapist, I married the use of my modality with the context and constrains of the process, which for me elevated the information accessed and enhanced the process. The use of drawing within the interview provided a means for assessing information that directed the interview structure and helped curate the process. As an art therapist, information was acquired and transmuted within the context of developmental spheres. Acquisition of this information was processed, translated and applied to support a child's interactive and communication patterns and facilitated engagement.

Premised upon attributes of art therapy, information was procured through the inclusion of free drawing to assist with the process. Information was shared with the team after the interview to clarify and explain a child's dynamics if not apparent to team observers. Forensic relevance as well as suggestibility and accuracy were areas addressed through the child's depictions in conjunction with the child's associations (verbalizations). This in turn contributed to the determination of further investigative measures and supportive interventions that were conjointly addressed. Drawing offered understanding and clarity with regard to evidentiary information disclosed, including situational and contextual material. Details that may not have been provided solely in a verbal context may have manifested via graphic imagery that promoted additional exploration, which contributed to fact-finding and cultivation of elicitation of additional material.

At the time of inception, with the emergence of an agency dedicated to integrated investigations, individual disciplines were not schooled in conducting and facilitating conjoint processes. With an increase in lead interviews, a common interview guideline was considered prudent to advance the mission aimed at fostering a multidisciplinary approach predicated upon cooperative and collaborative investigations. The guideline itself developed from my practice and use of the modality of art therapy as a means to foster fact-finding. The team was educated about the use of drawing to support the child, the investigative process and the team overall. The intent was not to convert team members into art therapists (after all, that entails a two-year master's program encompassing didactic and practicum experience as well as a thesis). Drawing when incorporated as an open-ended prompt in the investigative interview format assisted in facilitating the process and eliciting evidentiary material while empowering a child in a supportive and forensically compliant process that was child friendly and child centered.

As previously discussed, a multidisciplinary team is composed of individuals from diverse disciplines and fields, including law enforcement, mental health, medicine, prosecution and social services, that represent an array of backgrounds, experience and expertise. It is the combination and integration of these diverse resources that contribute to comprehensive investigations by the systems that intervene. The disciplines that comprise the multidisciplinary team have distinct and specific investigative needs that are pertinent to their respective purview (burden of proof). Often, desired information is essential to more than one, if not all, of the respective disciplines. An interview format that addresses the respective needs of each discipline is practical and pragmatic and ensures that everyone involved has a consistent method and a collective approach. Thus, the process is a shared and mutual language of sorts that incorporates and establishes the standard for the team. A common interview guideline is essential for three reasons: to improve the fact-finding process, to eliminate secondary victimization by minimizing repetitive interviews and to ensure the process is known to each discipline and affords consistency.

Common Interview Guideline

The premise of a collaborative investigative protocol or guideline was to streamline and improve both the investigative and prosecutorial processes. Investigative measures are directed at minimizing the need for repetitive interviews and multiple interviewers while maximizing the information provided by a child. Overall, the guideline had to satisfy the investigative objectives associated with the various investigative entities, maintain forensic integrity and allow for optimum elicitation of information from a child within a supportive context. Fundamental to achieving these goals and objectives was the concept of a developmental framework that included a basic understanding of maturational spheres as well as best practice with regard to interviewing (Cohen-Liebman, 2002).

Premised around the belief that the information gathered from a comprehensive process would serve all parties engaged in investigation while safeguarding a child, a Common Interview Guideline (CIG) based upon the process I had developed, implemented and was using in my role as a child interview specialist evolved. The investigative interview process I created was based upon my experience, background and training as an art therapist and a CIS (Cohen-Liebman, 1996, 1997a, 1997b, 1997c), and it was responsive to the lead interview role. Elements that factored into the subsequent guideline included exposure to other guidelines that were populating at the time, best practices, contemporary research and study related to investigative interviewing and engagement in professional development. Collectively, these factors contributed to the guideline that emerged from the interview process I crafted, which reflected my respective orientation(s) as a CIS and an art therapist (Cohen-Liebman, 1999). Ultimately, a forensically sound investigative interview process with therapeutic overtones resulted, given the adherence to forensic standards coupled with the supportive nature emanating from the principles and practices invoked that were based upon art therapy.

The CIG was developed for multidisciplinary team investigations of child sexual abuse allegations. The CIG incorporates free or nondirected drawing as an integral part of the interview process in the capacity of an open-ended prompt. The guideline was developed to provide the multidisciplinary team with a common language and a consistent method for investigating allegations of child sexual abuse. The CIG is composed of five phases that are fluid and not static. Each phase of the interview guideline is designed to refute the argument of suggestibility. This means that the interviewer is not leading the child to say or give a particular response, nor is the interviewer suggesting a given response. Each element incorporated into the interview process, whether with or without drawing, is included for a specific reason and is conceived with the idea that everything within the process must be legally defensible in a court of law. The interviewer must be able to defend every action and interaction within the process if requested to do so in court as well as be able to explain the process and the use of aids, tools and media if invoked.

Common Interview Essential Factors

The guideline was designed to be comprehensive and informative. The guideline emanated from exploration of methods and means to obtain information. In deference to the community that fostered the need for a common language, a guideline that incorporated the material requested by the various agencies to help in their respective investigations was conceptualized. This process ensured that a child would not be unnecessarily subjected to additional discipline-specific interviews or a mix of interviewers.

As conceptualization materialized, I realized that the guideline necessitated several components prior to and in correspondence with development, including a concomitant training program. In and of itself, a guideline meant that team members had to be educated and introduced to the process so that cohesion was promoted. Without instruction and explanation, the underlying components and the composition of the process would not necessarily be comprehensible. Devised as a team concept, the interview process and accompanying guideline necessitated dissemination in a format that was conducive for collaboration and interaction (Cohen-Liebman, 1999). Knowledge-based modules were identified that highlighted the areas intrinsic to the guideline and were vital to conducting forensic interviews. To be forensically acceptable, the process dictated consistent and sustainable elements.

Additionally, as the guideline was solidified, the interview was essentially one aspect of the entire investigative interview process, which eventually crystalized into six essential aspects or steps, with the investigative interview being only one part of the process. It was preceded by and succeeded by team processing to develop a comprehensive and dedicated process that was responsive for meeting the needs of all investigative entities. Finally, the guideline was designed to place the child at the center of the process. Safeguarding the emotional well-being of child victims and witnesses was a primary objective; as such, the process had to be child friendly and child centered.

In order to make this process a reality, several objectives had to be met: identifying what information was needed by each system for its respective investigation and identifying what material was needed to meet the respective burden of proof of each system. Interagency and cross discipline matters required addressment to break down barriers and instill trust and maintain respect among team members. Through cross disciplinary training, understanding of the roles and mutual appreciation for each discipline contributed to understanding the expectations associated with partner agencies. A coordinated process that was supportive and respectful of the various agency cultures and inherent diversity of the distinct disciplines contributed to shared and impactful interaction in the service of children and families which was fundamental. Creating a carefully crafted process that was all-inclusive demanded cooperation and collaboration and "buy-in" from the participating agencies, including administrators and front-line investigators. The sharing of information was critical to the process, as was cross training. Multiple perspectives were important to the process. Being able to take on someone else's perspective was important and helped maintain integrity and support within the team. Understanding child sexual abuse and forensic interviewing practices as well as familiarity with the list of competencies ensured that everyone, whether actively or passively participating in an interview process (leading or observing), would comprehend and understand the elemental features, including what (was happening), when (something or some aspect was incorporated) and why (something was introduced or included) within the process. All of this factored into the development of a common interview guideline and a corresponding training program.

A corresponding training program was created to enhance knowledge and provide opportunity for skill building for team members. Experiential exercises, many art therapy-based, were developed to reinforce learned material. Education surrounding interagency and interdisciplinarity was embedded within the training curriculum to promote interactive exchange among team members as well as to desensitize the process. Instruction on diverse topics relative to child sexual abuse investigations was provided. Investigators from child protection as well as law enforcement might be assigned to child abuse units within their respective agencies, sometimes without prior experience and exposure to the population. Training exercises, including interview scenarios simulating the process of interviewing, were incorporated to educate and foster cooperative investment.

Child sexual abuse prompts language and dynamics that may not be understood outside of the context of investigation. As such, exercises were developed to overcome barriers that might cultivate a lack of understanding or misunderstanding when speaking to children in the real world about experienced events. The words a child uses to speak about body parts and interactions that are sexual in nature are critical to understanding a child's experience. In addition, this information is considered with regard to assessing forensic relevance and credibility assessment. Investigators are not educators, and the role is not to provide language for a child or to ascribe meaning to what a child conveys. Through facilitating the elicitation of information in an interview, the fact-finder uncovers evidentiary material to assist in understanding a child's experience that is rooted in the child's ability to relate facts, including details. This may entail comprehending how a child communicates and expresses information. To appreciate a child's words or disclosure, an interviewer may need to explore how information, knowledge and material related to an experienced event were obtained or acquired.

As noted earlier, cooperative and collaborative investigations were considered state of the art in the 1990s as a method for reducing repetitive interviews and multiple interviewers while maximizing fact-finding. In response to the implicit diversity that permeated the various disciplines that were part of the investigative team and the respective investigative purviews, the CIG had to incorporate distinct goals and purposes while meeting associated specified criteria. The CIG had to satisfy the investigative objectives of each discipline, predominantly law enforcement, child protection and prosecution. In addition, it had to maintain forensic integrity and allow for optimum elicitation of information within a supportive and child centered environment. Underlying these goals and objectives was the need for a developmental framework that included a basic understanding of maturational spheres (including cognitive, psychosocial, expressive-receptive, linguistic, psychosexual, artistic and emotional), as well as best practice with regard to investigative interviewing (Cohen-Liebman, 1999).

To ensure a cohesive and inclusive process, a guideline that crossed disciplinary boundaries and eliminated systemic barriers and impediments was necessary. The goal was to develop a guideline that would integrate the objectives consistent with the various systems that respond to allegations of sexual abuse at the initial stage of investigation. To make this process a reality, several objectives had to be met: identifying what information was needed by each system for their respective investigations, determining what information was needed to meet the respective burden of proof of the different systems, developing a process that was inclusive of each agency's mandates and creating a child-centered process that safeguarded the child's welfare while maintaining forensic integrity.

The process merited interaction with the targeted agencies that constituted the multidisciplinary team to understand what information was essential and integral to the development and implementation of the interview guideline so that it was inclusive of agency mandates and would be acceptable in court. The format was designed to incorporate the use of drawing, since that was my primary mode of engagement and interaction with children. The use of drawing within the process was premised upon my background and experience as an art therapist. Within the context of the interview, drawing as an open-ended prompt provided information through the child's imaginal and verbal expression. Ultimately, the guideline originated from the investigative interview format that I had developed (as noted earlier) and was a consistent and familiar practice to investigators who (for some routinely) accessed the service.

The guideline and subsequent training curriculum derived from and were reflective of the interview format I created and corresponded to the way I conducted interviews. Art therapy and the use of drawing were central to my approach of interviewing. When required to testify about a case, I would be asked to explain and describe the interview practice and the use of drawing as well as art therapy, which was part of the qualification process as an expert in court.

Through instruction and training on the component elements of the interview in concert with understanding the essential features associated with each phase, team members were positioned to appreciate and understand the process as observers and, if need be, participants. Members were able to determine what was happening in the interview and understand why, which enabled participants to contribute to the team process. Through the development of a guideline, members of the team could potentially take the lead and conduct the process, although not as an art therapist and not by using drawing as an art therapist however, drawing(s) fostered understanding for the team. The information that was gathered assisted team members with decision making and determination of findings, as well as burdens of proof with respect to their agency mandates. In consultation with the team, the interviewer facilitated post-processing in which recommendations were collaboratively discussed and recommendations were collectively identified. The need for additional investigative measures and interventive strategies were considered within the team context so that information was relevant, timely, concurrent and supportive.

The two main systems that intervene on the front line of investigation are child protection and law enforcement. These two systems must make determinations that impact the safety and well-being of a child. In addition, potential prosecution, depending upon whether or not a crime is determined to have been committed, is predicated upon law enforcement's findings, which are addressed with the district attorney. The processes are separate but parallel, and the information is obtained from the same source: a child who is potentially a victim or a witness.

The interview process had to be configured to provide law enforcement and child protection with discernable information relative to their respective investigations. These two systems traditionally investigate the same allegations but with different burdens of proof, meaning that different outcomes might result. Law enforcement is focused on determination of whether or not a crime has been committed and, if so, by whom. Child protection's burden of proof revolves around the safety and protection of a child. Law enforcement is compelled (depending upon jurisdiction) to meet a 99.9 % burden, while child protection has a lower burden of proof to meet, which might contribute to the removal of a child from the home if the child is thought to be at risk.

CIG Training

The CIG emerged out of the need to provide a common language and bridge the communication gap that was existent at the time. Charged with the task of creating a process dedicated to fulfilling the respective mandates of each agency, including the investigative needs ascribed to child protection, law enforcement and prosecution, the guideline had to be not only comprehensive but all encompassing. It had to be predicated upon communicating with children in a developmentally, congruent manner while also directed at facilitating fact-finding in a supportive environment. Building trust and rapport had to be ingrained within the process and were central features that were to be maintained throughout the duration of the interview process.

I realized that supplemental to the guideline was the need for a compatible training program. The training program had to correspond with the competencies interviewers/team members needed to be familiar with in order to understand, appreciate and benefit from and, if the occasion were to avail itself, even conduct the multifaceted process. Also, what was at the core of the guideline needed to be instilled in team members in order for the process to be effective: trust – trust in each other, trust in the various systems and the respective roles of each agency and multidisciplinary team members, trust to share and support each other, trust to offer opposing points of view, trust to work together and trust that the guideline would be a practical method for fact-finding and be responsive to the needs of the investigative community as well as victims and witnesses.

It was not sufficient to just have a process without having a plan for training and educating team members. Competency-based modules or areas of knowledge were identified to support interviewers in conducting developmentally sensitive and comprehensive interviews. The curriculum incorporated modules dedicated to team building and cross disciplinary issues. A more effective and coordinated response is propagated if everyone shares the same knowledge base. Modules were devised that highlighted fundamental competencies that were intrinsic to conducting investigative interviews that were forensically sound, developmentally congruent and culturally sensitive. Competencies were identified as necessary for credibility and sustainability. Interviewers and team members are also advised to receive continuing education on competencies as well as supervision and to be knowledgeable and familiar with relevant (i.e., current) literature, research and publications.

Five key components were identified as inherent to the development of a comprehensive and dedicated process (Cohen-Liebman, 2002). These features addressed cross discipline and interagency training, interview techniques, team building and diversity, which encompassed an array of topics. Throughout the conceptual development, it became increasingly apparent that each component was integral for a successful outcome. These elements were defined as follows (Cohen-Liebman, 2002):

1. Forensic interview, component phases
2. Interview techniques
3. Training curriculum, competency-based modules
4. Cross discipline, interagency issues as well as cultural awareness and diversity
5. Team building and the issue of teaming

Cross discipline training merited attention because it provided a platform for each agency/discipline to explore and share information related to their specialty while comprehending the respective roles, processes, protocols and procedures associated with counterparts. Through the exchange of this information, team members understand and appreciate the mandates associated with their partners and understand what responsibilities and actions are congruent as well as what is not specific to another agency. Often, this information is vital in understanding systemic expectations and cultivating working relationships that are productive, genuine and authentic. Even though team members may have preliminary guidance on what is associated with the investigative team, often clarity of roles and responsibilities helps to eradicate misperceptions or misunderstandings that might be based upon erroneous assumptions or false notions that may have been procured through personal, professional or societal influences.

Six-Step Team Process

In addition to the need for a training component, the interview structure was recognized as a six-step process. Each step was team based, with the investigative interview being only one aspect in accord with pre- and post-interview concerns. Specific tasks were ascribed to each step.

History and Observation

The case facts are gathered and reviewed. Each team member is responsible for sharing his or her respective involvement and engagement with the child and family. The allegations, including the sequence of events that led to a report being filed, are examined, including what has been disclosed by the child, nonoffending caretaker and anyone else who may have had contact or who may possess information about the allegations or situation that yielded a report such as a medical examination. Identification of individuals and information acquired by anyone who may have talked to the child are discussed. Individuals who are central to the investigation, including child victims and child witnesses, nonoffending caretaker(s) and alleged perpetrators, are identified.

Information possessed by the respective agencies participating in the process is shared. Intake information is provided so that all representatives share the same contact information and understand who is involved from each agency. Introductions are made if representatives are unfamiliar with agency counterparts. In essence, this step consists of two parts: team and child.

Team members establish lines of communication and familiarize themselves with the agencies and representatives involved in a particular case. Second, information pertinent to the case is outlined, including previous professional contacts and cursory interviews that may have been conducted prior to the investigative interview process such as a line squad officer (perhaps police were contacted and the responding officer may have talked with the child before the matter was referred to sex crimes or the special victims unit depending upon the jurisdiction for a full investigation including an investigative interview).

The exchange and sharing of case history, current information and background material promote a unified response; everyone is on the same page, and movement is orchestrated with shared knowledge. Through discussion of what each agency has uncovered and what actions have been enacted prior to the team gathering, a partner agency might discover new information or address a lack of awareness of some form of evidence.

Case specifics are addressed, including whether additional agencies or resources have been invoked relative to the investigation or intervention or previous engagement. For example, whether the child has received a medical exam might be explored. Child protection might be asked if the family has had prior involvement with the agency and, if so, what was the extent of the interaction, by whom and the outcome. This meeting is prudent for the team and contributes to next steps with regard to the interview or investigative sequence. If prior agency history is uncovered, additional sources may need to be contacted to gather data. Such information may provide context and inform current interaction and provide clarity about previous investigation and subsequent interventions, which may factor into the approach and garner understanding as to whether or not the allegations are new or related to a previous report.

The nonoffending caretaker is invited to meet with the team at this point and share information pertaining to the allegations and disclosure. Identifying information is clarified with regard to family dynamics (who lives in the household, the individuals responsible for caretaking, who else the child may have had contact with), the circumstances surrounding the allegations and the individual's knowledge about the circumstances that gave rise to either disclosure or suspicion that resulted in a report. The team discusses their respective roles if this information has not been explained to the nonoffending caretaker. Questions and concerns are addressed with respect to the circumstances. The process is explained and the nonoffending caretaker is escorted out of the meeting at the conclusion.

Pre-Interview Planning

Once team members are aware of the status of the respective investigative agencies, and after the nonoffending caretaker meeting, planning for the child interview commences as a collaborative endeavor. The individual child and the original allegations are discussed so that a group decision is made to determine who should take the lead. The choice is a team decision so that the best interests of the child are considered. Specifics surrounding the allegations that merit additional exploration are determined to provide context; however, the interview is not predicated upon a script, and a question-and-answer format is not predetermined. Identification of pertinent information that merits examination is discussed in relation to individual agency mandates. Fact-finding as it relates to next steps is also considered.

Everyone contributes to decision making with regard to the semantics of the interview: who should take the lead, presence of another interviewer in the room, how the team will communicate with the interviewer, what type of media might be present in the interviewing room, memorialization (documentation) of the process, team logistics and where the team might observe along with other concerns.

Depending upon whether or not the child has been previously interviewed and by whom and in what capacity, the same individual may be identified as the appropriate person (from the team) to conduct the interview on behalf of the team. The interviewer selection is symbiotic such that the child will feel comfortable and supported and trust will be formulated within the process. Often, a nonoffending caretaker may request a certain agency conduct the interview or suggest a particular type of individual speak with a child. As a team, considerations are addressed; however, parents are informed that the process is contingent upon who is assigned to a case and that certain requests may not be fulfilled. Whoever interviews the child will conform with the interview structure and adhere to multidisciplinary standards, including engagement and interview protocol. Typically, the lead interviewer is the CIS unless otherwise determined as noted.

In essence, the team encompasses the assigned agents, and ultimately the team will determine who will take the lead in a process unless the structure of the interviewing location has a lead interviewer that is tasked with conducting interviews on behalf of the multidisciplinary team. If each member is properly trained and subscribes to the process, impediments and barriers will hopefully not be factors. In many instances, the interviewer is designated when a team process is consigned to an interview site. This may be the reason a process is scheduled at a particular setting, for instance, because of the presence of a forensic (lead) interviewer who is trained to conduct these processes.

Interview Considerations

Physical setting
- orientation of the space to promote comfort and minimize vulnerability
- eliminate excess stimulation and minimize distractions
- arrange sitting stations and media so accessible and minimal
- organize interviewing aids ahead of time to minimize distractibility
- these items are used to assist in fostering the child's communication and engagement

Note about the use of anatomically detailed dolls within the interview structure:
There is an entire body of literature devoted to the use of the dolls which exceeds the scope of the text. The use of dolls is briefly considered in the literature review in Part V.

Investigative Interview

The forensic investigative interview, specifically the CIG, proceeds with the lead interviewer facilitating. The child is escorted to the interviewing room by the lead interviewer. Rapport building begins upon arrival to the facility and continues until the child and nonoffending caretaker exit the building. The team gathers to observe via the methods available, either sitting in a room with a one-way mirror or perhaps in a space with a monitor. If the team has decided upon the presence of a secondary interviewer, this individual is present in the interviewing room with the child and lead interviewer. The presence of a second individual will be explained to the child, as is the process including the standard operating procedure (SOP) or interview instructions. I personally do not like to use the term "rules" (of the interview), which I think connotes an authoritarian tone, which is to be avoided as far as I am concerned (just my personal belief). The term "expectations" is also something I try not to use because I do not want the child to feel pressured to do something or say something. In conjunction with the child's developmental presentation, these elements are addressed age appropriately. The child is also informed that the process is being observed and documented. This information is conveyed in a nondescript fashion so as not to encumber the process or hamper the child's focus.

Caveat

> I share with the reader my approach to investigative interviewing. Please appreciate that I am not saying that my way is the only way or the right way or that my beliefs are sacrosanct. Rather, I share with the reader how I approach the process. I try to structure the process in concert with the needs, presentation and coping skills of a child, including orienting the child to the process and being transparent with regard to the interview context (Cohen-Liebman, 1999).

Depending upon the interview and team protocol, the interviewer may check in with the team at a certain point in the process. The idea of a break is discussed briefly and again without fuss so as not to disrupt the process. Team check-in provides an opportunity to ascertain if additional information merits investigation or if a certain avenue warrants exploration. A child may have suggested something that the interviewer was unaware of but another team member may have made a connection to something previously stated or something that was omitted. This interlude may be construed as giving the child a break during the interview wherein the interviewer exits the space and checks in with the team to see if there are areas that merit further exploration or if there is something that merits follow-up – perhaps a response made by the child. Sometimes the interviewer is not cognizant of something a child has revealed and may miss an opportunity to delve deeper into a topic. The check-in is conducted to provide the interviewer with objective information from the vantage point of external observation and a collective or shared perspective. After all, this is a team process and the interviewer is conducting the process on behalf of the team, so it is incumbent upon the interviewer to address the respective mandates associated with each of the investigating entities. Sometimes stepping out of the process may provide the interviewer with insight as to approach. It must be stated that there is no such thing as a perfect interview or a process that cannot be improved. As such, the opportunity for a brief check-in may redirect or reorient an interviewer to an area or a topic that may yield unexplored evidence or offer an additional avenue to examine.

Team Check-In

A check-in may be a determinant that is at the discretion of the interviewer. It may not be productive or probable in every situation and should be considered in deference to the process.

Considerations

A check-in offers advantages for the interviewer as well as the team and might provide a quick exchange that induces a change in direction or follow up of something previously provided or perhaps something that was missed, avoided or omitted. The way a break is explained to the child deserves attention, however, because an abrupt break may negatively impact the child or the process; the interviewer must make a judgement as to how to introduce this and follow through. The child may be surprised by a sudden change in communication pattern. The way in which the break is introduced may be considered beforehand in conjunction with the team and in all reality should be a standard part of the process but with modification to the progression of the interview and in response to the interaction of the child. It is not intended to be disruptive and, in some cases, may not be appropriate given pacing, timing and dialogical interaction. At the beginning of the interview, the child should be informed that at some time a break may be initiated by the interviewer. If that happens, the interviewer will step outside of the room and the child will remain possibly for a few minutes alone (of course, the child is not alone, as the child is being observed; however, it may be appropriate to let the child know that observation will continue even if the interviewer exits at some point to check in with the team).

Exemplar

In one case, a child who was very hostile toward law enforcement was very angry about being interviewed. When the interviewer exited the space, the child turned to the mirror, aware that the officer was situated behind it with other members of the team observing. The child proceeded to make an offensive hand gesture and mouthed some unflattering sentiments to accompany her gesture. The officer, not one to be intimidated, wanted to confront the child about the behavior exhibited, which regrettably she did. Needless to say, that was not the best response by a member of the team. Post-processing included discussion surrounding the need not to personalize, engage or invoke reactionary behavior; however, this, of course, is difficult to hear when one is under personal attack for doing one's job. Confronting a child about observed behavior while in the midst of the interview by a team member watching the process

---

Exemplar

---

is not contributory or an effective strategy even if the child's behavior is disconcerting. The child's presentation changed and became antagonistic when the interviewer departed the space for team check-in with the child expressing her anger directly and deliberately toward the officer.

Mechanisms that predated current trends

The concept of a check-in was predisposed to new ideas that proved to be distractive and disruptive early on. These novel techniques were intended to permit communication between the interviewer and the team; however, for the most part, they were deemed to be insufficient for the purpose and typically seldom repeated. Examples included a telephone (perhaps a push-button) in the room (pre–cell phones). Anticipating the ring tone and watching the phone on the table was distracting for the child as well as the interviewer. When the phone was activated and it rang, the sound was jarring. It was difficult to conceal the conversation from the child, who might disengage once the distraction occurred. The interviewer had to answer the phone and speak with the caller and receive instructions, which were to be translated accordingly and then the child had to be re-engaged.

Another device that was unsatisfactory was the "bug in the ear" in which a listening device was worn by the interviewer and the team was able to communicate thoughts or ideas from the observation room. The device made it difficult to maintain that voices were not being heard during the interview, as often the sounds coming from the microphone were audible to the child. Explanation to the child of what they were hearing, of course contributed to a break in the process and a need to refocus attention.

Eventually, stepping outside of the interview room seemed to offer the least troublesome avenue. The team had to determine if a knock was necessary to alert the interviewer to the need for a check-in versus the interviewer determining when and if a break was most fruitful.

Investigative interviewing techniques have evolved, as they have been subjected to scrutiny and study rendering transformation, adaptation and modification resulting in alterations in style, approach, practice and implementation.

Interview/Interviewer Debriefing

Once the interview has concluded and the child has been returned to the nonoffending caretaker, the interviewer is able to communicate his or her thoughts, positive and negative, about the experience. This provides an opportunity for the interviewer to decompress and express thoughts and even feelings about the process, such as did the interviewer feel positive or negative, were there additional avenues that merited exploration, did the interviewer feel there were missteps or pitfalls. From the interviewer's perspective, what went well in the process and what were potential areas for improvement are addressed. Questions by the interviewer and feedback as well as observations are brought forth from the participants/observers regarding the process. This is intended to be constructive, although at times given the circumstances it may not always be interpreted as such. Overall, feedback and critique are intended to be offered in a supportive manner. This piece of the process enables the interviewer to share impressions and to receive feedback. Learning and skill enhancement are ongoing with regard to investigative interviewing.

Essentially, this interactive segment provides a means for discussion surrounding best practice as well as areas that lend themselves to improvement or augmenting one's skills through exposure and experience. Topics may address why something was productive or why something was not, and suggestions may be offered in an effort to provide the interviewer as well as the observers with alternative approaches that are applicable to everyone. To restate, no process is perfect. Everyone benefits from sharing thoughts and offering as well as hearing differing perspectives. Self-assessment (as well as team assessment) and reflection on what went well and what did not are meaningful exercises.

There is no perfect process, and learning from one's mistakes, mishaps or just focusing on skill enhancement will provide a catalyst. I do not recall ever witnessing or being privy to the perfect interview process or someone volunteering that an interview was perfect or was absent any hitches. Invariably, during post-processing an interviewer will acknowledge something that was asked and say, "I shouldn't have said that or the question should have been asked differently".

Analysis of Interview and Information

Information from the interview is reviewed and compared with material presented and discussed during the pre-interview. Information gathered that precipitated the team process, perhaps emanating from a previous interaction depending upon how the report was received, is included in the discussion. Information is assessed to determine congruency with what was known to what was uncovered to identify what might be new information or what may differ. The facts of the case as initially presented are reviewed and evaluated within the context of what a child may or may not have disclosed in the interview. Discussion ensues with the team surrounding new facts as well as information previously revealed. Information gleaned in concert with the allegations is ruled out or ruled in, and forensic relevance is addressed. The facts of the case are considered, and patterns are examined in relation to the information as presented in the original report, uncovered through discussion with the nonoffending caretaker and other parties, what the child has or has not revealed prior to the interview and during the process. As such, evidence is examined with congruencies identified and paucities determined.

Discussion informs next steps regarding investigation. If the child identified unrealized victims and witnesses, and even perpetrators, additional interviews may be deemed necessary. Investigators discuss who is the primary for conducting such interviews (not investigative interviews, such as what the child just experienced, but information-gathering processes conducted by the respective agencies). Depending upon what a child has revealed in the interview, the team begins to outline and devise a plan for what happens next, with responsibility for actions assigned to each agency so that accountability and follow-up measures remain in the forefront.

If the child was reticent to communicate in the interview or provided limited information or confirmed salient facts without substance, discussion may focus on the need for an extended interview process, which blends with the next step. Concerns are identified with regard to whether or not an extended interview process may be necessary based upon how a child presented and what was discussed and/or disclosed. The facts of the case obtained prior to the interview, as well as those gathered during the interview, are revisited and examined to determine consistencies and inconsistencies as well as acquisition of new, additional or previously unknown facts. Everything is considered within the context of the allegations and the safety and well-being of the child. Whether the respective agencies are situated with regard to meeting mandates and determining purviews, as well as the direction of the case, are additional matters that factor into the discussion.

Multiple perspectives are garnered given the array of viewpoints from the diversity implicit. As a team, next steps are determined from analysis of the information. The multiplicity inherent in a shared process has a direct impact and can influence the process, especially if a singular point of view is not shared by everyone. A system of checks and balances exists which contributes to an expansion of ideas and will contribute to determination of a collaborative plan of action in the next phase of the process. Ideally, everyone is on the same page and sharing points of view that cultivate a comprehensive and coordinated plan of action that will be brought to fruition in the next step.

6) Recommendations/Plan of Action

Recommendations/Plan of Action/Team Assignments

This step is a two-prong process in that a plan of action is conceived and recommendations are generated because of the interview in conjunction with the overall facts of the case. The safety of the child is paramount. Interventions are determined that may assist the child and the family. A plan of action is drafted, and a coordinated response is outlined. Identifying next steps is a shared process, including the need for collateral interviews.

Although the CIG is not a therapeutic process, therapeutic overtones are infused within the construct. As such, recommendations are provided that address the welfare of the child. Supportive measures are identified for the child as well as the family. Recommendations for therapeutic or other interventive services may be presented. Issues identified related to the case or stemming from the need for additional fact-finding or acquisition of information may promote the need for an extended interview process. Conflicts, concerns and issues may lead to targeted recommendations surrounding medical, legal, child protection, mental health and familial support.

Step five merges with the recommendations and plan of action, as stated earlier. As a unit the team must make decisions based upon the facts that have been gathered and evaluated. Together, the team must decide what the next steps are and what is in the best interest of the child and the family. If the team determines that more information pertaining to the allegations is needed, then an extended interview process might be advocated. If investigators determine that another single-session interview might be enough to address unresolved issues or to obtain additional case-specific information that will assist in the next steps that is a possibility as well. An extended process may not then be necessary.

Exploring additional information with the child may provide relevant facts that may direct external pursuits such as interviews or search warrants or other matters surrounding the gathering of evidence that may contribute to investigation and/or prosecution as well as child protection. Examples may be witness identification contributing to exploration of additional persons of interest, including additional or unnamed perpetrators, and the existence of additional victims.

Whether or not additional professionals or agencies need to be brought in is a matter to consider, including a child advocate, or perhaps a medical exam is suggested. Referrals for services are discussed among the team and then the nonoffending caretaker is invited to meet with the team to discuss findings and recommendations. It is at the discretion of the team to inform the nonoffending caretaker about what the child may or may not have disclosed, depending upon the case as well as the safety and protection of the child. If there is concern that the nonoffending caretaker is not able to protect the child or maintain the child's emotional well-being, the team may formulate a plan of action to address such concerns that may merit immediate attention.

If sufficient evidence has been obtained and meets the mandates as stipulated by the respective agencies, the case may not demand additional investigation or interviews. If the investigating agencies have met their respective burdens, they may proceed as indicated. The case dynamics may be presented to prosecution by law enforcement (if prosecution was not present during the interview and or pre/post-processing). These are decisions to be made after the interview and in view of the larger case context.

The team may decide to present the case at a team review, which is an expanded conference to include additional parties that may not have been present for the interview, since they are not included in the team of primary investigators assigned to a particular case. Additional insight may contribute to next steps that might not have been previously envisioned or considered. External representatives from associated agencies that intervene but are not front-line investigators may be invited to case review in an effort to widen the scope of discussion and to gather additional perspective that may contribute to recommendations related to investigation or intervention. This gathering provides a forum for exchange of ideas and affords insight from external representatives. Investigative measures may be reviewed and examined with the intent of identifying issues or concerns associated with the case, and input regarding next steps may be procured with the assistance of expanded team representation.

The child's capacity as a witness in court and the need for preparation may merit consideration depending upon determination of next steps. Not everyone in attendance will be actively participating in every case brought forth for discussion. As such, the inclusion of external participation may afford perspectives and ideas not previously addressed. Typically, prosecution is present for these meetings, which also provides dialogue regarding next steps with regard to whether or not a case may proceed in the legal domain, which is determined from the facts of the case as presented by law enforcement to the prosecutor and may not be shared in this context. Child welfare issues are considered, as are recommendations for intervention such as therapeutic services and support services within the home.

In summary, a team meeting or a conference wherein the addition of individuals from external agencies or professions that have a vested interest may be convened (depending upon the case, there may be a child advocate, for example, or a medical professional) to clarify or educate, share information, review allegations and address treatment needs. Interdisciplinary collaboration continues through this venue to support the child, the team, the process and the investiture of services that extend beyond the initial investigation. These may include therapeutic intervention or participation in court school in anticipation of a judicial hearing, as well as a range of other offerings pertinent to the individual case.

Proviso

It was my experience that team members often relied upon the interview to identify which box to check with regard to determination of allegations (was a child sexually abused or not). Education regarding the scope of my role was often repeated. It was not my purview to make the assertion that a child was or was not sexually abused; rather, that decision was for the individual agency representatives to determine in relation to their respective mandates and burdens of proof based upon the information procured from an interview.

The reports that were generated after an interview detailed the process and included recommendations, which encompassed a range of interventions to address the needs of a child, including social and emotional supports. The recommendations were provided in response to the allegations and/or the investigation and with respect to the child's presentation during the interview. Recommendations addressed forensic and clinical issues given the nature of the process, which has been explained. The recommendations extended beyond evidentiary material and included suggestions that encompassed a range of interventions specific to each case.

Services to assist families were also identified, as was the need for further evaluation. The CIG, being a hybrid process, was not restricted to investigative recommendations but included interventive and supportive recommendations to address issues identified either during

---

(*Continued*)

pre- and post-processing or derived from the fact-finding process. As such, recommendations addressed both investigative and supportive measures that were intended to safeguard the emotional well-being of the child and maintain forensic integrity. The process was not a clinical one, but it had clinical overtones given the underlying art therapy orientation, and as such, recommendations were made to address investigative findings as well as supportive measures.

CIG Training Workshop

As part of the task to create and develop a CIG for team investigations of child sexual abuse, a corresponding training program was created and implemented. An orientation regarding the development and purpose of a training program, as well as an overview of the training, was initially presented to representatives of the multidisciplinary team and consisted of a two-and-a-half-day workshop. Through this gathering, the core components of the CIG were presented and the underlying principles that comprise it were explained. The workshop was intended to promote an appreciation and understanding for the CIG as well as provide interactive opportunities (Cohen-Liebman, 2002). This platform introduced the rationale behind the coordinated and collaborative interview process to representatives from each of the participating investigative agencies, including administrators.

The format presented the five phases of the CIG to familiarize participants with the interview structure. Thus, the agenda included experiential exercises, many art therapy-based, to emphasize team building as well as interagency collaboration, the component phases of the CIG and interview best practices (Cohen-Liebman, 2002). Specific art therapy tasks were utilized throughout the workshop to engage the participants, build trust, engender appreciation of agency-specific roles, develop respect, dissolve boundaries and promote the development of collaborative and collegial relationships. Becoming acquainted beyond disciplines was integral to a successful outcome. The workshop was structured to encourage interaction among participants to foster relationships across disciplines by promoting interagency interaction, which was essential for collaboration.

The implicit diversity inherent in a multidisciplinary team composed of individuals from an array of professions was examined with regard to differences in worldviews. Developing respect, building trust and eradicating misnomers, as well as examining preconceived ideas, were elements that factored into the workshop. The array of mandates, missions and creeds associated with the diverse and often not complementary systems required sensitivity. Recognition of the role of unconscious bias and erroneous perceptions and stereotypes contributed to breaking down barriers and fostered appreciation of the various roles and responsibilities that each agency/discipline/profession contributes to the team milieu. This in turn fostered awareness, respect and a shared commitment to learning and working together.

- educating prospective team members on how to conduct investigative interviews that were comprehensive and compatible with state-of-the-art practice
- interactive opportunities to dissolve barriers that might hinder collaborative investigations
- introduction to the interview structure
- exposure to training curriculum and knowledge-based competency modules
- exposure to the benefits afforded using drawing within the process
- participation in art therapy tasks designed to facilitate interaction and engagement and foster working relationships

The workshop provided the springboard for a modified training program that was later implemented on a consistent basis for front-line investigators. The individuals who participated and the investment by each agency was salient for a team process that was dedicated to streamlining and improving investigation, advocating interagency collaboration and promoting cooperative working relationships in the service of child victims and witnesses as well as nonoffending caretakers and families.

References

Aldridge, J., Lamb, M. E., Sternberg, K. J., Orbach, Y., Esplin, P. W., & Bowler, L. (2004). Using a human figure drawing to elicit information from alleged victims of child sexual abuse. *Journal of Consulting and Clinical Psychology, 72*(2), 304.

Allen, B., & Tussey, C. (2012). Can projective drawings detect if a child experienced sexual or physical abuse? A systematic review of the controlled research. *Trauma, Violence, & Abuse, 13*(2), 97–111.

American Academy of Child and Adolescent Psychiatry. (1990). *Guidelines for the evaluation of child and adolescent sexual abuse.* Author.

American Academy of Child and Adolescent Psychiatry. (1997). Practice parameters for the forensic evaluation of children and adolescents who may have been physically or sexually abused. *Journal of the American Academy of Child and Adolescent Psychiatry, 36*(10), 37S–56S.

American Professional Society on the Abuse of Children. (2002). *Practical guidelines: Investigative interviewing in cases of alleged child abuse.* Author.

American Professional Society on the Abuse of Children. (n.d.). *Mission and vision statements.* www.apsac.org/mission-and-vision

American Psychological Association. (1994). Guidelines for child custody evaluations in divorce proceedings. *American Psychologist, 49*, 677–680.

Bourg, W., Broderick, R., Flagor, R. Kelly, D., Ervin, D., & Butler, J. (1999). *A child interviewer's guidebook.* Sage Publications, Inc.

Brooks, C. M., & Milchman, M. S. (1991). Child sexual abuse allegations during custody litigation: Conflicts between mental health expert witnesses and the law. *Behavioral Sciences and the Law, 9*(1), 21–32. https://doi.org/10.1002/bsl.2370090104

Brown, D. A., Lamb, M. E., Lewis, C., Pipe, M. E., Orbach, Y., & Wolfman, M. (2013). The NICHD investigative interview protocol: An analogue study. *Journal of Experimental Psychology: Applied, 19*(4), 367–382.

California Attorney General's Office. (1988, October). *California child victim witness judicial advisory committee, final report.* Author.

California Attorney General's Office. (1994, July). *Child victim witness investigative pilot project, research and evaluation final report.* Author.

Carnes, C. N. (2000). *Forensic evaluation of children when sexual abuse is suspected.* National Children's Advocacy Center.

Carnes, C. N., Wilson, C., & Nelson-Gardell, D. (1999). Extended forensic evaluation when sexual abuse is suspected: A model and preliminary data. *Child Maltreatment, 4*(3), 242–254.

Ceci, S. J., & Bruck, M. (1995). *Jeopardy in the courtroom: A scientific analysis of children's testimony.* American Psychological Association. https://doi.org/10.1037/10180-000

Chadwick, D. (1999). A national call to action. *Child Abuse & Neglect, 23*(10), 955–956.

Cheit, R. (2014). *The witch hunt narratives: Politics, psychology and the sexual abuse of children.* Oxford University Press.

Cheung, K. F. M. (1997). Developing the interview protocol for video-recorded child sexual abuse investigations: A training experience with police officers, social workers, and clinical psychologists in Hong Kong. *Child Abuse and Neglect, 21*(3), 273–284.

Cheung, M. (2012). *Child sexual abuse: Best practices for interviewing and treatment.* Lyceum Books, Inc.

Child Welfare Information Gateway. (2014). *Definitions of child abuse and neglect.* U.S. Department of Health and Human Services, Children's Bureau.

Cohen-Liebman, M. S. (1991). *The art therapist as expert witness in child sexual abuse litigation.* Master's Thesis, Hahnemann University.

Cohen-Liebman, M. S. (1994). The art therapist as expert witness in child sexual abuse litigation. *ARTherapy: Journal of the American Art Therapy Association, 11*(4), 260–265.

Cohen-Liebman, M. S. (1996, November). *Nontraditional settings: Art therapy in the investigation and treatment of child abuse.* Oral Presentation, The American Art Therapy Association Annual Conference.

Cohen-Liebman, M. S. (1997a, March). *Draw and tell: Drawings within the context of child sexual abuse investigations.* Oral Presentation, American Orthopsychiatric Association, 74th Annual Meeting.

Cohen-Liebman, M. S. (1997b, March). *Nontraditional settings: Art therapy in the investigation and treatment of child abuse.* Oral Presentation, thirteenth annual Symposium on Child Sexual Abuse.

Cohen-Liebman, M. S. (1997c, November). *Forensic art therapy.* Preconference Course Presented at the Annual Conference of the American Art Therapy Association.

Cohen-Liebman, M. S. (1999). Draw and tell: Drawings within the context of child sexual abuse investigations. *The Arts in Psychotherapy, 26*(3), 185–194. https://doi.org/10.1016/S0197-4556(99)00013-1

Cohen-Liebman, M. S. (2002). Intro to art therapy. In A. P. Giardino & E. R. Giardino (Eds.), *Recognition of child abuse for the mandated reporter* (3rd ed., pp. 227–257). G.W. Medical Publishing.

Cohen-Liebman, M. S. (2003). Drawings in forensic investigations of child sexual abuse. In C. Malchiodi (Ed.), *Handbook of art therapy* (pp. 167–179). Guilford Press.

Cohen-Liebman, M. S. (2007). Parent support group: A non-traditional use of art therapy. In D. Spring (Ed.), *Art in treatment: Transatlantic dialogue* (pp. 68–85). Charles C. Thomas.

Cohen-Liebman, M. S. (2016). Forensic art therapy. In D. Gussak & M. Rosal (Eds.), *The Wiley Blackwell handbook of art therapy* (pp. 469–477). Wiley-Blackwell.

Cohen-Liebman, M. S. (2017). *Drawing and disclosure of experienced events in an art therapy investigative interview process with school aged children: A qualitative comparative analogue study* (Doctoral dissertation). Retrieved from ProQuest Dissertations and Theses database.

Cohen-Liebman, M. S. (2021). Drawing to disclose: Findings from an art therapy-based investigative interview process. In V. Huet & L. Kapitan (Eds.), *The art of practice & research: Art therapy international practice research conference proceedings'* (pp. 77–85). Cambridge Scholars Publishing.

Cohen-Liebman, M. S., & Gussak, D. (1998). *Investigation versus intervention: Forensic art therapy versus art therapy in forensic settings.* Paper presented at The American Art Therapy Annual Conference.

Conte, J. R., & Vaughan-Eden, V. (2018). Child sexual abuse. In B. Klika & J. Conte (Eds.), *The APSAC handbook on child maltreatment* (4th ed., pp. 95–110). Sage Publications, Inc.

Cronch, L., Viljoen, J., & Hansen, D. (2006). Forensic interviewing in child sexual abuse cases: Current techniques and future directions. *Aggression and Violent Behavior, 11*(3), 195–207. https://doi.org/10.1016/j.avb.2005.07.009

Davies, D., Cole, J., Albertella, G., McCulloch, L., Allen, K., & Kekevian, H. (1996). A model for conducting forensic interviews with child victims of abuse. *Child Maltreatment, 1*(3), 189–199.

Drake, B., & Jonson-Reid, M. (2018). Defining and estimating child maltreatment. In B. Klika & J. Conte (Eds.), *The APSAC handbook on child maltreatment* (4th ed., pp. 14–33). Sage Publications, Inc.

Elders, M. J. (1999). The call to action. *Child Abuse & Neglect, 23*(10), 1003–1009.

Everson, M. D., & Boat, B. W. (2002). The utility of anatomical dolls and drawings in child forensic interviews. In M. L. Eisen, J. A. Quas, & G. S. Goodman (Eds.), *Memory and suggestibility in the forensic interview* (pp. 383–408). Lawrence Erlbaum Associates.

Faller, K. C. (2003). *Understanding and assessing child sexual maltreatment.* Sage Publications.

Faller, K. C. (2014). Forty years of forensic interviewing of children suspected of sexual abuse, 1974–2014: Historical benchmarks. *Social Sciences, 4*(1), 34–65.

Faller, K. C. (2016). Disclosure failures: Statistics, characteristics and strategies to address them. In W. T. O'Donohue & M. Fanetti (Eds.), *Forensic interviews regarding child sexual abuse: A guide to evidence-based practice* (pp. 123–139). Springer International Publishing.

Friedenberg, G., Hansen, D., & Flood, M. (2013). Epidemiology of child and adolescent sexual abuse. In D. S. Bromberg & W. T. O'Donohue (Eds.), *Handbook of child and adolescent sexuality: Developmental and forensic psychology*. Elsevier.

Goodyear-Brown, F., & Myers, J. E. (2012). Child sexual abuse: The scope of the problem. In P. Goodyear-Brown (Ed.), *Handbook of child sexual abuse; Identification, assessment and treatment* (pp. 3–28). Wiley-Blackwell.

Goodyear-Brown, P. (Ed.). (2012). *Handbook of child sexual abuse; Identification, assessment and treatment*. Wiley-Blackwell.

Gould, J. W., & Stahl, P. M. (2009). The art and science of child custody evaluations. *Family and Conciliation Courts Review, 38*(3), 392–414.

Gussak, D. (2013). *Art on trial: Art therapy in capital murder cases*. Columbia University Press.

Gussak, D. (2020). *Art and art therapy with the imprisoned: Re-creating identity*. Routledge, Taylor & Francis Group.

Gussak, D., & Cohen-Liebman, M. S. (2001). Investigation vs. intervention: Forensic art therapy and art therapy in forensic settings. *American Journal of Art Therapy, 40,* 123–135.

Haralambie, A. M. (1999). *Child sexual abuse in civil cases: A guide to custody and tort actions*. American Bar Association.

Harris, S. (2010). Toward a better way to interview child victims of sexual abuse. *National Institute of Justice Journal, 267*, 12–15. www.ncjrs.gov/pdffiles1/nij/233282.pdf

Home Office. (2007). *Achieving best evidence in criminal proceedings: Guidance on interviewing victims and witnesses and using special measures*. Home Office.

Jenny, C., Crawford-Jakubiak, J. E., & Committee on Child Abuse and Neglect. (2013). The evaluation of children in the primary care setting when sexual abuse is suspected. *Pediatrics, 132*(2), 558–567.

Kalichman, S. C. (1993). *Mandated reporting of suspected child abuse: Ethics, law & policy* (1st ed.). American Psychological Association.

Kalichman, S. C. (1999). *Mandated reporting of suspected child abuse: Ethics, law & policy* (2nd ed.). American Psychological Association.

Katz, C. (2014). The dead end of domestic violence: Spotlight on children's narratives during forensic investigations following domestic homicide. *Child Abuse & Neglect, 38*, 1976–1984.

Katz, C., Barnetz, Z., & Hershkowitz, I. (2014). The effect of drawing on children's experiences of investigations following alleged child abuse. *Child Abuse & Neglect, 38*(5), 858–867.

Katz, C., & Hamama, L. (2013). "Draw me everything that happened to you": Exploring children's drawings of sexual abuse. *Children and Youth Services Review, 35*(5), 877–882.

Katz, C., & Hershkowitz, I. (2010). The effects of drawing on children's accounts of sexual abuse. *Child Maltreatment, 15*(2), 171–179.

Kelley, S. J. (1984). The use of art therapy with sexually abused children. *Journal of Psychosocial Nursing and Mental Health Services, 22*(12), 12–18.

Kemp, A. R. (2017). *Abuse in society: An introduction*. Waveland Press, Inc.

Kempe, A. R. (2007). *A good knight for children: C. Henry Kempe's quest to protect the abused child*. Booklocker.com, Inc.

Kempe, C. H., & Helfer, R. E. (1968). *The battered child*. The University of Chicago Press.

Kempe, C. H., & Helfer, R. E. (1972). *Helping the battered child and his family*. J.B. Lippincott.

Krugman, R. (1997). Child protection policy. In M. E. Helfer, R. S. Kempe, & R. D Krugman (Eds.), *The battered child* (5th ed., pp. 627–641). The University of Chicago Press.

Krugman, R. (1999). The politics: A national call to action: Working toward the elimination of child maltreatment, *Child Abuse & Neglect, 23*, 963.

Krugman, R. (2005). Brandt F. Steele. *Child Abuse and Neglect, 29*(3), 207–208.

Krugman, R. (2018). The more we learn, the less we know: A brief history of the field of child abuse and neglect. In B. Klika & J. Conte (Eds.), *The APSAC handbook on child maltreatment* (4th ed., pp. 1–13). Sage Publications, Inc.

Lamb, M. E., & Brown, D. A. (2006). Conversational apprentices: Helping children become competent informants about their own experiences. *British Journal of Developmental Psychology, 24*(1), 215–234.

Lamb, M. E., Hershkowitz, I., Orbach, Y., & Esplin, P. W. (2008). *Tell me what happened: Structured investigative interviews of child victims and witnesses* (Vol. 36). Wiley-Blackwell.

Lamb, M. E., Orbach, Y., Hershkowitz, I., Esplin, P. W., & Horowitz, D. (2007). A structured forensic interview protocol improves the quality and informativeness of investigative interviews with children: A review of research using the NICHD investigative interview protocol. *Child Abuse & Neglect, 31*(11), 1201–1231.

Lippmann, J. (2002). Psychological issues. In M. Finkel & A. Giardino (Eds.), *Medical evaluation of child sexual abuse: A practical guide* (2nd ed., pp. 193–211). Sage Publications Inc.

Lyons, S. (1993). Art psychotherapy evaluations of children in custody disputes. *The Arts in Psychotherapy, 22*(2), 153–159.

MacFarlane, K. (1995). Who's on first? Roles and responsibilities of team members. In *MDIC Handbook: A guide to the establishment of multidisciplinary interview centers for the intervention of child sexual abuse* (Vol.1, Chapter 8, pp. 2–15). Children's Institute International & Giarretto Institute.

Macleod, E., Gross, J., & Hayne, H. (2013). The clinical and forensic value of information that children report while drawing. *Applied Cognitive Psychology, 27*(5), 564–573.

Malloy, L. C., Brubacher, S. P., & Lamb, M. E. (2011). Expected consequences of disclosure revealed in investigative interviews with suspected victims of child sexual abuse. *Applied Developmental Science, 15*(1), 8–19.

Mannarino, A. P., & Cohen, J. A. (1992). Forensic versus treatment roles in cases of child sexual abuse. *The Pennsylvania Child Advocate Protective Services Quarterly, 7*(4), 3–7.

Mathews, B., & Collin-Vézina, D. (2017). Child sexual abuse: Toward a conceptual model and definition. *Trauma, Violence, & Abuse*, 1–18. https://doi.org/10.1177/1524838017738726

Melinder, A., Alexander, K., Cho, Y. I., Goodman, G., Thoresen, C., Lonnum, K., & Magnussen, S. (2010). Children's eyewitness memory: A comparison of two interviewing strategies as realized by forensic professionals. *Journal of Experimental Child Psychology, 105*, 156–177.

Milchman, M. (2011). The roles of scientific and clinical epistemologies in forensic mental health assessments. *Psychological Injuries and Law, 4*, 127–139.

Miller-Perrin, C. L., & Perrin, R. D. (2012). *Child maltreatment: An introduction* (3rd ed.). Sage Publications, Inc.

Monteleone, J. (1996). *Recognition of child abuse for the mandated reporter.* G.W. Medical.

Myers, J. E. B. (1998). *Legal issues in child abuse and neglect practice* (Vol. 1). Sage Publications, Inc.

Myers, J. E. B. (2019). *Mental health law in a nutshell.* West Academic Publishing.

Myers, J. E. B. (Ed.). (2011a). A short history of child protection in America. In *The APSAC handbook on child maltreatment* (3rd ed., pp. 3–15). Sage Publications, Inc.

Myers, J. E. B. (Ed.). (2011b). Criminal prosecution of child maltreatment. In *The APSAC handbook on child maltreatment* (3rd ed., pp. 87–99). Sage Publications, Inc.

Myers, J. E. B. (Ed.). (2011c). Legal issues in child abuse and neglect practice. In *The APSAC handbook on child maltreatment* (3rd ed., pp. 361–375). Sage Publications, Inc.

Naitove, C. (1980). Arts therapy with sexually abused children. In S. M. Sgroi (Ed.), *Handbook of clinical intervention in child sexual abuse* (pp. 269–308). Lexington Books.

National Children's Alliance (NCA). (n.d.). www.nationalchildrensalliance.org

National Children's Alliance. (2010). Standards for accredited members. www.national childrensalliance.org

The National Network of Children's Advocacy Centers. (1994). *Best practices manual: A guidebook to establishing a children's advocacy program* (2nd ed.). Author.

O'Donohue, W. T., & Fanetti, M. (2016). *Forensic interviews regarding child sexual abuse. A guide to evidence-based practice.* Springer.

Office of Juvenile Justice and Delinquency Prevention (OJJDP). (April, 2022). *InFocus; Children's Advocacy Centers.* Retrieved from ojjdp.ojp.gov.

Olafson, E. (2012). A call for field-relevant research about child forensic interviewing for child protection. *Journal of Child Sexual Abuse, 21*(1), 109–129.

Orbach, Y., Hershkowitz, I., Lamb, M. E., Sternberg, K. J., Esplin, P. W., & Horowitz, D. (2000). Assessing the value of structured protocols for forensic interviews of alleged child abuse victims. *Child Abuse & Neglect, 24,* 733–752.

Patterson, T., & Hayne, H. (2011). Does drawing facilitate older children's reports of emotionally laden events? *Applied Cognitive Psychology, 25,* 119–126.

Pence, D., & Wilson, C. (1994a). Reporting and investigating child sexual abuse. In *The future of children* (Vol. 4, No. 2, pp. 70–83). The Center for the Future of Children, The David and Lucille Packard Foundation.

Pence, D., & Wilson, C. (1994b). *Team investigation of child sexual abuse.* Sage Publications, Inc.

Pennsylvania Psychological Association (PPA). (2015). *Pennsylvania child abuse recognition and reporting.* Act 31 Home Study Continuing Education Program.

Pennsylvania, The Child Protective Services Law 23 Pa. C. S. A. §6311 (b)). (23 Pa. C. S. A. §6340 (a).

Perry, N. W., & Wrightsman, L. S. (1991). *The child witness: Legal issues and dilemmas.* Sage Publications, Inc.

Poole, D. A. (2016). *Interviewing children: The science of conversation in forensic contexts.* American Psychological Association.

Poole, D. A., & Lamb, M. E. (1998). *Investigative interviews of children: A guide for helping professionals.* American Psychological Association.

Poole, D. A., & Lamb, M. E. (2003). *Investigative interviews of children: A guide for helping professions.* American Psychological Association.

Poole, D. A., & Lamb, M. E. (2009). *Investigative interviews of children: A guide for helping professions.* American Psychological Association.

Raskin, D. C., & Esplin, P. W. (1991). Statement validity assessment: Interview procedures and context analysis of children's statements of sexual abuse. *Behavioral Assessment, 13,* 265–291.

Reed, L. D. (1996). Findings from research on children's suggestibility and implications for conducting child interviews. *Child Maltreatment, 1*(2), 105–120.

Runyan, D. K., Dunne, M. P., & Zolotor, A. J. (2009). Introduction to the development of the ISP-CAN child abuse screening tools. *Child Abuse and Neglect, 33*(11), 842–845.

Sadler, B. L. (1999). The vision: Why a national call to action. *Child Abuse & Neglect, 23*(10), 955–956.

Sadler, B. L., Chadwick, D. L., & Hensler, D. J. (1999). The national call to action: Moving ahead. *Child Abuse & Neglect, 23*(10), 1011–1018.

Salmon, K., Pipe, M. E., Malloy, A., & Mackay, K. (2012). Do non-verbal aids increase the effectiveness of "best practice" verbal interview techniques? An experimental study. *Applied Cognitive Psychology, 26*(3), 370–380. https://doi.org/10.1002/acp.1835

Salmon, K., Roncolato, W., & Gleitzman, M. (2003). Children's report of emotionally laden events: Adapting the interview to the child. *Applied Cognitive Psychology, 17*(1), 65–79.

Sapp, M. V., & Vandeven, A. M. (2005). Update on childhood sexual abuse. *Current Opinion in Pediatrics, 17*(2), 258–264.

Saywitz, K., Lyon, T., & Goodman, G. (2018). When interviewing children: A review and update. In B. Klika & J. Conte (Eds.), *The APSAC handbook on child maltreatment* (4th ed., pp. 310–329). Sage Publications, Inc.

Sgroi, S. (1982). *Handbook of clinical intervention in child sexual abuse.* Lexington Books.

Shapiro, L. R., & Maras, M. H. (2016). *Multidisciplinary investigation of child maltreatment.* Jones & Bartlett Learning.

Sorenson, E., Bottoms, B., & Perona, A. (1997). *Handbook on intake and forensic interviewing in the children's advocacy center setting.* Office of Juvenile Justice and Delinquency Prevention.

Steele. L. C. (2012). The forensic interview: A challenging conversation. In P. Goodyear-Brown (Ed.), *Handbook of child sexual abuse; Identification, assessment and treatment* (pp. 99–119). Wiley-Blackwell.

U.S. Advisory Board on Child Abuse and Neglect. (1990). *Child abuse and neglect: Critical first steps in response to a national emergency.* U.S. Government Printing Office.

Van Eys, P., & Beneke, B. (2012). Navigating the system: The complexities of the multidisciplinary team in cases of child sexual abuse. In P. Goodyear-Brown (Ed.), *Handbook of child sexual abuse; Identification, assessment and treatment* (pp. 71–97). Wiley-Blackwell.

Vieth, V. (2006). Unto the third generation: A call to end child abuse in the United States within 120 years. *Journal of Aggression, Maltreatment and Trauma, 12*(3/4).

Ward, T. (2006). English law's epistemology of expert testimony. *Journal of Law and Society, 33*(4), 572–595.

Wilson, C., & Pence, D. (2018). Multidisciplinary teams and child maltreatment. In B. Klika & J. Conte (Eds.), *The APSAC handbook on child maltreatment* (4th ed., pp. 385–403). Sage Publications, Inc.

Yuille, J. C. (1991). *The step-wise interview: A protocol for interviewing children.* Unpublished manuscript, University of British Columbia. Author.

Yuille, J. C. (2002). *The step-wise interview: A protocol for interviewing children.* Unpublished manuscript, University of British Columbia. Author.

Yuille, J. C., Hunter, R., Joffe, R., & Zaparniuk, J. (1993). Interviewing children in sexual abuse cases. In G. Goodman & B. Bottoms (Eds.), *Child victims, child witnesses: Understanding and improving testimony* (pp. 95–116). Guilford Press.

Part II   The Art of Interviewing
The Common Interview Guideline

The Common Interview Guideline (CIG) emerged from my practice as a forensic art therapist. Forensic art therapy (FAT) is a sub-specialization of art therapy (Gussak & Cohen-Liebman, 2001). It is a distinct and complex investigative practice (Gussak Cohen-Liebman, 2001; Gussak, 2013) that adheres to forensic standards and has therapeutic overtones. FAT is predicated upon the juxtaposition of art therapy principles and practices with legal and judicial tenets.

My background and training as an art therapist were central factors in developing the CIG. The CIG, a FAT investigative interview procedure, was developed for multidisciplinary team investigations of child sexual abuse allegations (Cohen-Liebman, 1999, 2003). Drawing was incorporated in a supportive capacity and assisted in the investigative interview process. Although team members were not expected to function as art therapists or use drawing in the same manner, they were educated about the usefulness and integrity that drawing afforded when incorporated within the investigative format as an open-ended prompt.

Drawing serves various functions within the process and offers inherent advantages and benefits for the child, the interview and the team. As described earlier, the CIG emerged out of the interview process I developed and implemented in my capacity as a child interview specialist. The interview I created provided the basis for a common language for investigators and subsequently, the development of the CIG and subsequent training components. This emergence as well as my process, including the juxtaposition of art therapy within a forensic context have been addressed in the literature (Cohen-Liebman, 1999, 2002, 2003, 2007, 2016, 2017, 2020, 2021).

Drawing as an open-ended prompt serves to enhance the process and contribute to fact-finding. However, some information cultivated via a drawing may not be understood or elucidated if art therapy principles and practices are not shared or explained. The knowledge, experience and background that accompany education surrounding art therapy are essential to comprehending the use of drawing within this context (Cohen-Liebman, 2017).

Although the CIG is accepted in court as a valid investigative method (Cohen-Liebman, 1999), empirical study on the guideline is a recent endeavor (Cohen-Liebman, 2017, 2021). The use of nondirected drawing as a primary resource in an art therapy investigative interview process as a means to stimulate recall (memory) to facilitate fact-finding or evidentiary disclosure was explored in conjunction with the encoding of trauma and the corresponding role of imagery. Study findings will be discussed in Part V.

The CIG incorporates nondirected or free drawing in the capacity of an invitational prompt within the investigative interview format to facilitate recall, enhance memory and promote elicitation of information. As such, drawing functions as a primary rather than a secondary or an ancillary support, wherein drawing is used as a means to confirm

DOI: 10.4324/9781003225041-3

a verbal statement. The use of drawing as an open or invitational prompt provides a child with an opportunity to convey information in an ego-syntonic manner through graphic or pictorial imagery which in combination with a child's associations, may promote a narrative regarding personal experience. In cases where a child is unable to verbally convey experience, the use of drawing may provide a child with a mechanism to "say what they cannot speak" and may promote verbal elaboration.

Multidisciplinary Team Response to Use of Drawing

Multidisciplinary team (MDT) members have recognized the benefits of integrating the use of free or open-ended drawing within the interview process and support the practice as a means of gathering information relative to the experience of a child (Cohen-Liebman, 1999). As such, existing systems incorporate the use of art therapy in a supportive capacity. The increased acceptance of art therapy is due to an expansion and collaboration with other disciplines (Smart, 1986). Furthermore, drawing functionally supports the child, the team and the process (Cohen-Liebman, 1999, 2002).

Proponents of the use of drawing within multidisciplinary team investigations also caution about assessing meaning and extracting information from drawing in isolation and minus contextual material. Robert Hugh Farley, a police officer schooled in the multidisciplinary investigative arena and who worked within this milieu, wrote that the interviewer that is typically not trained in art therapy must not attempt to analyze drawings, but rather defer to the professional trained in such matters (Farley, 1987).

The Office of Juvenile Justice and Delinquency Prevention (OJJDP) developed a manual to assist law enforcement and other justice system officials in the investigation of physical abuse and sexual exploitation of children. The manual included guidelines on investigating child abuse, interviewing techniques and legal issues relative to child abuse cases. It was intended to benefit investigators at the local, state and federal levels. The use of drawing within the interview process by investigators was discussed as follows.

> Once an initial assessment of the child's developmental level has occurred and rapport and trust have been established, a transition can be made to gathering critical information. Because this phase of the interview can be awkward for the investigator as well as the child, it can be helpful to use an interview aid. One popular aid involves the use of a plain piece of paper and crayons (Shepherd et al., 1995, p. 151).

> The investigator will ask the child to write their name and then draw a picture of themselves and complete it before asking questions. Referred to as the "drawing of yourself" picture this may then be utilized for a body inventory in an effort for the investigator to obtain the child's words for specific body parts. The investigator may ask subsequent questions to delineate additional information through the use of nonleading and nonthreatening questions (Shepherd et al., 1995, p. 152).

The manual states that there are many investigative tools to help facilitate a discussion.

> It is recommended that these aids be employed only as necessary by a qualified investigator. The manual also states that mental health professionals and child therapists can provide MDT members with training, information and tools required to collect evidence in this manner (Shepherd et al., 1995, p. 154).

These pictures make excellent pieces of evidence, and they can serve also as a non-traumatic vehicle for initiating a progressively probing line of questioning. The investigator should refrain from attempting an in-depth analysis or interpretation of the drawing(s); exceeding his or her level of training and competency can seriously jeopardize the credibility of the investigator and the case (Shepherd et al., 1995, p. 152).

Caveat Re: Drawing and the Multidisciplinary Team

Specific to the CIG, the guideline had to be inclusive and address the mandates associated with each agency and be comprehensible, as well as legally defensible. Anyone, whether active (facilitating) or passive (observing), would invariably understand the process and, if need be, take the lead, although as an interviewer not an art therapist, and thus the use of drawing might be modified. Interviewers were not to interpret a drawing or determine an allegation solely in response to one. Interviewers not trained as art therapists were not encouraged to use drawing in the same manner and would most likely not procure information (such as developmental and maturational) derived from the process-oriented approach, given the knowledge that an art therapist acquires through education, experience and training. Drawing was incorporated as a primary component due to the inherent advantages associated with the integration. Interpretation rested with the child, not the interviewer.

Guidelines and Multidisciplinary Investigation

Investigative interviews foster practices and procedures that require specially trained and highly skilled interviewers. The CIG provided a consistent method for investigating allegations of child sexual abuse for the investigating agencies that responded to reports of child sexual abuse allegations. The disciplines that comprise the MDT have distinct and specific investigative needs that correspond to their respective burdens of proof. Often, desired information is relevant to more than one, if not all, of the respective disciplines. A CIG is essential, as noted previously, for three reasons: to improve the fact-finding process, eliminate secondary victimization by minimizing repetitive interviews, and the process affords consistency because it is known to each discipline.

Although stated before (if the previous section was not perused), an MDT is composed of individuals from a host of disciplines that represent a myriad of backgrounds, experience and expertise. Representatives from diverse fields and specialties, including law enforcement, mental health, medicine, prosecution and social services, work together and blend their respective skills (Cohen-Liebman, 1999). It is the combination and integration of these diverse resources that contribute to comprehensive investigations by the systems that intervene. An interview format that addresses the respective needs of each discipline is essential. A collaborative investigative protocol or guideline streamlines and improves investigation and is directed at maximizing the information provided by a child.

As such, the guideline had to satisfy the investigative objectives associated with the various investigative entities, maintain forensic integrity and allow for optimum elicitation of information from a child. Fundamental to achieving these goals and objectives was the concept of a developmental framework that included a basic understanding of maturational spheres as well as best practice with regard to interviewing (Cohen-Liebman, 2002).

Forensic Art Therapy Investigative Interview Process

Charged with the task of creating a CIG, the process that evolved was predicated upon the interview format I had developed as a child interview specialist who was also an art therapist. The CIG is an investigative/forensic interview guideline. Free drawing is incorporated in the capacity of an open-ended or invitational prompt to generate a responsive and interactive process that is child centered. Drawing is used to facilitate free recall and elicit event-specific information in a nonthreatening manner. Artistic skill or talent is not necessary.

The CIG is a supportive relational process, given the interactive nature that ensues between the interviewer and child. Thus, the CIG is predicated upon rapport building, attunement to a child's developmental capabilities, fact-finding and minimization of re-traumatization (Cohen-Liebman, 2017). Rapport is facilitated and maintained throughout the process. Rapport building is not just a component phase; rather, this aspect of the process is ongoing and continuous throughout the interview and concludes when the child exits the setting.

Three central principles underlie the CIG:

- an open invitational drawing process
- the dialogical and relational process
- the encoding, storage and recall of (traumatic) memory in image form

Conceptually, the CIG embraces foundational ideas, including a dialogical or relational process, the use of nondirected drawing to facilitate fact-finding and the use of imagery as a means to elicit information and promote verbalization of an experienced event. The CIG is not a scripted interview process; rather, it is a semi-structured process that is comprised of phases that are fluid, not static and may overlap. It is not a step-wise process or a structured protocol wherein phases are to be adhered to in a predictable pattern. The phases are not necessarily sequential; rather, the phases progress or meld in concert with the child's presentation and in response to the dialogical process. The guideline consists of five phases that are fluid and flexible: rapport building, developmental assessment, anatomy identification, fact-finding and closure.

Each phase of the interview guideline is designed to refute the argument of suggestibility. This means that the interviewer is not leading the child to say or give a particular response, nor is the interviewer suggesting a desired response. Each element incorporated into the interview process, whether with or without drawing, is included for a specific reason and is conceived with the idea that everything within the process may be scrutinized in court, and as such the interviewer is responsible for defending actions and activities incorporated or invoked within the scope of the interview.

The CIG is a guideline for investigative interviewing that is predicated upon art therapy principles and practices juxtaposed with forensic tenets. Free drawing is used in the CIG as an open invitational prompt within the five phases of the interview. The phases are identified as rapport building, development assessment, anatomy identification, fact-finding and closure (Cohen-Liebman, 1999). Drawing assists in attaining the specified goals and objectives affiliated with the interview process.

Drawing assists the interviewer in assessing information in a quick and direct manner. Information derived from drawing guides the process as information is obtained and then translated. The flexibility which underlies the process enables the interviewer to utilize the information communicated and expressed by the child through drawing and associated verbalizations to configure and sequence the interview. The CIG is not a standardized process. It was conceived as a guideline rather than a protocol. The latter is described as a structured process with designated steps or phases that are followed in a prescribed manner. A guideline, in contrast, provides freedom and flexibility with regard to the inherent phases and movement within the process.

The guideline promotes maneuverability, given the nature of the child-centered process. The interviewer follows the interactive patterns of the child while maintaining control of the process. By moving in and out of the interview components, the interviewer follows the child's lead yet still directs the process (Cohen-Liebman, 1999). For example, if a child sits down and launches into a discussion concerning what brought them into the interview, the interviewer does not stop the child and contaminate what is being communicated. Rather, the interviewer will respond to the child and orchestrate the process accordingly. As such, the phases of the guideline dovetail and overlap and may even occur concomitantly.

Although the CIG is presented here in a linear fashion, it is not intended to be a stepwise protocol, meaning that it is not intended to be conducted one phase after another. Rather, the phases blend and merge and the interviewer has the flexibility to move in and out of the phases in response to the child's presentation. The phases are not adhered to in a specific order, although they are presented as such for educational and informational purposes. The phases are discussed separately and independently, but again, this is not a format that dictates adherence to a pattern or a specific course of action.

CIG

- forensically sound investigative interview with therapeutic overtones
- developmentally sensitive, forensically defensible, comprehensive interviews
- minimizes the need for repetitive interviews
- designed to improve fact-finding process and eliminate secondary traumatization
- guideline addresses investigative needs of the various systems that intervene at initial stage of investigation
- incorporates drawing in the capacity of an open-ended prompt

---

The discriminating features associated with each phase of the guideline, as well as the corresponding attributes associated with the integration of drawing within each phase, are highlighted. Identified concepts are discussed as they pertain to the process, including forensic relevance, credibility assessment and competency.

Drawing in the CIG (Cohen-Liebman, 1999)

- integral component
- incorporated in a supportive capacity
- assists in the investigative interview process
- complements the process
- can be used in a parallel manner
- may serve as a stimulus for both the interviewer and the child to explore material both manifest and latent

---

(*Continued*)

Drawing in the CIG (Cohen-Liebman, 1999)

- drawing can be retained and used later to explore material previously uncovered or not yet disclosed
- functions as a bridge within the investigative process
- may later serve as a judiciary aid
- helps the interviewer assess information quickly in a nonthreatening manner
- drawing provides information in a quick and direct manner that can be transferred into structure and process
- helps the team comprehend the child's developmental capabilities
- provides the team with insight into the level of functioning of the child
- insight into the level of trauma
- provides concrete and objective evidence

The process in combination with drawing tasks provides the team with insight into a child's coping skills, level of trauma, emotional reaction to the abuse and in many cases abuse-specific information (Cohen-Liebman, 1999).

CIG and Use of Media

Upon entering the interview setting, preselected media or art materials are available. White drawing paper, usually the size is 8" × 11", is placed in advance on the table along with two choices of structured media either crayons, craypas or markers, which may be thin or thick. The child is invited to choose where they want to sit, so the process begins with the child procuring a seat or a chair and choosing art materials instead of being told where to sit or what to use. This informal introduction and orientation to the setting hopefully instills a sense of trust with the interviewer. The selection by the child pertaining to seat and media fosters empowerment from the onset of the process, denoting the child-friendly nature.

Structured Versus Unstructured Media

Media or art materials exist on a continuum from structured to less structured. Structured media include materials that have a fixed shape and make a definitive mark. These materials are two-dimensional and include pastels, craypas (a combination of crayons and pastels), markers and pencils. Unstructured media (sometimes referred to as three-dimensional art materials) include paint and clay, of which a variety of types exist, and are subject to gravity or manipulation by the user. These materials are fluid and do not make a definite mark.

Media evoke different responses by the user. Art therapists are versed in the inherent properties of media, as well as the stimulus potential of the media since materials may evoke a different response. For example, media can be used to release or contain, cover or uncover. The choice of media will impact structure and process and possible outcomes. The art therapist will introduce media and tasks that are congruent with the client's coping skills and needs. Without prior knowledge about a child's presentation, typically structured media is provided, since not knowing how one might respond to the use of materials that require physical energy, meaning kinesthetic or tactile engagement, may be met with resistance. Structured materials tend to avoid such issues since the media is contained, usually wrapped, or encased in some way. These materials are familiar on some level and easy to manipulate and control. They do not invoke unintended anxiety, but rather offer a socially acceptable means to discharge underlying anxiety or stress.

A note about the use of clay sticks. Clay is available in various forms and with varying characteristics. At times, the use of clay sticks, which are more structured and less loose than other forms of clay, is introduced in a process and serves an intended purpose. An example is provided a bit later. The use of clay may invoke a sensory response in that the user has to manipulate the clay, which may signal an interactive and energetic action. At times, clay sticks are used to engage a child nonverbally when resistance is high or another reason precludes interaction. The working of the material may promote a dynamic reaction or interaction, which may transfer to the dialogical process. Often, clay sticks are incorporated within a process with an adolescent who may be reticent to communicate as a way to initiate the interactive process in a nonthreatening way and to instill trust. The creation of an object, whether representational or abstract, by an individual is informative and may generate an avenue for initiation of conversation as well as activate participation.

Given the nature of the interview process, a child is encouraged to self-select from two types of materials so that choice and empowerment are cultivated, signaling that the process is child oriented, not punitive, and the child has some measure of control with regard to engagement and interaction. Choice extends to subject matter. Interviews may be stress inducing especially if a child has been interviewed multiple times or by multiple interviewers. The use of the media allows for discharge of underlying thoughts and feelings in a socially acceptable manner. A child may be conflicted to express a personal experience or event associated with abuse or trauma. An alternative method of expression may promote disclosure of material that a child cannot express verbally. Researchers have concluded that after drawing a related picture, verbalization is enhanced (Kelley, 1984). Information derived from a drawing can assist in the total process of assessing the child when employed with other evaluative processes (Falk, 1981; Landgarten, 1987; Malchiodi, 1990; Miller et al., 1987; Powell & Faherty, 1990).

The purpose and the process are clarified so that the child comprehends that they are not present because of something they did, nor are they in trouble. Empowerment is central to the process and is initiated upon entering the interview room, which is why choosing where to sit and selecting art materials a child may wish to use if he or she decides to draw is part of the introductory or rapport building, which is sustained throughout the process. The empowerment dynamic connotes that the interviewer is an ally, not an authoritative figure, and the meeting is child centered.

Children are typically not in a position of power when interacting with an adult. The locus of control is shifted such that the child understands that the dialogical process is intended to be conversational, not adversarial. The imbalance of power is reduced, which is not something that children are always exposed to, especially when an abusive situation exists. Child friendly and child centered are key facets of the process, conveyed by the presence of art materials and the invitation to draw. This helps to ensure comfort, lessen anxiety and minimize the power differential. Anxiety, if a child presents as such, is distilled given the presentation of the art materials and the invitation to use what they like from the selection on the table while they talk with the interviewer.

Children are invited to draw at will as the interview commences. They are informed that they may draw throughout the process. A set number of drawings is not requested or implied. Many children provide information as to who may have prepared them for the interview and why they are meeting with someone. A child may have unreal ideas or erroneous expectations as to their presence. Art materials and an invitation to draw during the conversation promote engagement, empowerment and encouragement to dialogue and interact.

Task directives are unstructured. Follow-up prompts may be used similar to a verbal process. A child may be asked to explain something they may have said or to clarify something drawn. If the associations to a drawing merit elucidation, a child may be asked to explain the drawing, and they may be asked if there is anything else they wish to draw or say about the content depicted. They may be asked to discuss information if they depict something related to the allegations. If they volunteer information verbally rather than pictorially, they may be asked if they can show the interviewer what they are talking about if they do not initiate a pictorial depiction providing another opportunity for free recall and narrative.

The child's associations (verbalizations or verbal explanations) are always procured so that the interviewer is not projecting onto the child's graphic or imaginal content. The interviewer may inquire through verbal cues by asking if there is "anything else" the child may wish to share. Often a child may say they cannot tell but they may say they can "draw it" or they may ask specifically to show by drawing. Since drawing functions as an open-ended prompt or invitation, the child is encouraged to show what they mean or what they cannot say. A child might be asked to draw what they are discussing, or they may be prompted to draw if they are unable to verbalize. Sometimes a child might describe details associated with an experience that are difficult to articulate or comprehend given limitations in developmental knowledge, such as language or cognition. Perhaps they display an inability to process what they experienced and as such they lack the vocabulary to explain an experienced event. As such, a child might be invited to use the drawing materials if they so choose to show the interviewer what they are trying to communicate or express.

Drawing Within the Art Therapy–Based Process

- free drawing
  - invitation to draw promotes engagement
  - unstructured task directives
  - a subsequent drawing may be structured as a follow-up to something drawn, depicted or described for clarification purposes
  - if a child is in need of an alternative method for personal expression
  - to assist with communication efforts
- selection of media
  - provides control, choice and empowerment
  - connotes child-friendly process

Inherent Advantages of Drawing Within the Interview

Free drawing is used to support the child and as an open-ended prompt within the interview process. Drawing assists with the objectives ascribed to the interview and renders inherent advantages. Drawing may serve as a stimulus for both the interviewer and the child to explore material that is manifest (overt) as well as latent (covert). Additional advantages associated with the use of drawing in this manner include:

- children respond in a variety of ways to art materials/media
- drawing provides an ego-syntonic discharge of underlying thoughts and feelings
- provides an alternative method of communication by allowing nonverbal expression
- often a child will explain, "I can't say it but I can draw it", perhaps due to developmental discrepancies (lack of understanding, developmentally incongruent knowledge, language deficit, lack of vocabulary)
- after drawing, verbal elaboration may follow signifying free recall which may contribute to a narrative

- child's associations or explanations surrounding the drawing provide insight and understanding
- drawing is a concrete, objective record made by the child to represent an experienced event
- supplements and complements the format in a manner that is forensically sound, child friendly and nonthreatening (Cohen-Liebman, 2002)

CIG Component Phases

CIG Investigative Interview Guideline/Component Phases

- rapport building
- developmental screening/skills assessment
- anatomy identification/body parts inventory
- elicitation of abuse-specific information/fact-finding
- closure

The CIG is a five-phase format that conforms with interview practices that were common when developed yet continues to evolve as practice and research dictate. Within each phase, integral aspects associated with investigative interviews are embedded. It must be noted that component parts and phases may vary with regard to reference depending upon the protocol or guideline. For example, a rules component may be independent or integrated within a designated phase. The process depends upon the interview subscribed to by a given community; however, fundamental features underlie the process. There is no standard or preferred method, as was previously discussed. Phases may differ in name and presentation; however, the content is comparable even with regard to international formats (Cheung, 1997).

The CIG includes essential elements with the addition of drawing integrated in a primary function rather than a secondary or adjunct support. The guideline was designed to integrate exploration of the discipline-specific information that is required by the respective agencies. Typically, the process is conducted as a single interview unless the team decides otherwise.

Rapport drives the process and is cultivated throughout from start to finish even though it is identified as a phase. It does not end, but rather develops throughout the process and is maintained so that the process is supportive as well as interactive. Rapport is a central factor within the process as it promotes trust with the interviewer, with the process and for encouraging personal expression. The development of trust is incumbent upon the interviewer, who cultivates a relational and receptive environment. The setting is conceived to be a welcoming environment. The use of art materials as well as the ability to draw convey that the process is child friendly, which is reflective of the atmosphere. "An investigative interview is predicated upon the willingness of the child to participate in concert with the child's expressive communicative ability" (Cohen-Liebman, 1999).

As noted previously, the guideline is not a protocol, which adheres to a sequential progression; rather, it allows for fluidity and flexibility regarding the phases. The phases are not intended to be rigid, and they may occur in any order, as well as

(Continued)

overlap. They are presented singularly for discussion purposes; however, the interviewer meets the child where the child presents and adapts the process in response to the child's needs and presenting behavior. Goals and objectives associated with the phases presented here are identified.

The integration of drawing within each phase is considered as well. For explanation and teaching purposes, the phases are demarcated with specific examples of drawing. Integration of the use of drawing is explained within the synopsis of each phase. An example of how each phase is presented during a workshop, class or professional training is also included to offer insight into how experiential exercises are employed to provide hands-on learning and application within the investigative interview guideline that is art therapy-based.

Examples of training exercises are included to showcase how the CIG is taught through experiential and didactic means. Although professionals and students are offered materials in the form of Skittles (fruit-flavored individual candies) and small packs of crayons to use for the exercises, this is not the case with children in an interview. No incentives or gifts of any sort are provided to children, lest they be considered bribes or rewards within the interview context. Inclusion of such would mitigate interview strategies, compromise forensic integrity and potentially influence a child. At the very least, such exchange would be construed as leading, which is contradictory to the process. To be clear, children are not given takeaways such as stickers or food products during the interview process and candy, treats or juice boxes are not provided. Art materials remain in the interviewing space and are not sent home with the child.

Rapport Building

In the rapport building phase, children are engaged, empowered and encouraged to participate and communicate. Rapport building begins at the commencement of the process and concludes when the child leaves the setting. It is not limited to a particular segment of the interview; rather, rapport is built and sustained throughout and contributes to the development and maintenance of trust. Comfort is promoted with the interviewer, as well as within the setting. The standard operating procedure is addressed in a developmentally congruent manner. This entails explanation of the setting, task and premise (such as we will be talking but not playing a game) and memorialization of the process, as well as introduction to the interviewer. Children are informed at the onset of the process that they are being observed and that information will be shared with the team so that surprises or deception leading to mistrust are avoided. A child is asked to explain their presence and who may have prepared them for the meeting in accordance with their ability and developmental presentation. The child will be asked to explain their understanding of why they are present to clarify misperceptions and eradicate erroneous claims.

A child's explanation for meeting varies depending upon how they were prepared for the interview. Some may present as anxious while others are circumspect. Still others are intrigued by the media and the interview room. Others may not be concerned with why they have been asked to speak with a stranger. It is important that the child understand that they are not present for anything other than to talk with the interviewer. Clarity regarding the nature of the process is offered so that children understand that they are not being engaged for punitive reasons. Children are not traditionally in a position of power when interacting with an adult and as such the initiation of the process promotes mastery while garnering a measure of control. This again is intended to reaffirm that the child is not in trouble and to let the child know that the process is oriented to be favorable and friendly. Power dynamics as such are suspended, which is incongruent with the dynamics of child sexual abuse, in which a child may be subjected to the will of a person who is in an authoritative or an established or implied position of power.

In the rapport building phase, the concept of accuracy is emphasized. Accuracy is defined by the child and discussed, and children are instructed that the interview is not play time; rather, discussion will focus on experienced or real events, not make-believe. These constructs are presented within the confines of a developmental approach so that children comprehend the significance of the content to be addressed. Practice and role play are incorporated to explore a child's understanding and comprehension of relative terms.

Furthermore, to emphasize the focus on accuracy, children are encouraged to challenge authority, acknowledge confusion and clarify misperceptions. As an example of challenging authority, a question might be posed in which a child is asked, if called by the wrong name, how might they respond. The interviewer will provide an example and engage with the child so that the child understands that they are part of a dialogical process and as such are being empowered and given permission to correct the interviewer at any time. This factors into assessment of suggestibility and provides insight regarding how a child might respond to suggestion given the importance of this concept within the investigative interview process and possible subsequent judicial engagement.

Resistance to suggestion is central throughout each phase and is assessed, practiced and demonstrated via role play, as opportunity to practice allied tasks is extended during rapport building and developmental assessment. This is important especially when fact-finding ensues. The interviewer may need to provide explanation on the witness stand with regard to why certain tasks or skills were addressed or presented as part of the interview process. Everything that is done within the context of the interview must be defendable in court and as such the interviewer will need to be cognizant of behavior, tasks, skills and techniques. The interviewer must be able to articulate the premise and explain the purpose of potentially everything employed during the interview, including verbal, and nonverbal interactions, tools, techniques and strategies.

Children are engaged through the use of open-ended questions. Dialogue is initiated around an innocuous topic unrelated to the allegations in the hope of instilling in the child an example of interactive conversational patterns which may promote a narrative rejoinder. The interviewer may introduce a topic to a child and encourage the child to respond and include details, facts and relevant information, perhaps about a daily activity or routine or some other nondescript topic, to establish the kind of dialogical repartee. The interviewer may also practice this by providing the child with an example. The hope is that through practice and example, the child will provide information based upon free recall about something of interest as a means of role play that extends to fact-finding. This type of conversational engagement is especially relevant when discussing material specific to the allegations or the child's experience that prompted the interview. Research demonstrates that the use of open-ended questions supports a narrative telling of an event, including associated details (Lyon & Ahern, 2011). Unlike leading questions, which direct a response, open-ended inquiries are used to elicit free recall or a narrative.

THE COMMON INTERVIEW GUIDELINE
RAPPORT BUILDING

Engage

promote comfort, trust, active participation

Empower

provide choice – locus of control

Encourage

foster interaction

give permission to challenge authority/interviewer

promote correcting, disagreeing, questioning, dialoguing

clarify misperceptions and misnomers

Establish

standard operating procedure

documentation, observation

Explain

no guessing, free to say "I do not know" or "I do not understand"

Demonstrate

role play and give examples

responsive listening and mirroring

Emphasize

accuracy, reliability, truth (in developmental construct)

Assess

suggestibility

resistance to suggestion

Rapport Building

- engage
- empower child
- promote comfort
- promote dialogue/communication
- emphasize accuracy
- assess suggestibility
- assess resistance to suggestion
- promote trust
- activate participation
- address standard operating procedure (setting, task, documentation, observation)
- provide choice
- challenge authority
- acknowledge confusion rather than guess
- encourage child to disagree or correct
- give permission to decline to respond if too difficult or anxiety provoking
- clarify misperceptions
- find out who prepared child
- ascertain child's understanding about the interview
- role play and mirror responsive listening
- practice dialogical interactions

Rapport Building	*Drawing*

- ice breaker
- develop/promote trust
- engagement
- stimulate conversation/interaction
- choice = empowerment
- control
- stimulus to explore
- bridge to fact-finding
- media as stimulus

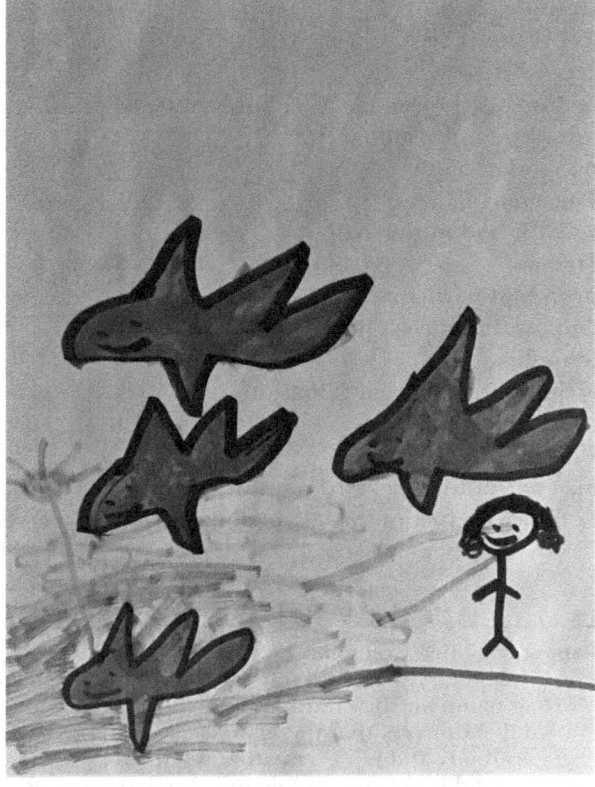

Figure 2.1 Drawing made to establish rapport by an eight-year-old. Child's description of his drawing: "Someone getting splashed by dolphins at Sea World".

Integration of Drawing

Children are provided with a choice of media. The very nature of the media connotes that the process is child friendly. Through the integration of drawing, a child can be engaged verbally or on a nonverbal level. The selection of media promotes choice, which is empowering for a child, given that most children lack control in abusive situations. Often children will engage in spontaneous art activity because the media is openly displayed. Within the context of the various phases the children may respond pictorially. The use of drawing materials may stimulate conversation and help establish trust while building rapport with the child. Drawing content and the associations provided by the child regarding imagery and pictorial depiction may serve as a catalyst for disclosure of information that may be salient to the allegations as well as the investigation. Drawing may serve as a stimulus for discovery of material previously unknown. Drawing may activate free recall and personal narrative.

INTEGRATION OF DRAWING IN COMMON INTERVIEW GUIDELINE RAPPORT BUILDING

Develop Comfort

icebreaker

promote trust

connote child friendly and child-centered process

invitation not command

non-judgmental support

Engagement

verbally and nonverbally

Media

promotes participation, encourages interaction

empowerment via choice

Stimulus

active not passive participation

locus of control

Bridge to Fact-Finding

may promote disclosure of information

graphic production may contribute to enhanced verbalization

Rapport Building Exemplar

I might explain the need to please correct me if I make a mistake such as using the wrong name for the child. I might role play and ask the child to do the same so that I can demonstrate that the child is allowed to correct me. This also is used to refute suggestibility and is a theme that is addressed throughout the process by demonstrating that a child is not susceptible to being led to say something. The child is given permission to challenge the interviewer and speak up when a purposeful mistake is presented. This lends credence to the child not being suggestible, which is important in discerning the information that may be disclosed during fact-finding. It is also important to be able to refute in court the argument of suggestibility by demonstrating the child's capabilities and resistance to suggestion through the various strategies and techniques employed within the interview.

Art materials are set out ahead of the child's arrival on the table in the interview room. Rapport building is initiated upon greeting the child in the waiting area and while accompanying the child to the interview space. Upon arriving at the interview room, the child is asked to select a chair and to please feel free to use the art materials as they wish. I might invite the child to use the drawing supplies while we talk. I will explain who I am and ask if they know why they are present. If the child begins a drawing during this phase of the interview, I will use it to get to know more about the child and their level of functioning. The free choice topic that is initiated by the child will be explored and the child's associations to the drawing will contribute to how the interview evolves. The conversation will be formulated in conjunction with the child's depiction, associations and use of the materials. The interview is process oriented, meaning that it is dynamic. What the child draws and what is said about the picture is a stimulus for conversation perhaps directed at the reason the child is present, or the drawing may contain information that merits exploration about what is depicted and the relationship (if any) between the content and the interview process. The interviewer must be receptive to what the child is expressing or not saying, both verbally and nonverbally as well as pictorially, and pursue information accordingly in line with forensic practice and procedure.

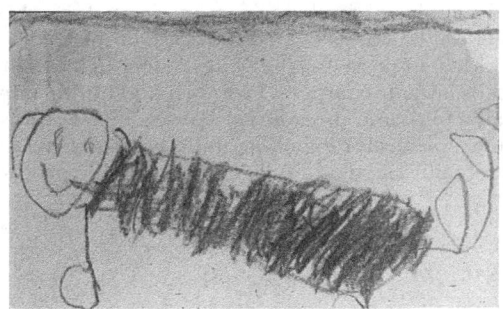

Figure 2.2 Five-and-a-half-year-old child drew a picture of her dog and discussed her family of origin as well as her responsibilities for the family pet.

Child spontaneously drew a picture of her dog while developing rapport with the interviewer. Child spoke at length about her dog and how the dog's name was determined. In addition, she disclosed that she is allowed to walk her dog on a leash in the company of her older siblings. She also discussed that it is her responsibility to feed her dog when she gets home from school. Child provided information pertaining to her family of origin as well as afterschool activities she participates in with her siblings.

TRAINING EXERCISE: Clay sticks are presented and distributed. Participants choose a single color. They are encouraged to manipulate and play with the clay as they choose while rapport building is discussed. This is a way to promote engagement verbally as well as nonverbally. In relation to a child, if the child is anxious about speaking with someone, they do not know about something they may not quite comprehend or are embarrassed to discuss, the clay provides a way to expend energy in an ego syntonic manner. The clay provides an individual with the opportunity to discharge underlying anxiety. Discussion centers around how each individual used the clay in a nondirected fashion. Did the clay provide a means of stress reduction, did it enable the release of underlying anxiety or energy? Was it used as a means to stay focused? Did the clay stick trigger creative engagement? Did it motivate one to stay in tune with the information being presented? Was it calming or soothing? Did it spark a negative response and, if so, what is that attributed to by the manipulator or creator. All of these thoughts are ones that have been identified by participants as well as students.

Clay sticks are distributed as a way to engage and begin building trust, yet it affords so much more within the context. Typically, children in an interview are not provided with clay. Clay may be provided when a child or a preteen or adolescent is resistant to interacting with the interviewer. The discharge of underlying emotions can provide the impetus for eventual engagement. Perhaps the interviewer might pick up a piece of clay as well and mirror the child's movements as a way of engaging with the child nonverbally. This reflective interaction may stimulate conversation by shifting the focus onto the engagement with the media. Kinesthetic connection may be made or provide a way to engage via a tangible interaction. Perhaps a child or teenager may make something representational with the clay. This may bridge to a larger discussion. It may provide the overture for the beginning of a discussion. Perhaps even situating the individual pieces together and discussing concrete elements such as position, color and feel of the clay may lead to conversation.

Sometimes representational as well as abstract clay figures or items are produced. The clay has the potency to inspire creativity. The use of the material provides participants and students with an understanding about the possibilities of developing rapport through nonverbal means and as an outlet for underlying thoughts or feelings that may be stress provoking and may inhibit engagement or interaction.

Speaking to someone unfamiliar about something that happened may promote stress. The clay sticks offer a means to discharge the anxiety so that focus can be directed to the interview. I often use clay sticks with adolescents in interviews for these purposes. Younger children who may need to release energy so that they can focus and remain seated may use a stick of clay to allow for discharge of kinetic energy and as a bridge to move through the interview.

An example of clay providing a bridge:

Child aged 8 exhibited anger and resistance at the beginning of the interview. Child was unable to remain in the interview space. To maintain the integrity of the process and encourage the child to stay in the interviewing room and participate, I taped a piece of paper

(*Continued*)

to the wall and drew a circle. I gave the child a choice of modeling clay and invited the child to make a ball and throw the clay at the target on the wall. The manipulation of the clay into a ball required physical energy and provided a release for the child's anger in a socially acceptable manner, as did the throwing of the clay at the target. Once the child hit the target a few times with the clay ball, the child was able to sit and the interview proceeded. For this child, meeting him where he was by providing a means for expelling underlying anxiety, anger and excessive energy enabled him to focus, remain seated and fully engage with the process.

Developmental Screening/Skills Assessment

The developmental assessment phase provides the interviewer with information pertaining to a child's level of functioning and skill set. This information is used by the interviewer to accommodate a child's abilities and support and maintain rapport. To engage a child and facilitate the fact-finding process, the interviewer has to communicate in a developmentally congruent manner that is responsive to the child's level of function. The interviewer assesses the child's cognitive, linguistic, social, emotional and artistic capabilities. The latter is in reference to developmental level, not talent. Artistic development occurs in tandem with other developmental phases and will be addressed. How the child processes information and the child's expressive-receptive capabilities are also considered.

During this phase, competency is assessed as well as congruency of concepts such as truth and lie. The information will factor into the fact-finding phase and perhaps support a child's resistance to suggestion. All of this information is important for the interviewer to assess in an effort to comprehend how a child communicates and interacts. This is important so the interviewer can modify and adapt language and tasks to be commensurate with a child's interactive and communication patterns; otherwise, there is a disconnect between what is being expressed and what is received, which may contribute to an unproductive and frustrating process (for both the child and the interviewer). Ideally, the interviewer modifies and adapts language and concepts to communicate in a developmentally congruent, culturally respectful and sensitive manner with the child.

Interviewers incorporate exploration of various concept dyads such as good and bad, truth versus lie, real versus pretend to ascertain a child's understanding of terms that may factor into the interview. Understanding how a child understands congruency of concepts, including definitions, is a factor especially with regard to truth and lie. Asking a child to explain what it means to tell a lie will often result in an explanation associated with telling the truth or not telling the truth. One must realize that just asking and receiving the opposite response does not necessarily impart the child's level of comprehension; instead, it illustrates that the child is familiar with the duality of the concept. For example, if a child is asked, what is the opposite of truth, the response typically may be "a lie". If a child is asked, what does it mean to tell the truth, a response often offered is "don't tell a lie". The interviewer has to demonstrate through active engagement and exploration what the child understands. "Interviewers want to avoid questions with cognitive demands that exceed a child's knowledge base and reasoning skills" (Saywitz et al., 2018, p. 319). For example, "number and time are concepts common in investigative interviewing that develop gradually and are difficult for young children to understand and use accurately in verbal conversation" (Saywitz et al., 2011, p. 346) when ascribed to personal experience. This is best achieved by asking the child to explain the concept through description rather than definition. Depending upon the age of the child, it may be best to discuss examples and have the child provide a vignette to illustrate comprehension and concept confirmation or to practice and role play.

How the child provides explanation showcases that the child has a developmentally appropriate understanding of a concept dyad. This information is important during fact-finding in an effort to offer support for what a child might disclose about an experienced event. If a child has no understanding of opposing concepts or lacks age-appropriate developmental knowledge and skills, credibility may be challenged in court. It is incumbent upon the interviewer to use various tactics to explore how a child describes and explains the duality of concepts. It is best to try to get the child to provide a narrative or an example rather than a one-word response. It is important to be able to demonstrate the child's skill level. This is relevant in the event a child is questioned on the witness stand and attempts are made to discredit a child. Establishing the foundation to offset such an approach by demonstrating the developmental capabilities of a child that were exhibited in the interview, such as how the child handled various tasks, will be productive for illustrating the child's capabilities and may merit explanation in court by the interviewer.

Understanding a child's developmental spheres, skill level, comprehension and dynamic processes contribute to managing what may be disclosed with respect to the allegations. Typically, core details related to an experienced event remain constant, while peripheral details may change in accordance with a child's developmental capacity such as memory. Research has demonstrated that even very young children can provide accurate information pertaining to experienced events; however, the need for cues or prompts may be necessary in light of recognition versus recall with regard to memory retrieval (Hewett, 1999; Lippmann, 2002).

THE COMMON INTERVIEW GUIDELINE
DEVELOPMENTAL SCREENING/SKILLS ASSESSMENT
Assess
skill level in various maturational spheres
cognitive, social, emotional, linguistic, psychosexual, artistic
interactive patterns of engagement
expressive-receptive communication
patterns of speech/sentence structure
comprehension
ability to attend
strengths/weaknesses
ability to follow tasks
focus/maintain engagement
Concept Formation
spatial relationships
prepositions
color/number identification/other age-related tasks
developmentally congruent tasks (mastery or inability to demonstrate)
Congruency of Constructs
truth/lie, real/pretend, good/bad, right/wrong, comfortable/uncomfortable
Address
issue of mistake/misunderstanding
Permission
to clarify, correct or ask for assistance, to admit lack of understanding
Demonstrate
role play, practice, narrative, dialogical exchange
Adaptation

developmental capabilities, speech and language patterns,
communication and interactive style
Appraise
competency

INTEGRATION OF DRAWING IN COMMON INTERVIEW GUIDELINE
DEVELOPMENTAL SCREENING/SKILLS ASSESSMENT
Artistic Developmental Level
comprehend developmental capabilities and level of functioning
Media
use and engagement
practice and role play
demonstrate skill level with regard to maturational spheres
Adaptation
patterns of interaction so congruent with child
meet child where child is at developmentally
responsive engagement and listening
communication at the child's level
enhance engagement
verbal and non-verbal interaction

Developmental Screening/Skills Assessment

- assess child's skill level

  - cognitive, social, linguistic, emotional, psychosocial, psychosexual, artistic

- modify and adapt communication style
- assess expressive (used by speaker) and receptive (understood by listener) skills
- evaluate comprehension of prepositions

  - spatial relationships

- assess congruency of concepts

  - truth vs. lie; real vs. pretend; right vs. wrong

- information assists interviewer in comprehending child's level of functioning
- allows for modification and adaptation of language, tasks, communication patterns
- interviewer is developmentally sensitive
- ascertain type of questions child can answer
- assess ability to interact
- mirror sentence structure, choice of words
- responsive listening
- repeat back to child to reduce risk of misconstruing
- receptive – words understood by listener
- expressive – words used by speaker
- errors of commission (add) and omission (leave out)
- congruency of concepts
  - real vs. pretend
  - something that happened vs. something made up
  - right vs. wrong
  - truth vs. lie
- concepts
  - spatial relationships
  - prepositions
  - developmentally congruent tasks

- practice and role play

  - provide concrete examples rather than request a definition
  - address and demonstrate issue of mistake
  - assess concepts separately
  - for example, if use color and numbers to establish developmental level, do not use to ascertain truth vs. lie

Developmental Assessment and Drawing

- drawing and use of media assist in assessing skill level, mastery of developmentally congruent tasks, spatial relationships, congruency of concepts
- information assists in adaptation of interviewer communication style
- artistic developmental level provides information on cognitive, social/emotional functioning
- maturational spheres are assessed via drawing to assist in adaptation of communication patterns to foster synchrony between the interviewer and the child
- artistic development is sequential, similar to other developmental stage theories

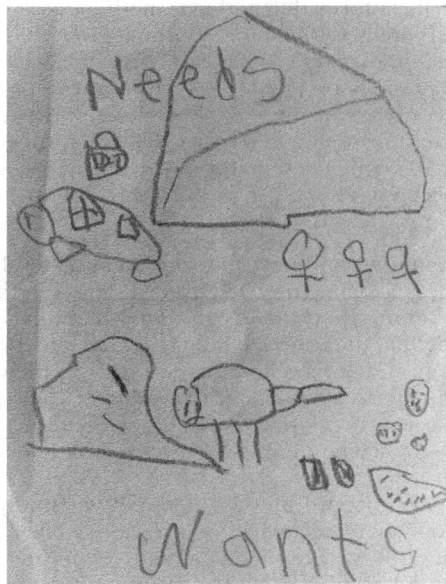

Figure 2.3 Six year old child split image horizontally to illustrate needs (family, a car and groceries) versus wants (a cat, chocolate chip cookies and snacks) demonstrating developmentally congruent tasks, and maturational spheres.

Integration of Drawing

Assessment of a child's artistic developmental level assists the interviewer in comprehending the child's level of functioning. Drawing and the use of the media provide information in conjunction with identified maturational spheres, including cognitive, linguistic, social and emotional. Skill level, mastery of developmentally congruent tasks, comprehension of spatial relationships and congruency of concepts are factors that may be considered via artistic developmental level. Artistic ability develops incrementally just like other developmental spheres. Artistic talent is not relevant to the process.

In an interview, a child may be given specific tasks designed to provide information relevant to the process, including the ability to comprehend and follow directives, stay on task and concept associations. This information supports the interviewer in relating to and speaking with the child. The interviewer modifies and adapts communication patterns to reflect those of the child so that the interviewer and the child are speaking on the same level and expressive receptive capabilities are compatible. Artistic developmental levels provide additional information about a child's functioning that will help guide the process and the dialogical interaction. Sometimes in the absence of words or comprehension of a developmentally incongruent activity, a child may use drawing materials to put marks on paper and describe an experience kinesthetically, as described next.

I might ask a child to identify colors through the use of the media. I may also ask a child to count items or spell his or her name. I will use a crayon or marker box and ask a child to demonstrate comprehension of prepositions so that if later a child explains that something happened to them and they use descriptors such as inside, next to or on top of, suggestibility is decreased because the child is able to differentiate spatial from prepositional concepts. These tasks are used to defeat the argument of suggestibility, which will be a factor with regard to disclosure of abuse-specific or event-specific information and may merit defense in a court of law.

In an interview process, a purpose is ascribed to everything given that the process, the content and the interviewer and the interviewer's behavior may be subjected to scrutiny in court and merit defending. Every task that is invoked, every interaction, must be translated so that forensic standards and integrity are maintained. Every action invoked within the interview proper must be included for a reason and be explicable and justified in the event the interviewer is subpoenaed and compelled to testify about the process, including a child's statements in relation to what was said, asked or exchanged in the interview.

Exemplar:

Artistic levels were a factor in understanding a 10-year-old child's level of functioning. The child alleged that a sibling had touched her (on her privates); however, the child's communicative patterns were delayed, including speech and cognition. It was through the graphic productions the child made that the team was able to appreciate the disconnect between the child's chronological age and her level of functioning. Her pictures were reflective of the artistic developmental patterns associated with a younger child, perhaps five years old. Explanation surrounding artistic developmental levels assisted the team in understanding how to engage with the child so that communication patterns were matched and interaction was congruent.

The child's disclosure was understood within the context of her ability to communicate and express herself. Her developmental delays had not previously been identified despite the fact that she was 10 years old and she was enrolled in a regular education classroom. As evidenced in her interactions and her delays in speech and cognition, her needs were not being met. Evaluation, intervention and services were advocated to provide assistance to the child and family in addition to the issues stemming from the child's disclosure pertaining to abuse.

The child provided information regarding ongoing sexual abuse by her biological sibling. The case was multilayered given the child's presentation, her developmental delays and ongoing victimization due to regular visitation with the alleged perpetrator who lived outside of the home with another relative. The team identified several areas of concern, including the lack of intervention and services and blurred family boundaries. The mother appeared to exhibit cognitive delays as well. The father was not responsive to the need to maintain separation between the two households and specifically deny access to the victim child by the older sibling.

Drawing was central in assisting the team with understanding the child's developmental deficits. Information procured from the child's drawings within the context of the process factored in to the determination of next steps, including addressing the child's welfare and safety in addition to further assessment, investigation and support services.

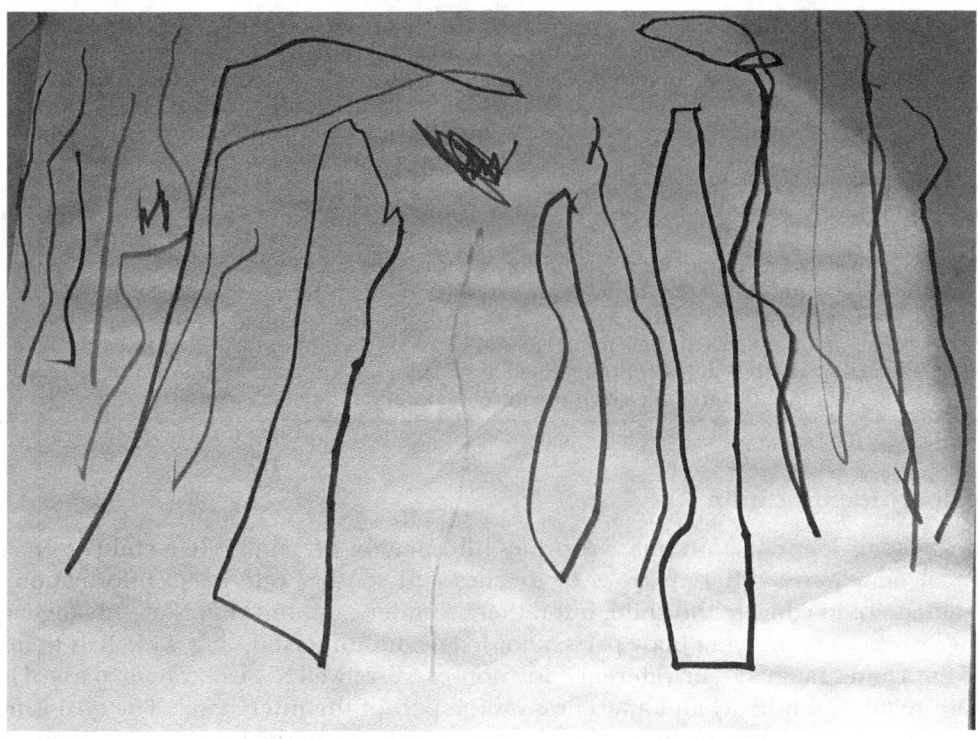

Figure 2.4 Drawing made by 10-year-old who was developmentally delayed to show color identification by drawing individual shapes while naming colors.

TRAINING EXERCISE: When training team members I distribute snack-size Skittles candy and Crayola four packs (each box holds four crayons in primary colors). Team members break into dyads and take turns role playing as interviewer and child. Each dyad practices and role plays developmental screening tasks such as color identification and counting using the candy and the crayons. Although I never give a child candy or gifts of any sort during an interview, for training purposes I believe that candy is very useful for motivational purposes and for demonstrating tasks relevant to the process. The use of these items engages team members, and the objects offer a means to assess color identification, counting and spelling, which provide tangible ways to evaluate skills. This type of exercise also places team members within a childlike activity, which is grounding for the type of process invoked, which in turn is important for supportive purposes. It is up to each dyad to develop the role play with regard to interviewer and child as they explore skills.

With regard to the use of the crayon box, it provides a small and useful tool for exploring prepositional knowledge in the training or teaching environment. When considering sexual abuse allegations, which are sensory based, a child may disclose that something happened to them or someone did something that involved insertion, penetration or placement. To refute the argument of suggestibility, by demonstrating that a child has knowledge of what it means to insert something inside of something or place something on top of something through the use of the media packaging (crayon or marker box – using what is available in the interview setting which is streamlined), the interviewer can establish that the child possesses awareness and understanding of prepositions which manifest in relation to sexual abuse and may factor in the allegations.

Reflection
I accompanied a group to a baseball game where I believe the stadium was filled almost to capacity. Although I do not recall the exact number of attendees, the group I was seated with

(*Continued*)

sat in the nosebleed section. At one point, I left the seating area and while walking around the upper level, I heard my name being called. I thought I must be hearing things, realizing the voice was not from someone in the group. I was mistaken, as a detective who had attended one of my trainings several years back, caught up to the small group I was walking with at the time. This person proceeded to pull out his small box of crayons and said to the group, "I never leave home without this little box of crayons". It was an amazing moment because essentially, he was validating the usefulness of the media, including the box itself and the four crayons inside. As he explained, he said that he wanted to be prepared in the event he had to respond to a situation where he might need to talk to a child. He offered that the crayons and the box provided a myriad of applications that he found useful in his day-to-day interactions as an officer. He identified that he had utilized the crayons and the box as an ice breaker, as a means to establish and gain trust, to engage children and to let kids know that he was approaching them on and at their level. He said it was the best and most useful item he had ever received in all his years of training. Such a nice memory and validation for the inclusion of the crayons and the container given the implicit potentialities.

Anatomy Identification

The anatomy identification phase provides information pertaining to a child's perception of body parts, different types of touches and sensory reference. Information is obtained not to educate the child, but rather to understand the child's use of language with respect to identifying body parts, knowledge and understanding, as well as to mirror the child's language or reference for nonsexual as well as sexual body parts. This phase requires sensitivity and awareness on the part of the interviewer. The goal is not to promote stress or stimulate anxiety. Care must be taken in the handling of this phase; when to introduce it and how to approach the topic. Discussion centering on one's own body and the manner in which such discussion is elicited may trigger a negative response given the circumstances that have brought a child into an interview.

The use of a drawing may distill apprehension associated with self-reference, given that a drawing is an external object, although reflective of self. As a result, the discussion of a picture is less threatening than talking about one's body directly. Drawing can serve as a demonstration tool and provide evidentiary evidence that may factor in a court proceeding. A drawing is self-created and self-referential. It is an objective and concrete representation.

THE COMMON INTERVIEW GUIDELINE
ANATOMY IDENTIFICATION
Identification
body inventory
sexual and nonsexual body parts
Assess
different kinds of touch
Sensory Reference
senses/function

INTEGRATION OF DRAWING IN COMMON INTERVIEW GUIDELINE
ANATOMY IDENTIFICATION
Demonstration aid
Client generated product
Externalization
Objectification
Concretize

Anatomy Identification
- identification of body parts, including sexual and nonsexual (within a developmental continuum, many children, especially older ones, are not asked to identify body parts through demonstration or self-reference)
    - location, function
- sensory reference
    - see, smell, hear, taste, touch
- explore different types of touch
    - good, bad; comfortable, uncomfortable; safe, not safe
- demonstration tool
    - provides externalization/distance
    - confirmation of identification pictorially and verbally
    - demonstration aid/depiction

Anatomy Identification and Drawing

- demonstration aid
- client-generated product
- externalization/distance
- evidentiary material
- confirmation of verbalization
- objective

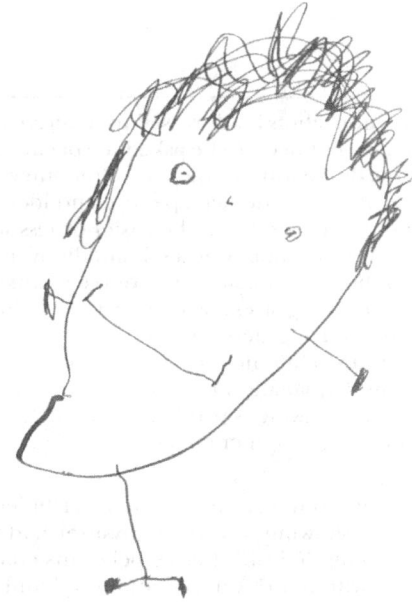

Figure 2.5 Self-portrait by a four-year-old used to identify body parts including location and sensory reference.

Integration of Drawing

A client-generated drawing provides a child with distance when discussing and identifying body parts. A drawing empowers a child to talk about and depict a picture of a person that is self-referential but enables externalization and lessens the focus on one's own body. As a result, the discussion of a picture is less threatening. The depiction is representative or demonstrative of one's self, yet, for a child, it may be easier to talk about a picture of someone in the picture as opposed to talking about one's own body. Pointing at one's body and saying what each part is called may be a trigger or it may be stress inducing for some individuals. Drawing can serve as a demonstration tool in this manner. A body inventory self-created (not a template or a preconceived drawing) in which nonsexual and sexual body parts are indicated and identified minimizes concentration on sexual body parts. This alleviates concern that the interviewer is only addressing certain areas on the body, which may be construed as leading the child to say something specific.

Body templates or schematics do exist that include images of unclothed figures representing all ages, including very young children up through elderly individuals. The images are depicted to represent different genders, races and cultures. I prefer to have children create their own drawing for many of the reasons listed earlier and noted throughout the text. Templates like anatomically detailed dolls have a history within the realm of investigative interviewing and are considered to be tools, props or aids. The reader is advised if interested in acquiring additional information about anatomically detailed drawings or dolls to consult the relevant literature, as these topics are not addressed beyond cursory mention in this text as noted previously.

Anatomy identification is addressed in deference to a child's developmental level. Older children may not need to be asked to specifically identify nonsexual and sexual body parts. This merits discretion on the part of the interviewer as well as sensitivity. A child might use the drawing materials to depict a picture and identify body parts. The use of drawing provides a means for distancing. It may be easier or less stress provoking to discuss a picture of a person rather than speak about one's self and body in particular, especially with regard to a topic that might be embarrassing or a source of anxiety. The use of art materials provides a way to manage underlying stress. Even very young children can identify body parts on a self-directed drawing that is congruent with their developmental level. The interviewer may write the name provided by the child next to the specific body part referenced and document the child's associations. Explanation as to why the interviewer rather than the child wrote the associated names on the drawing is prudent (in court), given that many children may not be able to spell in relation to developmental level.

EXAMPLAR

A four-year-old drew a circle and then scribbled over it repeatedly. The child explained that she was showing how the babysitter had rubbed her on her privates. Her kinesthetic movement coupled with her associations enabled the child to provide information that was congruent with her developmental level and was later corroborated through investigation. The use of the art materials in conjunction with her associations provided the child with a kinesthetic way to depict her experience, which rendered an image that was consistent with her artistic developmental capability. Without knowledge about the manner in which the drawing was made and the circumstance in which it was drawn, the graphic image in isolation does not offer explanation as to what the child said or what her experience was. In combination with her words, the imagery and use of media, she was able and empowered to disclose what she experienced in a manner that was credible and age appropriate.

TRAINING EXERCISE: For training and teaching purposes, an exercise devoted to desensitizing discussion about sexual body parts is incorporated. For some not familiar with the population and the vernacular associated with it, a discussion surrounding the terms children, preteens and adolescents use to refer to sexual body parts varies and may provoke shock or discomfort. An interviewer must remain neutral and objective. Addressing the terminology that may be heard during an interview affords an opportunity for practice and also acceptance of what words a child or teen may say, as well as pursuance of where the term may have originated.

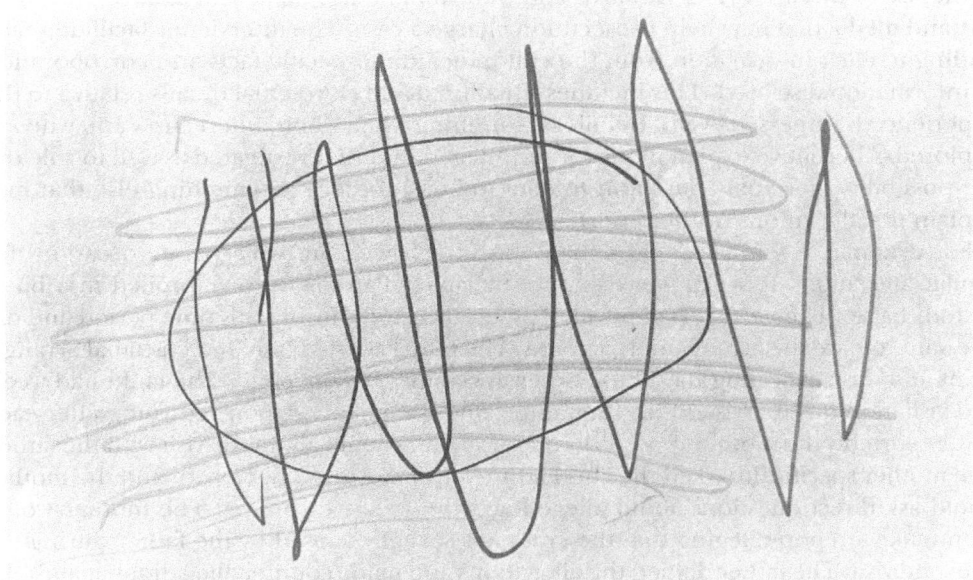

Figure 2.6 Kinesthetic drawing made by a four-year-old to show how she was touched (rubbed) on her private part. Child's associations were important to understand what the child's experience was and what she was trying to convey through her graphic depiction.

An interviewer has to be cognizant that they do not want to respond or react in a way that may cause a child to shut down or become withdrawn or feel embarrassed. The interviewer does not want to give a negative impression or react in a manner that may convey judgement. Reference to body parts is far ranging, from commonly used words to real terms to made-up words and beyond.

For training purposes, team members are broken into small groups and asked to make a list of the names they have heard in interviews by children to identify both male and female private parts. This is definitely an ice breaker, but it also promotes respect for how difficult the task may be for children, prepubescents and adolescents to describe and talk about body parts with people they do not know and because of less-than-ideal circumstances. The lists range from known words to nonsensical terminology that investigators have encountered. The lists are written on large post-its which are positioned so that the group is able to see and respond to the terms. Often explanation is provided to clarify how and why a child may have utilized an identified term for self-reference of a body part. Although some terms are graphic, the lists or the activity is meant to demystify and desensitize the language children may use. The exercise is an opportunity for interviewers to discuss how they have reacted in various situations in response to children applying terms and associations to body parts. Feedback is provided as to how to handle disconcerting disclosure, and desensitization is actively practiced, as is nonjudgmental support.

Team members have to accept whatever a child may disclose during an interview and not react in a negative or non-neutral way regardless of the nature of the term appropriated. The interviewer will, of course, want to know from the child in the interview where the body reference was acquired. The interviewer will explore the names children associate with their body parts and investigate where or how they acquired information.

Fact-Finding

In fact-finding, abuse-specific information is explored, including information that may contribute to charge enhancements and forensic elements. Charge enhancements refer to the use of threats, bribes, rewards and punishment, as well as sexual aids, pornography and media that may help prosecution charge a case. The interviewer facilitates fact-finding to elicit information from the child, including specific facts and corroboration of information disclosed. This includes situational and contextual details relative to the experienced/witnessed event. Details surrounding what, when, where, how and who are explored. Alternative explanations for the allegations are investigated as well to rule out the possibility of sexual abuse and to comprehend if there is something else that may explain the allegations or the report.

For example, a seven-year-old female was interviewed on two separate occasions for similar allegations approximately six months apart. Parents were embroiled in a bitter custody battle. The mother had primary physical custody during this time period and did not want to have the arrangement altered. The father wanted a shared custodial arrangement and was advocating that the mother was abusive to the child. The child had weekend visitation unsupervised with the father, who lived alone. Upon returning after each visit, reportedly the mother repeatedly questioned the child about the visit with the father. The mother specifically asked the child if the father had given her a bath and the mother would ask direct questions about alleged activity to derive context. The mother would then make a report alleging that the child was sexually abused by the father during the weekend visit. The father denied the allegations and made counter-allegations against the mother for emotionally abusing the child and for making false statements.

The child denied being sexually abused by the father. When the child was interviewed, she explained that when she took a bath at the father's house, he was the only adult. He helped her get dressed, bathe and brush her teeth. She explained that the mother asked her if the father had touched her on her private parts when she was in the bath. The child reported that she told her mother that her dad helped wash her using a cloth from her head to her toes and that he did not touch her any different anywhere on her body. The child reported being confused as to why the mother kept asking her the same questions. She stated that her dad took good care of her, just like her mother, and that she did not understand why her mother always asked about bath time. The child denied that her father touched her in a way that made her uncomfortable or that he touched her in a bad way. She provided details about bath time and disclosed that her father assisted her with bathing as she described. The mother reported that the child disclosed that the father had touched her during the bath on her private parts. The child reported that her dad helped her in the bathtub, and he only touched her with a washcloth because she could not reach all of her body parts, including her back and behind.

In summary, the mother reported sexual abuse on more than one occasion following unsupervised visits with the father in his home. The child denied abuse and disclosed that her father helped her bathe, just like her mother did, when she took a bath at home. With each subsequent report, investigation was pursued. The child was being interviewed on multiple occasions and appeared to be decompensating. The team determined it was not in the best interest of the child to be repeatedly interviewed, given the custodial situation, although each report necessitated an investigation, which included the investigative interview and often a medical examination.

Given the custodial issues, recommendations included a court-ordered custodial evaluation (which was described in the previous chapter), support services for the child as well as for the parents singularly and within parent and child dyads and assessment of the child with each parent in their respective home. Although the allegations of sexual abuse were not substantiated, the magnitude of the situation coupled with the emotional and psychological impact on the child given the counter-allegations, as well as additional stressors, including repeated investigations and the ongoing custodial battle, contributed to identification of recommendations (some noted earlier). Others addressed intervention and therapeutic measures. Cases in which custody is an issue such as the one described here can be very complex and may require additional processes and professionals in addition to the primary investigative team members.

THE COMMON INTERVIEW GUIDELINE
FACT-FINDING
Inquiry
question continuum
open-ended, focused, direct
non-leading to leading
general to specific
fact-finding
Details
core, peripheral, contextual, situational, idiosyncratic
who, what, where, when, how
Facts
information gathering
corroboration of information
explore alternate hypothesis
Assess
credibility
competency
Merge
developmental assessment with fact-finding so interaction is congruent
Maintain
rapport
nonjudgmental support
acceptance through neutrality and objectivity

INTEGRATION OF DRAWING IN COMMON INTERVIEW GUIDELINE
FACT-FINDING
Drawing
facts/details
disclosure
corroboration of information/facts/details
Charge enhancements
collateral material
threats, bribes, rewards, punishment, coercion, media, exposure
Imagery
may lead to enhanced verbalization
may stimulate information gathering and fact-finding
child may relate what cannot say
bridge to disclosure
clarification/explanation
confirmation

- fact-finding process
- contextual and situational information
- specific facts
- collateral material – multiple vs. isolated incidents
- explore alternative hypothesis/explanations for the allegations
- reverse continuum of questioning
- open-ended, less focused (less suggestible) to more focused/direct (more suggestible)
- explore details
- who, what, when, where, how
- no "why" questions
- corroboration of information
- charge enhancements – pornography, media, sexual aids
- coercion/threats/bribes/rewards/punishments/force/promises

Question Typology and Continuum

In the fact-finding phase information pertaining to the allegations is addressed. By defeating the argument of suggestibility from the onset of the process, as well as demonstrating the child's developmental capabilities, the interviewer can explain and, if necessary, defend in court the type of questions and the tasks incorporated within the process. The interviewer can also discuss the exchange of information or the dialogical process, including the use of open or invitational prompts to elicit a narrative response as well as question typology. The typology is a continuum of question types that may be construed as less suggestive to more suggestive.

The more focused the question, meaning the more specific information that is included, the more it may be construed as adulterated due to the element of suggestibility, which is a factor associated with a question continuum. Responses to more open-ended questions appear less suggestible than leading or focused questions, especially when person, place and activity are included or combined. For example, when two or more elements factor into the question, such as, "Did your father touch you on your pee-pee with his hands in the bedroom" (person, place, activity), this is highly suggestible and may be considered to be leading, as a response to the question may be closed or limited to a yes or no response. This type of question does not promote free recall or narrative.

Question Typology

Question typology and attention to how and when to introduce various types of questions are topics that can occupy an entire text and often absorb large chunks of training. Questions exist on a continuum with regard to open ended, leading, direct, specific, focused and follow-up (sometimes referred to as cues or prompts). Questions may include a range of types from multiple choice to yes/no (which are less encouraged), as well as open-ended which are intended to stimulate free recall.

Questions are related to development as well and have to be considered within the context of the dialogical process. For instance, a young child may not respond to an open-ended question with free recall, or the child may simply provide a closed response necessitating a follow-up question or cue to narrow the focus for a child.

Training is so vital in this area as well as practice. Like any skill, preparation, practice and patience are required to master how to ask questions and move through the continuum when conducting fact-finding processes and when interviewing child victims and witnesses as well as adolescents about experienced events.

Confidence decreases as questions go from nonleading to leading. Researchers have discussed types of questions versus confidence of response. Less suggestive questions have a higher level of confidence, while more suggestive types of questions are associated with less confidence. As such, interviewers try to minimally use suggestive types of questions. Free narratives are elicited through the use of open-ended or invitational prompts, which are considered best practice.

Even though open-ended prompts are preferred, such invitations are not always practical or pragmatic, and as such it is contingent upon the interviewer to "step in and step out" of the question continuum, meaning an open-ended question may require a more focused follow-up question or prompt that is more direct or specific because more structure may be required with regard to question format or in relation to a child's developmental level. When such a prompt is utilized, the interviewer should follow up with a more general or nonspecific question such as "anything else" or "what happened next" in an effort not to lead the child or suggest a response. This movement, stepping in and out of the typology creates an opportunity to facilitate fact-finding or information gathering.

There is a continuum of suggestiveness with regard to questions, with open-ended at one end and coercive at the other. Myers (1992) states that definitions of different types of questions are useful to a point, yet there is not a "definitional yardstick" per se to compare against. The thought is to consider how a question might invite a child to provide a particular response as the interviewer moves in and out of the continuum.

- open-ended – least suggestible but may not yield a response if too general and unfocused

  - especially with a younger child
  - used to stimulate free recall, perhaps leading to a narrative response

- general, open ended – more confidence since no assumptions or specifics
- focused questions may be needed with younger children, and caution is warranted in directing a child to a particular topic

  - more specific than open-ended and may draw attention to a particular action, event, person, etc.
  - include only one area of focus to lessen the degree of leading or suggestibility
  - rather than integrate elements or aspects such as person and action, address person or activity or some other element individually or independently
  - also exist on a continuum – from less specific to more
  - have been identified as necessary to elicit information but should be followed up with a less focused question

- direct questions

  - more suggestive than focused
  - combine elements such as person and activity

- leading questions are close-ended

  - may suggest a given response
  - may influence a child to say something or agree with something (implied or suggested)
  - child may feel pressured to provide a response that may or may not be accurate

- follow-up strategies are nonleading and may address contextual or situational material related to what the child has provided
- follow-up may invite narrative or clarification (repeat what the child said or using what child stated, "You said your brother . . .)
- follow-up

  - Anything else?
  - Uh huh.

(*Continued*)

(Continued)

- o And then what?
- o What happened next?
- o I am not sure if I understand . . .

- specific follow-up

  - o Help me understand
  - o Was it night or day?
  - o Where were you?

- coercive questions are to be avoided

  - o may influence or intimidate a child into saying something that may not have happened

- questions that are less preferred for interviewing but are not necessarily unavoidable

  - o misleading questions – introduce something that is incongruent with the facts being described
  - o presumptive – include known material or presume something that is offered or introduced prior to the child saying anything about what is asked
  - o non-neutral – "Can you tell me . . ." implies something happened rather than asking if something happened
  - o assumptive – the more elements combined will influence the level of suggestion

    - Tell me everything you remember about what your dad did . . .
    - Tell me everything your dad did to you when you went to visit . . .

- it is not plausible to only rely on open-ended questions for a variety of reasons, some of which may be attributed to a child's developmental level, which may be incompatible with open-ended or general or relatively unfocused questions
- without focus, a child may be unable to narrow or direct a response, resulting in a lack of synchrony between the interviewer and the child
- skills and abilities may preclude a child's ability to be responsive to a follow-up prompt or cue
- research and the literature indicate that free recall tends to be more compatible with accuracy
- minimizing interviewer influence is ideal, so awareness of sentence/question structure is necessary
- questions to avoid include compound or complicated and obtuse syntax that will only serve to confuse a child or generate a response not directed at the entirety of what is asked
- interviewers must be cognizant of tone of voice and pacing, which can impact a child, who may misinterpret what is being asked
- a child may become distracted and confused with regard to why the interviewer sounds a certain way which may make a child think that they are in trouble or have done something wrong which may influence or suggest a particular response

Myers offers strategies for interviewers to defend against attacks in court regarding question typology
- explaining situational and developmental reasons for the use of different types of questions with a particular child
- prudent use of focused and even mildly leading questions (questions typically beginning with are, is, do, did and were)
- understanding of memory and suggestibility

The American Professional Society on the Abuse of Children (2002) guidelines provide that
- (highly) specific questioning be used only when other questioning methods have not yielded information
- when previous information warrants concern
- when a child's developmental level precludes more nondirective approaches

Interviewer Note-Taking/Documentation

Questions, including how to formulate, pose and articulate, invoke a learning curve. Highly skilled interviewers as well as beginners will be challenged due to the nature of the process and the interactions that are predicated upon maintaining engagement and focus with a child or adolescent. The process itself requires quick thinking and immediate mental processing such that an interactive and engaging exchange is cultivated. This leads to concerns pertaining to documentation by the interviewer.

When confronted with taking notes and documenting in real time, one learns to write without looking at one's notes and developing a quick and resourceful way to record without interrupting the flow and distracting from the process. This is a skill and technique that one must develop in response to the process. It must be stated that documentation in any form, including handwritten notes, may be subpoenaed and as such, records must be clean and free of extraneous information, including doodles, personal remarks, thoughts unrelated to the process and other personal notations.

When asked to observe interviews conducted according to agency mandates, investigators might write while talking with a client or a nonoffending caretaker the exact question followed by the respondent's answer, which would be recorded verbatim. This process is labor intensive and stilted. There is no natural ebb and flow due to the time that elapses while waiting for the questioner to record on paper each question and every answer, question, answer. Documentation attained in this manner is at times slow and delayed and contributes to a break in the conversation. Although at times and in accordance with discipline specific mandates, this is a fruitful endeavor, it is not the recommended procedure for an interviewer engaged in an investigative interview process for the reasons stated.

The interviewer has a multifaceted role in that:

1. a child's developmental level and skill level must be assessed in order to interact in a compatible fashion
2. questions need to be formulated and articulated in a manner that is facilitative
3. the interviewer must organize information received and respond effectively to what a child is communicating or expressing
4. it is the responsibility of the interviewer to engage with the child and engender trust and facilitate the process by attending to the child's presentation through a responsive manner while organizing the flow of the process and gathering information
5. if the interviewer is tasked with the responsibility of documenting the process, the interviewer must be able to manage and handle this task in a manner that is least offensive and distracting for the child and the process

Sample Interview Exchange

The following is a composite interview that demonstrates an aggregated conversation with a fictionalized nine-year-old child. This is provided to demonstrate how questions vary and how open-ended questions are followed, with more focused follow-up cues or prompts in response to the child's answers. Developmental screening and anatomy identification/screening are not included in the exchange, and orientation to the process is condensed (rapport building). This is an amalgamation of an interview scenario for demonstration purposes with the focus directed at fact-finding.

Interviewer: Hi Johnny. My name is Ms. M. (rather than Dr. since the goal is not to confuse the child about the role of the interviewer by thinking there is a medical component to the process).
Interviewer: It is nice to meet you.
Johnny: Okay.

Interviewer: Is Johnny your nickname?

Johnny: No. Everyone calls me that.

Interviewer: Shall I call you Johnny?

Johnny: Sure.

Interviewer: If I were to call you Jimmy would that be ok? (Assessing if amenable to suggestion.)

Johnny: No, but you can call me John if you want.

Interviewer: I am glad you said that it would not be ok to call you Jimmy. Thank you for saying that I may call you John.

Johnny: Whatever. What should I call you again?

Interviewer: I am so glad that you asked. If you do not remember something or if you forget anything, please feel free to just tell me that. You can just call me Ms. M.

Johnny: Ok, Ms. M.

Interviewer: Johnny, if I call you Jimmy by mistake because sometimes, I might forget or make a mistake, please tell me. Everyone makes mistakes.

Johnny: I do all the time.

Interviewer: Tell me something that was a mistake.

Johnny: Really? Well, I thought today was Tuesday instead of Wednesday. I thought I was going to basketball practice, but it's not until Thursday. I like going, so I guess I made a mistake.

Interviewer: No problem. We all make mistakes. So, if either of us makes one while we are talking, let's just say so.

Johnny: Got it.

Interviewer: How old are you?

Johnny: Nine.

Interviewer: Since I do not know you, tell me three things about you. (Avoid the words "can you tell me . . ." because that sets up a yes/no response rather than attention being paid to the prompt.)

Johnny: I don't know.

Interviewer: What do you like to do for fun? (More focused because a topic is introduced – fun.)

Johnny: Watch TV and play video games.

Interviewer: Thank you for sharing that with me (concrete). Anything else? (Invitational prompt – open ended or follow-up.)

Johnny: Not really.

Interviewer: What do you like to do at school? (More focused since a place is included in the question.)

Johnny: Nothing. I don't like school.

Interviewer: Okay. Can you tell me what you do not like about school?

Johnny: Everything.

Interviewer: Okay. Let's talk about something else.

Johnny: Whatever.

Interviewer: Can you tell me why you are here today?

Johnny: No.

Interviewer: Did someone explain to you what we do here?

Johnny: I don't remember.

Interviewer: Who brought you here?

Johnny: My mom.

Interviewer: What did you and your mom talk about on the way here?

Johnny:	I can't remember.
Interviewer:	Well, my job is to talk to people, mostly children.
Johnny:	What do you talk about?
Interviewer:	Different things. Whatever someone wants to discuss. I want you to know that the markers and the paper are here for you to use while we are in this space. I usually keep the pictures children make here. They help to remind me what we talked about.
Johnny:	Okay, I like to draw pictures of cars and dogs.
Interviewer:	Nice. Feel free to make whatever you like.
Johnny:	Okay.
Interviewer:	Is there something you want to talk about today.
Johnny:	I'm not sure.
Interviewer:	Did your mom tell you to talk today?
Johnny:	Yeah, she said I need to talk about what happened with my dad.
Interviewer:	Okay. Can you explain what you mean?
Johnny:	My mom said I have to tell what he did.
Interviewer:	Okay.
Johnny:	He did something.
Interviewer:	Who?
Johnny:	My dad.
Interviewer:	Your dad. Okay. (Responsive listening.)
Johnny:	He did something bad.
Interviewer:	Okay. Maybe you can help me understand what you are talking about.
Johnny:	About what?
Interviewer:	About your dad.
Johnny:	He said not to tell but my mom said it's okay to tell.
Interviewer:	Johnny, this is a safe space, which means you can talk about anything here. You are not in trouble.
Johnny:	But my dad will be in trouble. That's what my mom says, so I don't want to tell you about my dad.
Interviewer:	I want you to know that it is okay to talk with me about why you are here. I am not going to talk to your dad.
Johnny:	My dad doesn't want me to tell but my mom does.
Interviewer:	That is hard. What do you want to do?
Johnny:	Well, he did something bad. It hurt. So, I think I should tell but not because of my mom.
Interviewer:	Okay. What is the reason you think you should tell?
Johnny:	Because it's not right and my new little brother and sister live with my dad and his girlfriend.
Interviewer:	Uh huh (follow-up). When do you see your new little brother and sister?
Johnny:	I go to my dad's every weekend because my mom has a boyfriend and she works. I don't like going to my dad's house anymore because the babies cry a lot and my dad is always mad at me.
Interviewer:	What makes him mad?
Johnny:	I don't want to say.
Interviewer:	Okay. Maybe you can help me understand what you do when you visit.
Johnny:	I have to sleep on the floor because there are only two bedrooms.
Interviewer:	What about at your mom's house? Do you have your own room?
Johnny:	Kind of but I share it with her boyfriend's kids.

Interviewer:	Okay, Johnny. So, you do not have your own room at either place?
Johnny:	No, I don't. It's not fair. It is never quiet anywhere.
Interviewer:	Anything else about when you visit your dad's house?
Johnny:	Like what?
Interviewer:	You told me that you do not like to visit your dad. You also told me that he has two new babies. You said he lives with his girlfriend too. What do you do when you are there?
Johnny:	Now I have to be quiet. We used to play games or watch TV.
Interviewer:	What did you watch?
Johnny:	Sports. Stuff like that.
Interviewer:	What is your favorite show? (Anxiety is increasing so to provide Johnny with an opportunity to decrease anxiety, the focus is shifted.)
Johnny:	I don't really have one. Things are different over there now.
Interviewer:	How so?
Johnny:	I get into trouble a lot more.
Interviewer:	What happens when you are in trouble?
Johnny:	I have to stand in the corner or sit on the bottom step.
Interviewer:	Anything else?
Johnny:	Well, my dad makes me shower with him. I don't like doing that.
Interviewer:	What about that don't you like?
Johnny:	Because he sometimes touches it.
Interviewer:	Touches it? I am not sure I know what you mean.
Johnny:	You know.
Interviewer:	No, I don't think I understand.
Johnny:	Picks up a black marker. He proceeds to draw a picture, which he describes as his dad and him in the shower. He then shows the interviewer what he has drawn.
Interviewer:	Help me understand what you have drawn.
Johnny:	That's my dad and me in the shower at his house.
Interviewer:	Okay. I am wondering if you can describe the picture more.
Johnny:	He makes me wash his bird and then he says he is going to wash mine.
Interviewer:	Okay. You said his bird?
Johnny:	Yes, his private – what guys have. (Johnny points to the figure identified as his dad in his drawing.)
Interviewer:	Ok.
Johnny:	He uses his hands, and he doesn't stop. He just keeps rubbing it and he makes me do the same thing to him. I don't like it. It doesn't take that much soap or water to get clean.
Interviewer:	Okay. Anything else?
Johnny:	I don't want to say.
Interviewer:	I understand. Maybe you can show me in the picture what you do not want to say.
Johnny:	Yeah, ok. Johnny explains that he has depicted his father standing behind him, while they are in the shower. Johnny explains that his dad is touching his "bird" from behind. The figure identified as Johnny has his hands in the air. Johnny provides a narrative as he explains his drawing. Johnny says that his father's bird is touching his buttocks in the picture while his hands are on his (Johnny's) bird. Johnny explains that the picture shows them in the shower and what his dad does to him there.

Interviewer:	Repeats what Johnny has said about the picture to confirm what Johnny has disclosed (responsive and reflective listening). Anything else you want to share about what happens in the shower with your dad? (Focused because person and place are stipulated in response to Johnny's disclosure). Or about what you drew? (open-ended).
Johnny:	Not really. My dad makes me take a shower with him every time I go over there, so I do not want to go anymore. He says I can't take my own shower. He told me not to tell anyone about what he does in the shower to me.
Interviewer:	Did he say anything else to you?
Johnny:	He says he's allowed to do it since he is my dad.
Interviewer:	How did your mom find out?
Johnny:	Cause my butt was hurting and one time it was bleeding when I went to the bathroom. I think my mom saw blood in the toilet. That's how she found out. She said it was gross, but she wasn't mad at me, just my dad. Then she called the police, I think.
Interviewer:	Ok, Johnny. You told me some things about your dad and you drew a picture. Let me see if I understand – interviewer reviews drawing content using Johnny's narrative. Anything else?
Johnny:	I told you and I drew it. It's all there. I don't like what my dad does in the shower and besides I am old enough to take a shower by myself. He shouldn't do those things to me in there. That's why I don't want to go back there now. We never watch TV, and the babies are always crying or needing something. My dad says the shower is the only quiet place and he likes that it's just him and me. He said not to say anything about what he does to me, especially not to tell my mom and his girlfriend about it. He doesn't want anyone to know. He says it's guy stuff and that makes it ok. He said that since I'm older, I'm one of the guys and he can do that kind of stuff to me since he does it with other guys. (This disclosure would be pursued in a real interview).
Interviewer:	Johnny, what would you like to happen?
Johnny:	I do not want to go back there. Here, I'll tell you what I want. (Johnny is observed tapping the colored pencils on the table. Spontaneously, Johnny depicts two drawings, which he says show what he wants to happen.)
Interviewer:	Johnny, tell me about your drawings.
Johnny:	I think you know.
Interviewer:	Well, it would be helpful for me if you explain what you drew.
Johnny:	I put my dad behind bars. What he does is bad so I want him to stop. I really don't want him to go to jail because he has the babies, and his girlfriend will be mad at me if I ruin their lives but my dad is ruining mine. I just want him to stop doing those things to me so I made a picture of him and I wrote STOP because I can't tell him that. He would just get mad at me and say that I'm a kid and he's the grown-up and he can do what he wants. He tells me if I don't like something, that's just tough.

The use of art materials provided Johnny with an ego-syntonic means of expressing what he was unable to convey to his father. Although he provided that he drew his father behind bars, his ambivalence and divided loyalties are apparent via his associations. Johnny does not want his father to go to jail but he wants the touching to stop. He is clear that he is afraid to confront his father, and he feels powerless to stop the activity when he is with his father. The use of drawing enabled Johnny to express what he is unable to say to his father without fear of recrimination, and provided a means for control.

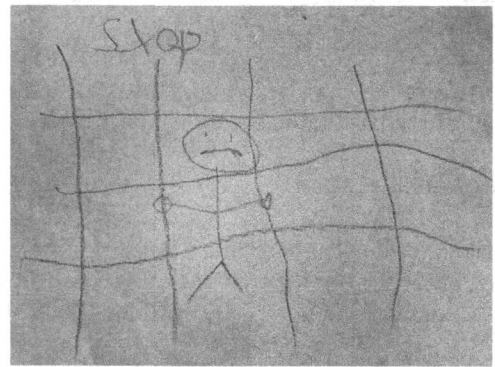

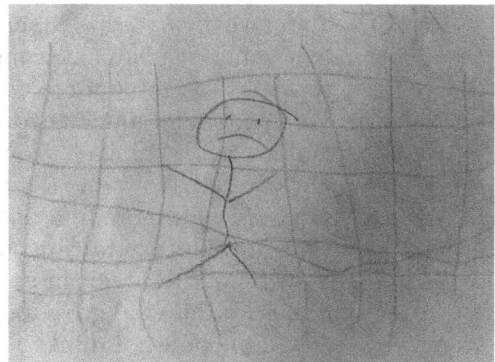

Figure 2.7 Johnny depicting what he wished he would have been able to say to his father.

Figure 2.8 Johnny's drawing showing what he wanted to happen to his father for doing the things he did to him.

Synopsis of Sample Exchange

The interview would continue; however, this is provided for explanatory purposes to demonstrate how a process might develop through the use of different question formats.

In the demonstrated exchange provided earlier, the interviewer is trying to remain invitational and provide the child with the opportunity to discuss why he is meeting with the interviewer. Initially, the interviewer is trying to ascertain the child's knowledge about the interview, including who may have prepared him and how that was done. The interviewer is attempting to glean material from the child by following the child's lead and mirroring sentence structure in an effort to find out if the child has been told what to say to the interviewer. The child exhibits a lack of knowledge with regard to why he is talking with the interviewer initially as well as a reluctance to explain why he is present. He does disclose that he does not want to talk about something that happened that involved his father. The interviewer is trying to remain open-ended, but because the child is limited in his response, the interviewer attempts to focus the questions in response to the information the child is offering. The interviewer asks follow-up questions. The dialogue demonstrates movement in and out of the question continuum. If only open-ended questions are asked, it is unlikely that every child will respond accordingly. The manner in which the interviewer phrases questions and poses inquiries should be configured in response to what the child is saying or not saying. Once the child offers that the father did something, the interviewer may narrow or focus questions to gather additional information and try to obtain additional event-specific information, including a narrative, by stepping in and out of the question typology, as was presented.

Using the information provided by the child, the interviewer can structure or focus questions and then follow up with more general or open-ended ones. In this manner, the interviewer is not leading the child to say that the father did something that may not be what the child experienced. Starting from general and open-ended to focused means that initially the child is invited to tell what brought him to the interview. Based upon the child's interactive patterns, the interviewer has to find another way to approach the topic. As the child engages and then discusses that his father did something but told him not to tell, the interviewer has obtained a piece of information that can be used in focusing questions. The interviewer has to be aware of not integrating what is known with what has not been uncovered. The child has not disclosed what may have occurred and has only stated that the father did something and the child does not like what the father did, nor does he wish to visit with the father and his family.

The interviewer has to elicit additional information or facts from the child and then try to corroborate that information as the interview progresses. Through incorporating the facts as they emerge in tandem with the use of drawing, the child provided information regarding person, activity, location and salient details that situate or corroborate the child's narrative. The interviewer is gathering information in an interactive and engaging manner that is responsive to the child's willingness to cooperate and share details. As such, it is not possible to ask open-ended questions in isolation. Follow-up and focused questions may be introduced in concert with what is being shared. The interviewer must abstain from proposing or introducing ideas or specifics before a child has elaborated about information disclosed or communicated corroborative facts. Although it is easy to ask outright "what did your dad do (to you)", it is not best practice to explore or fact-find with leading questions.

By collapsing information such as person, place and activity within the structure of questions, suggestibility may increase, depending upon the type of question. The goal is to have the child disclose the information rather than the interviewer outline it for the child, which is leading and decreases confidence associated with the type of questions. It may be necessary to integrate details as they are provided into the question format – for example, what did your dad do? What did your dad do to you? What did your dad do to you in the shower? When your dad was with you in the shower, where did he touch you? Questions become more focused and direct as more elements are incorporated.

Interviewers must be aware when questions may become leading or direct especially if the child has not supplied information to support the questioning, or the interviewer may be structuring and suggesting implicitly what information the child should convey. The more elements that the interviewer integrates, the more narrow the focus of the dialogue. It is incumbent for the interviewer to remain neutral and to try to utilize open-ended prompts, focusing as needed in response to what the child is communicating, and then step back and introduce a follow-up prompt or strategy to give the child the opportunity to provide additional corroborative information and to elaborate via narrative if possible. It is a process and a skill that takes training, practice and time to refine.

This example is not averse to improvement, refinement and discussion. As noted previously, there is no perfect process or way to conduct an interview. These processes are conducted in the moment and as such have to be responsive to the interaction taking place, which is impacted and correspondent to a child and the child's presentation and willingness to interact and engage as well as offer information. There are strategies, techniques and best practices, but even the most skilled and experienced interviewer will encounter road blocks, obstacles and impediments. It takes an arsenal of skill, training and education to do this work and do it well.

Interviewing is a skill, and question typology is a competency that factors into training. Question continuum is a source of consternation. As stated, there is no perfect process, and I think from doing this work, there is always room to improve and enhance skills. I think interviewers engage in self-reflection even without benefit of team post-processing and feedback. Revisiting and contemplating what went well and what did not will impact self-awareness and contribute to skill development and enhancement. The emphasis is on trying to facilitate free recall, which is believed to be more accurate. "Children are most suggestible about elements of their experience that they do not recall or are less sure of" (Steele, 2012, p. 104).

Fact-Finding, Drawing and Map Scene

The previous three phases as presented (rapport building, developmental assessment, anatomy identification) do not necessarily happen in isolation or in a specific sequence and may overlap. They provide a foundation for information gathering in the fact-finding phase. Drawing related to fact-finding may yield information that is significant for investigation and potentially prosecution. A child may make "a disclosure drawing" in which abuse-specific activity is detailed. A disclosure drawing is a picture in which the child depicts the experienced event or information pertinent to the allegations. Collateral material and corroboration of details and facts may be included. A drawing may contain contextual information such as who, what, when or where. Elements that may constitute charge enhancements or specific information related to chargeable offenses may be included. Through a drawing, a child may provide confirmation of verbal statements in a concrete and objective fashion. Drawing serves as a stimulus for free recall. As such, a child may depict pictorially what they cannot say (for whatever reason) which may stimulate verbalization or enhance verbal communication.

Fact-Finding and Drawing

- collateral information
- situational, contextual material
- details
- corroboration
- specific facts
- charge enhancements
- disclosure drawings
- map scenes
- objectification of experienced event

Fact-finding is especially responsive to the use of drawing. Drawing may be used in different ways, as a child might ask to draw rather than tell. Sometimes, when a child is unable to find the words or if the child lacks understanding of an experience, drawing may offer a way to help the child communicate. Verbalization may be enhanced. A child's associations as they pertain to a drawing are central to understanding what a child is expressing. It is not the interviewer's role to interpret a child's drawing. Rather, the interviewer elicits information to comprehend what the child is expressing and communicating both verbally and nonverbally as well as pictorially.

A child may draw a map scene that depicts multiple layers of information, which is consistent with nonlinear expression. A map scene may provide details such as who was present, including the alleged offender and the presence of additional witnesses. A map scene may include the setting and location as well as idiosyncratic information that may corroborate a child's statements such as details pertinent to the allegations.

Children are able to provide concrete details regarding their experiences. In a map scene, a child may provide salient information pertaining to what, where, who and how as well as information that is confirmatory, corroborative or forensically relevant. Children may provide a detailed narrative while drawing or provide additional facts as they discuss what they have depicted.

For example, a six-year-old boy related that he was abused in different rooms in a relative's home. In his drawing he split the picture into three columns in an attempt to indicate the different levels of the house, including the basement, the upstairs and the main level. The child described that there were bars on the windows which he represented in blue (basement) on the left and green (upstairs windows) on the right. In the center, the child's experience, which was described as being hurt by older teenage relatives and being made to do things that

Fact-Finding and Drawing

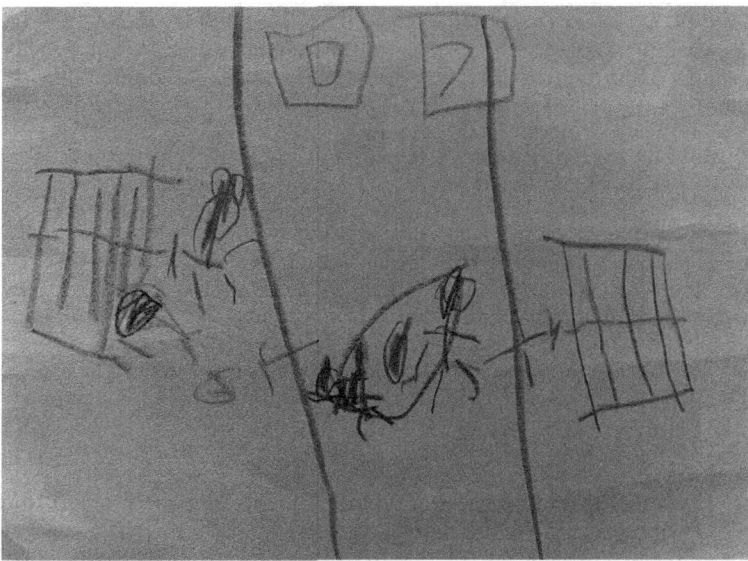

Figure 2.9 A map of the scene where the alleged abuse took place showing different levels within the home including different rooms as well as the perpetrators and the activity.

he did not want to do with them, was drawn and detailed. The child reported additional details about his experience, which included multiple acts of abuse by a myriad of perpetrators on each level of the house. His drawing provided a way for him to discuss and disclose the different acts perpetrated against him. The child provided information that had not been previously articulated. The child explained that he was abused on different occasions in various locations within the house, often during extended family gatherings. Due to the nature of the setting, the child revealed that doors were locked and he was unable to escape.

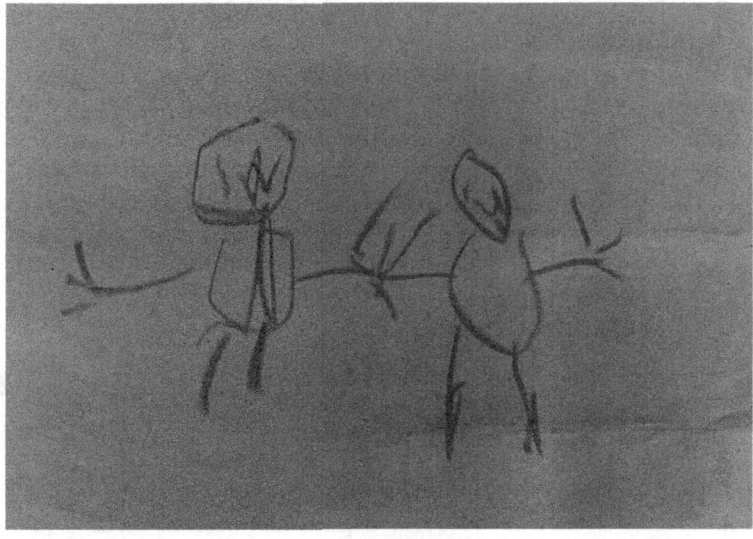

Figure 2.10 The child depicted himself in orange and drew one of the perpetrators in brown that he identified when he explained what was happening in the map scene on the other side of the paper.

(*Continued*)

(Continued)

Fact-Finding and Drawing

The child flipped his paper over and made a dyad that included himself and one of the individuals he described as abusing him. His ability to detail the scene and provide a map was enhanced by his verbalizations and explanations. He continued to disclose information and facts related to his experiences by providing information with respect to individual incidents as well as individual perpetrators.

TRAINING EXAMPLE: Team members are broken into small groups or dyads depending upon the number of participants. Abuse-specific scenarios are distributed and members are asked to role play twice: once as the interviewer and once as the child being interviewed. By switching roles each member is able to experience what it might be like to have to talk about an experienced event as well as practice interviewing skills. This provides the opportunity for team members to bring together the skills they have been practicing throughout the training and demonstrate fundamentals associated with interviewing and incorporate knowledge related to each phase of the process.

This exercise also invokes a bit of a peer-review component in that groups or dyads are asked to give feedback at the conclusion of the exercise with regard to what the experience was like both as interviewer and interviewee. Constructive feedback is shared and offered from and to one another. If time permits, volunteers will be asked to demonstrate or enact a piece of the role play for group review and shared insight. Team members may also be given a peer-review sheet to provide written feedback as part of skill building. Names are omitted, and comments are asked to be expressed constructively and with a positive tone. This is a constructive exercise, especially since this may be the first training or experience for participants conducting interviewing.

Closure

The closure phase is critical to the process and has ramifications for future interactions with the child. Several tasks are addressed in this phase, including establishing a context for a possible reinterview; bridging to what happens next (literally, which may mean informing a child that the interviewer will take him or her back to the parent); and addressing the child's questions, fears and concerns. The child's participation, and perhaps effort, is acknowledged (not what they may or may not have disclosed), and information from the interview, including if a drawing was made, may be reviewed, revisited or clarified. An interviewer may also ask if there is anything they may have forgotten to ask the child. Such an inquiry provides an opportunity for the child to indicate if there is something the interviewer might have overlooked, or a child may say "you forgot to ask me . . .". Sometimes, information may be disclosed at this point in the interview that was not shared previously, leading to pursuance of additional exploration and possible acquisition of factual material that may factor into the investigation.

THE COMMON INTERVIEW GUIDELINE
CLOSURE
Thank
for participation not information
Address
concerns/questions within a developmental and realistic manner
avoid false hopes
bridge to next steps
End positively
reconstitution

Transition
to what happens next
take away drawing
Conclude
leave door open for possible re-interview

INTEGRATION OF DRAWING IN COMMON INTERVIEW GUIDELINE
CLOSURE
Review
may trigger or stimulate recall of additional information
Revisit
flush out details
additional fact-finding
information not previously disclosed may emerge
Clarify
information and drawing content
Bridge
to what happens next
re-constitution
take away drawing
end positively

Closure

- leave door open for possible reinterview
- address child's concerns/questions
- respond truthfully but generally
- address personal safety
- bridge to what happens next
- end positively rather than negatively
- thank child for effort, not for information
- ask if there is anything forgot to ask
- avoid false hopes
- address fears, concerns, issues
- may address personal safety within developmental context
- allow child to reconstitute if child decompensated
- in certain circumstances, provide child with a means of contacting the interviewer
- very important piece of the interview

If the interview proved to be stress provoking for the child or if the child is unable to manage the emotional response, the child may need to regroup before leaving the interview room. If a child has decompensated during the process, the child may be invited to make a "take away" drawing. This picture is construed as non-investigatory and may provide the child with a means of support. The process is intended to conclude positively rather than negatively. This drawing may function as a transitional object and assist the child with closure. The drawing is self-directed and the child is invited to take the drawing. Sometimes, a child may ask to make a drawing at the end of the process to give to the non-offending parent (or the guardian that accompanied them). As such, a closure drawing may emanate out of a child's request or at the discretion of the interviewer at the conclusion of an interview process. In this respect, the drawing is not intended as a means for reconstitution and it is not relevant to the fact-finding process.

- review of information elicited
- clarification
- revisit information disclosed
- memory stimulus/trigger when reviewing (child may remember something additional)
- bridge to what happens next – concrete and literal
- reconstitute if necessary
- positive conclusion may impact child if another interview is warranted
- transitional object in the form of a drawing (made after the fact-finding piece of the process) may help the child conclude the process positively

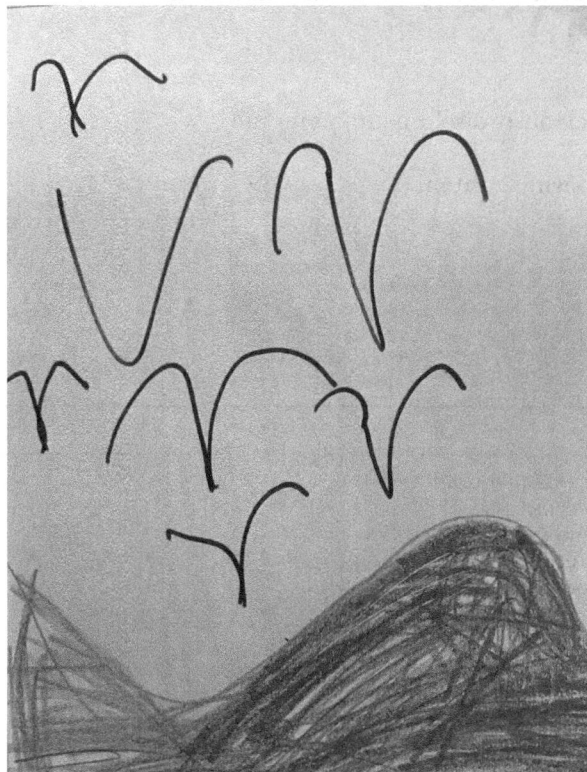

Figure 2.11 Drawing made by a nine-year-old female as a way to conclude the interview on a positive note. The child drew birds flying around the beach on a hot sunny day in anticipation of a weekend at the shore with her family.

Integration of Drawing

In the closure phase, drawing can be used to review or clarify information discussed. Drawing may also provide a positive means of concluding the process and help a child regroup, if necessary. Drawing may be used in a concrete manner as a bridge to what happens next. For example, I have had children make a card or a drawing to take with them that is unrelated to the interview process and is created with the intention of fostering closure. As such, if the drawing is not related to fact-finding or the allegations and if it is created after the interview is concluded per se, the drawing may serve in the capacity of a transitional object and the child may take it. Sometimes the child may ask the interviewer to keep it or they may give it to the interviewer. The use of drawing reaffirms the child-friendly nature of the process and contributes to receptivity in the event a re-interview is necessary.

The closure phase is critical to the process and for the overall well-being of the child in a myriad of ways. This phase has ramifications for future interactions with the child, specifically, if another interview is deemed necessary or if a child is to participate in a judicial proceeding. If the latter is a possibility, a child may need to be prepared for testifying and speaking about their experience in a courtroom. Concluding the interview on a positive note and in a supportive context will hopefully impact a child's subsequent engagement with investigation or prosecution. Furthermore, the child will hopefully feel supported and empowered from the interview process in such a way that the child will be able to address residual and impact issues through recommended interventive and therapeutic services.

EXAMPLE: Sometimes additional information may be revealed at the end of the process, meriting continuation of fact-finding. A five-year-old girl during the closure phase reported that she forgot to tell the interviewer something about her brother. She then proceeded to draw a picture of what she referred to as a bad touch. The interview was extended to explore the event that was disclosed via the drawing. The child stated that while reviewing her previous drawing that involved a nonfamilial individual, she recalled that her brother had also done something to her and she wanted the interviewer to know what he did and what happened after.

TRAINING EXERCISE: Participants in dyads assume the role of either interviewer or child. Within this context the interviewer is asked to begin to conclude the interview by reviewing what was discussed in a mock scenario. The dyad is asked to consider how to approach, inquiring if anything had not been broached earlier in the process that the child may wish to share. The interviewer might ask, "Is there anything I forgot to ask or is there anything you want to share?" This provides participants with the opportunity to experience disclosure statements that may occur at the conclusion of a process and how to address and process such information. Often when this happens a child might inform the interviewer that the interviewer did not ask about something, or a child may just say they remembered something additional or perhaps they just forgot to tell. Perhaps a child may inform the interviewer that they never asked so the child did not think to mention something. Structuring the interview and following the child's lead while maintaining control will help the interviewer to conduct a fact-finding process that will maximize the exploration of allegations. Sometimes, a child may be reluctant to disclose related or relevant information for whatever reason (threats, fear, etc.). In such situations, it may behoove the child as well as the investigation to consider an extended interview process or even a referral to therapy if the child is not able or ready to address the allegations. The investigative process may be impacted, which is a team or jurisdictional consideration. Therapy and investigation should not be conducted concurrently with regard to the allegations; however, an extended interview process which is not a therapeutic intervention may be in the best interest of the child as the child's needs take precedence.

In post-processing, the disclosure of information at the end of a process will be discussed, with the interviewer receiving feedback as to whether or not opportunities were missed for eliciting fact-finding earlier in the process. This is not a criticism – sometimes a child does not share information until the end because that may be when a child feels most comfortable to do so or when something surfaces, perhaps in response to something previously expressed or discussed, and when reviewed, a child may recall additional or new information.

(Continued)

(Continued)

Sometimes interviews take on a life of their own for whatever reason, and interviewers need to be prepared to gather information and address whatever is disclosed whenever it is offered during the process professionally and in accordance with the guideline; hence, flexibility and fluidity are central to the process. The phases are not sequential and may merit repeating as the process evolves.

EXAMPLAR

I have sat on the floor with a child or under the table to speak with a child. Sometimes the anxiety associated with the process or perhaps in response to how a child was prepared for the interview may impact how a child presents. Despite all good intentions, a child-friendly process and child-friendly setting and art materials, a child may just not be ready to engage. Sometimes when such is the case just being present with a child until they are comfortable is enough. I have had children sit on the floor with a crayon or a marker and reach up to the table and draw on a piece of paper. It is important to meet a child as they present and be respectful of their need to orient and engage. If that means sitting on the floor or under a table together and talking or working while exploring art materials, then so be it.

Three-dimensional art materials may also offer a means of discharging underlying anxiety or stress associated with the process or the unknown of speaking about one's personal experiences with someone they have never met. Clay sticks provide a child or a teenager with an outlet for managing anxiety or stress in a manner that is self-contained and manageable. Just working with the material, whether to create something representative or just manipulating the media, may offer a means of self-soothing that results in productivity and an ability to be engaged. Sometimes just enabling someone to explore the materials and spontaneously use them as they gain composure and reassurance is a benefit.

Use of Drawing Within the CIG Reviewed

Once again, the phases are listed as distinct; however, they are not intended to be sequential but to be addressed as they unfold in response to a child's engagement and participation.

Rapport Building

The use of drawing, although intended as an open-ended prompt, may also function similarly to the use of media, which is invoked for various purposes in interview contexts. As such, drawing may provide a dual purpose within the interview process. Tools, props and other aids have been utilized within interviews for differing reasons. They have provided support for developing rapport or to initiate conversation in the guise of an ice breaker.

The presentation of art materials connotes a child-friendly process. Engagement is welcome on a nonverbal level, which encourages the development of trust and fosters an atmosphere for rapport building and dialogical interaction. Suggestibility and accuracy, fundamental components within the interview process, can be addressed and clarified through a child's graphic depictions.

Developmental Assessment

Simple and basic tasks may be addressed or approached through the use of art materials. These include color identification and counting through use of the media (crayons, craypas or markers), which assist in determining a child's developmental level and providing additional maturational information. Drawing and artistic developmental levels help to cull information to assist in the comprehension of associated spheres, including social, emotional, cognitive and psychosexual. This information is integral for the interviewer in adapting and modifying interaction so that the interviewer and the child are working together rather than in a disconnected fashion. Attentiveness to the well-being of the child while adhering to forensic practice is vital to the process being productive and supportive. Modeling the communication patterns exhibited by the child promotes patterns of engagement that are correspondent.

Anatomy Identification

Regarding anatomy identification, drawing assists in providing the client with the opportunity to generate a demonstration aid, allowing for distancing or externalization. Body part identification, if warranted, is directed at a picture of a person (self) rather than physical demonstration, shielding one from potential embarrassment and stress. The use of a drawing provides for distance, negating the need to point to one's body to convey information that may be too personal and stress inducing. Identification of sexual and nonsexual body parts through a self-generated picture contributes to a developmentally congruent rendering. The use of a client-generated picture allows for distillation of anxiety and may serve as a concrete and permanent record that may later serve as a judiciary aid or provide evidentiary evidence.

Fact-Finding

Drawing within the fact-finding phase of the interview may help facilitate disclosure while at the same time it may potentially augment a child's verbal statements. A drawing may contribute to the disclosure of additional information or provide clarification about something discussed. It may provide a child with the ability to disclose information not previously shared. Corroborative material and collateral information depicted may provide or confirm details about an experienced event. Abuse-specific information may be revealed through a child's depiction, and material may emerge that contributes to investigative exploration. Drawing may contain details, facts and supplemental information, as well as information not previously disclosed, which may contribute to a narrative via the child's associations. The pictorial imagery may contribute to uncovering of pertinent information, which may impact potential prosecutorial decisions depending upon what may be drawn such as charge enhancements or details regarding what, where, who and how.

Closure

In closure, drawing is a means of bridging quite literally to what comes next and for ending positively rather than negatively. Drawing may also provide the opportunity for refreshing memory about topics discussed that may foster uncovering of additional information that may corroborate previously shared material or lead to discovery of new material. This may stimulate continued fact-finding and information gathering. Drawing in this phase may be used to prepare a child for possible courtroom engagement. The creation of a separate drawing at the conclusion of an interview may be requested by a child or considered by the interviewer as a means of transitioning out of the interview process. The child may take this picture out of the interview room and retain it as it is created for purposes not fundamentally associated with fact-finding. As such, this final drawing may assist the child with regrouping and leaving on a positive note. If another interview is necessary or deemed appropriate by the team, a positive conclusion will hopefully contribute to a child's willingness to participate in a follow-up process. An end or final drawing (or a take-away drawing) is not made in the service of the interview and is not forensic evidence as such and will not be considered evidentiary material or serve as a judiciary aid.

Free Drawing and the CIG

Drawing allows for an alternative method of communication (Cohen-Liebman, 1999). Information is conveyed via the creative process and allows for nonlinear, unrestricted communication. Drawing provides advantages. It allows a child to communicate and express thoughts without the threat of punishment or the fear of recrimination. Empowerment is promoted through the use of nondirected drawing, thus enabling a child to take a risk in order to be understood (Cohen-Liebman, 1999). Verbal elaboration often accompanies graphic telling (Kelley, 1984).

Free drawing may contain contextual and situational information that otherwise might not be disclosed. The imaginal content in concert with the child's associations promotes additional exploration. Idiosyncratic details that emerge lend credence to a child's disclosure and may assist in the uncovering of material previously not revealed or discovered. In a forensic interview free drawing may help a child organize, process and integrate experience even though the interview is not presented or conducted as a therapeutic process. As previously explained, an intrinsic therapeutic nuance underlies the process (CIG, when conducted by an art therapist), given the underlying juxtaposition of art therapy and forensic tenets. The process itself is predicated upon adherence to forensic standards to maintain judicial integrity and art therapy principles, which contribute to safeguarding the emotional well-being of the child.

CIG and Drawing

- integral component of multidisciplinary investigations
- incorporated in a supportive capacity
- assists in the investigative interview process
- complements the process
- can be used in a parallel manner to the guidelines
- serves as a stimulus for both the interviewer and the child to explore material, both manifest and latent
- helps the interviewer assess information quickly in a nonthreatening manner
- drawing provides information in a quick and direct manner that can be transferred into structure, process and technique
- the process, in combination with drawing tasks, provides the team with insight into a child's coping skills, level of trauma, emotional reaction to the abuse and in many cases abuse-specific information
- drawings can be retained and used to explore additional material previously uncovered or not yet disclosed
- functions as a bridge within the process
- serves as evidentiary material
- may function as a judiciary aid
- may provide information related to charge enhancements
- helps to safeguard the emotional well-being of a child, given the child-friendly nature of the process
- desensitizes the investigative aspect, which may be stress provoking

---

In the CIG, drawing provides the team with insight into a child's coping skills, level of trauma, emotional reaction to the abuse/experience and often abuse-specific information (Cohen-Liebman, 1999, 2017). Drawing complements the process, as it is used in a parallel manner to the guideline and may serve as a bridge between and among the respective phases.

Drawing may serve as a stimulus for both the interviewer and the child to explore material that is both manifest and latent. Moreover, drawings can be retained and used later in a court proceeding or as a means to refresh a child's memory if an extended amount of time has elapsed between the interview and the proceeding. The use of drawing aids a child to recall what was disclosed at a given moment in time. A drawing may be presented in court as evidentiary material and function as a judiciary aid.

Response to Drawing by Children

- children respond in a variety of ways
- ego-syntonic discharge for underlying thoughts and feelings
- alternative method of communication by allowing nonverbal expression
- "I can't say it but I can draw it"

Use of Interview Aids, Props, Tools and Strategies

In an effort to enhance children's abilities to provide information about personally meaningful experiences in investigative interviews, research studies have explored various aspects and ancillary strategies and techniques associated with the process of interviewing (Faller, 2014; Gee & Pipe, 1995; Poole & Bruck, 2012; Poole & Lamb, 2009; Salmon, 2006; Wesson & Salmon, 2001). Guidance for interviewers extends beyond the question format and includes use and introduction of props, aids, tools and various media (Faller, 2014; Lamb & Brown, 2006). The use of interviewing adjuncts has long been identified as contributory as well as controversial within the practice of forensic interviewing (Barlow et al., 2011; Faller, 2014; Kendall-Tackett, 1992; Poole & Bruck, 2012; Poole & Lamb, 2009). "Debate about the appropriate roles for props in interviews is ongoing and often heated" (Poole, 2016, p. 144).

Interview props have been associated with assisting children to communicate. Poole (2016) states that prop-based techniques satisfy one of four purposes: comfort techniques, assessment techniques, communication techniques and as clarification and documentation techniques (p. 144). Poole (2016) explores various research studies associated with these purposes or techniques. Additionally, research has examined various auxiliary strategies associated with interviewing (Faller, 2005, 2014; Poole, 2016; Poole & Bruck, 2012; Poole & Lamb, 2009), including the use of dolls, (anatomically detailed), puppets and other aids including schematic diagrams of human bodies. Many of these aids are considered controversial in the literature due to the way they are used within interviews; however, others have been determined to "appear valuable for assisting young children to provide forensically useful information" (Wakefield & Underwager, 1998, p. 177). It has been stated that "It is not the tool itself that makes for a powerful interviewing technique, but rather the skill with which the clinician uses it" (Hoorwitz, 1992).

Some of the discrepancies in the literature and research may be explained by the manner in which interview techniques and strategies have been studied with regard to enhanced reporting by children about personal experience (Gee & Pipe, 1995; Salmon, 2006; Wesson & Salmon, 2001). It has been proposed that interview aids came into practice when practitioners were responding to rapid changes in the number and complexity of abuse cases (Poole & Lamb, 2009) and empirical data were not secured. As a result, minimization of media within the structure of investigative interviews has been advocated by some researchers (Lamb et al., 2007) and discouraged by others. Still, some contend, "Techniques using images vary greatly as to whether they introduce potential error into the investigation or whether they are useful aids to accurate recall" (Wakefield & Underwager, 1998, p. 179).

The use of drawing has been identified as an ancillary support for interviewers (Poole & Lamb, 1998). Drawing has also been studied to assess effectiveness as a retrieval tool. Studies have considered drawing in relation to age of the child, type of event to be recalled and length of delay between the event and the retrieval, as well as the use of free recall prompts (Butler et al., 1995; Gross & Hayne, 1998, 1999; Jolley, 2010; Katz & Hershkowitz, 2010, 2013; Salmon et al., 2003; Wesson & Salmon, 2001). With regard to development of new interview techniques, "it is important that an increase in the amount of information that children report does not occur at the expense of accuracy" (Patterson & Hayne, 2011, p. 119).

- rapport building
  - ice breaker
  - development of trust and rapport
  - communication tool
  - engagement on a nonverbal level
- developmental assessment
  - skill assessment
  - maturational spheres
  - comprehension of this information factors into correspondence between interviewer and child
- anatomy identification
  - demonstration aid
  - client generated (drawing)
  - externalization process
- fact-finding
  - facilitation of disclosure
  - collateral information
  - confirmation of verbal statements
- closure
  - memory stimulus/referential trigger
  - bridge to what happens next
  - assists with positive conclusion

Drawing and Forensic Investigations

Drawing within the context of an investigative interview provides data for both investigative and prosecutorial purposes while minimizing subjective interpretation (Cohen-Liebman, 2003). Within a forensic context, drawing may function in one of three ways (Cohen-Liebman, 2002, 2003). The three ways drawing may function have been detailed, explained and explored (Cohen-Liebman, 2003).

- as interviewing tools
  - used in a supportive capacity in the investigative process
- as charge enhancements
  - provide contextual information that can contribute to the determination of charges, as well as the identification of additional arenas to explore
- as judiciary aids
  - provide evidentiary material that may be admissible in a judicial proceeding

Drawing as Interviewing Tools or Aids

Drawing may be used in a supportive capacity as an interviewing tool or aid to explain or clarify a child's experience such as in the guideline provided earlier. A drawing may support a child in the interview process by promoting engagement, development of rapport with the interviewer and empowerment. The use of drawing connotes that the process and, by extension, the interviewer are child friendly and the process is child centered. Drawing may provide the catalyst for the interviewer to pursue previously unexamined material stemming from a disclosure drawing in which a child depicts information pertaining to the allegations specific to an experienced event. Drawing may contain information that was unknown to investigators despite investigative measures simply because drawing has the potential to provide a child with a nonverbal means of expression that may contribute to uncovering of facts perhaps not yet disclosed or known by investigators. Often, a child may lack the capability to directly relate experience in any other form. The use of drawing has the potential to stimulate verbalization in conjunction with explanation of the imaginal depiction. Drawing in essence may support the child's ability to convey in a developmentally congruent manner what the child was exposed to or what the child may have experienced.

Drawing is not considered in isolation from the context in which it was created. Drawing supplements and complements the process, and as such, it is not detached from the process. The associations of the child in concert with the child's imagery provide the team with insight and understanding of a child's experience. An investigative interview which includes drawing may provide additional material with regard to an experienced event and reveal information that is related to a crime.

Additionally, drawing may signal or indicate a child's level of trauma in relation to the experience, which factors into post-processing and determination of further investigative, prosecutorial and interventive measures (Cohen-Liebman, 1999). As an art therapist, my role is not to interpret a drawing or to make meaning of the drawing for the child, but rather, through the dialogical process, the child's associations are sought to understand through a meaning making experience what the child is communicating.

As Interviewing Tool
used in a supportive capacity in the investigative process

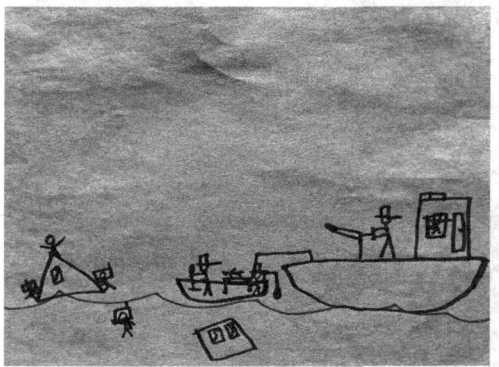

- ice breaker
- demonstrative tool
- discharge anxiety
- screening tool
- memory stimulus
- develop rapport
- build trust
- connote child-friendly process

Figure 2.12 Ten-year-old drew a scene depicting a water rescue by the Coast Guard of a family in distress as a metaphor for the child's perception of the interview.

As Charge Enhancement

Drawing can provide contextual information that may contribute to the determination of charges as well as the identification of additional arenas to explore within the interview context and externally as well. As such, drawing may include situational and contextual information that is relevant to a child's experience. Previously unknown material may come to light. Salient and significant information includes details pertaining to people, victims, witnesses and perpetrators; places, locale or setting of an event; or facts such as descriptive material.

Drawing and fact-finding may contribute to uncovering of information that may be used in the determination of criminal activity and may possibly be appraised as chargeable offenses. Examples include the use of force, punishment of some sort, rewards, bribes or the use of elements or items in connection to the abusive event. The latter may include sexual aids, devices, the use of media such as pornography and anything that may have been used within the context of the abuse, which may be assessed with regard to establishment of criminal activity. A few examples disclosed by children include a rope and a clothesline (use of force); not allowed to see friends, no dinner (punishment); Vaseline, pornography, tapes, alcohol (sexual aids); trip to the pet store and circus (bribe); and harm to the family and loss of pet (threats). Details including situational or contextual elements may contribute to the determination of additional investigation and possible prosecution (to be determined by law enforcement and presented to the prosecutor or equivalent).

For example, a child may indicate that they were threatened or bribed by an alleged offender to engage in some type of sexual activity. An interview with an eight-year-old girl resulted in disclosure of the use of force as well as an instrument to tie her up. The child disclosed through her drawing in tandem with her verbal explanation that a clothesline was used by the perpetrator, which resulted in additional charges being brought against the identified suspect.

Charge Enhancement

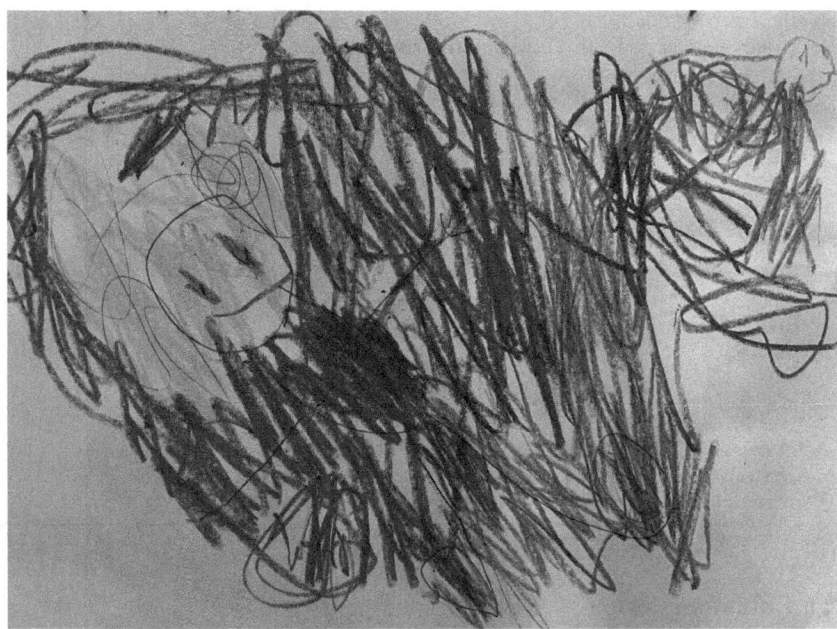

Figure 2.13 The child depicted her experience of being touched by a monster, the alleged perpetrator, the green figure located in the upper right-hand corner, while she was under the covers. She provided that the individual said he was playing monster with her and that the monster (the alleged perpetrator) said he was going to tickle her. The child reported being touched under her clothes in her "special area on her private parts".

A child can depict information that extends beyond a verbal (linear) configuration, resulting in a pictorial matrix (Wadeson, 2010) that may contain additional details and idiosyncratic information that extends beyond what the child is saying and encompasses a multitude of information, including facts, details and illustration of overlapping factors. The child will try to depict within the scope of the drawing information that is salient to the experience in accordance with artistic developmental level. Although the picture may not on first view make sense, as a child explains and describes or provides a narrative, the underlying meaning and understanding of the child's experience will emerge. A child may utilize a spatial configuration to depict details that occurred at the same time, which may be hard to verbally describe given that verbalization is a linear process. Graphic depiction can lead to disclosure of a myriad of aspects in the same picture, revealing events and associated details that may have occurred simultaneously or on different days or in different settings. So-called "disclosure drawings" convey the event(s) and experience of a child and may lead to enhanced verbalization to describe accurate and factual details.

Charge Enhancements – Considerations for the Interviewer

- provide investigators with enough information (facts) to support charges
- corroborative information is needed to establish that a crime was committed
- are there allegations that may enhance a penalty or increase a potential sentence
- the interviewer is obligated to address the elements associated with a crime within the interview context (and to meet the needs of the investigators, including law enforcement who will present to prosecution)
- to garner the information needed to help in determination of potential charges
- the interviewer will need to know what constitutes a crime according to the jurisdiction
- interviewer does not want to overlook or not explore the elements associated with a potential crime
- exploration may help uncover information relevant to determination of a crime that may result in charges being filed as well as uncover material not previously reported
- to prevent lack of exploration of elements that may be related to a crime
- interviewer must be aware and mindful of what a child is expressing or not saying in conjunction with allegations
- the interviewer is entrusted with the task of gathering information for the team, which includes law enforcement and the district attorney (depending upon jurisdiction – may be identified differently)

The interviewer using drawing must explore the details and the context as explained by the child to comprehend what the child experienced and ascertain relative information as to whether the child is depicting a single event or conflating events, setting(s), activity, witnesses, other victims, offender(s) and/or additional information.

Forensic/Charge Enhancements provide contextual information that can contribute to the determination of charges (as per law enforcement, who decides whether or not	Drawing in conjunction with verbal description or associations may contribute to additional information that may be relevant for fact-finding and next steps

---

(Continued)

(Continued)

to present evidence to prosecution, who will make the determination)	in the investigation; details and factors that emerge may provide or contribute to the basis for the acquisition of a search warrant by law enforcement, as well as identification of additional witnesses, victims or perpetrators, meriting additional investigatory measures and intervention
provide contextual information that can contribute to the determination of charges as well as the identification of additional arenas to explore	elements of secrecy
	situational or contextual information
	developmentally incongruent knowledge
details or elements of an event may be discovered	threats, bribes, rewards, coercion, punishment, pressure
may provide information that may contribute to additional investigation, as well as eventual prosecution	physical harm, restraints, force
	pornography
	sexual aids
	media, cable, Internet
depict salient and significant information or details pertaining to a child's experience	
additional information previously unknown such as additional victims, witnesses or perpetrators may be indicated/depicted	

As Judiciary Aids

Presentation of drawing in the courtroom is powerful and presents the child's experience affectingly. A drawing may be admissible in a judicial proceeding wherein the drawing is presented in court as evidentiary material (Cohen-Liebman, 2002, 2003; Gussak, 2013; Gussak & Cohen-Liebman, 2001). A drawing is a permanent and objective visual record of a child's experience at a given time. A drawing provides a concrete representation of a child's experience that, when presented in court, may offer corroborative evidence and clarification of a child's verbal statements. Children often draw what they cannot say, and in a court of law, a drawing truly can speak volumes, as I have discussed (Cohen-Liebman, 1999) and witnessed.

I have encountered judicial officers who were invested in understanding what a drawing made by a child expresses and how the drawing was produced within the context of the interview. I have encountered judicial officers who have literally left the bench to be able to experience a drawing made by a child without space, barriers or the need to be treated as the trier of fact wherein they have come over to view pictures made by victims and witnesses and ask questions to comprehend the content.

For one particular judicial officer, wanting to see each picture and understand the context from which each drawing emerged resulted in a visceral experience. The movement by the fact-finder, rising from behind the bench to walk over to view the drawings up close, connoted the reverence bestowed upon the artwork in that setting at that time. Speaking through each drawing, the child's experience was poignant and impactful. The judge engaged almost to the exclusion of everyone else in the room as more than one drawing was viewed, providing a visual narrative of one child's experience. The propensity of a drawing to effectively convey what the child was not present to say and communicate her experience (via imagery coupled with her associations as related by the author) was not lost on anyone in the courtroom. Evidentiary material in the form of drawing provided voice and expression enabling the child to communicate her narrative; to speak, to say, to be heard, to be present.

Drawing as Judiciary Aids

- drawing may focus on the effects of the abuse
- detail situational factors contributing to abuse
- content of abuse may be depicted
- who, what, when, where, how
- permanent record
- spatial matrix; information is provided outside of a linear configuration
- rule out alternative explanations
- objectification
- concretize behavior, thoughts, feelings at a given moment in time
- visual record
- detail situational factors contributing to abuse
- charge enhancements
- corroboration
- details of the abuse – setting, observers, participants
- a child may draw what they cannot say
- leading to enhanced verbalization and additional information communicated
- provide evidentiary material that may be admissible in a judicial proceeding
- imaginal speech conveys the child's experience

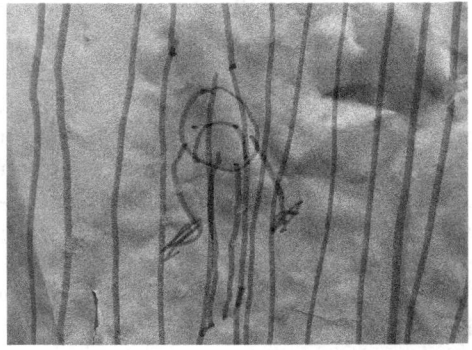

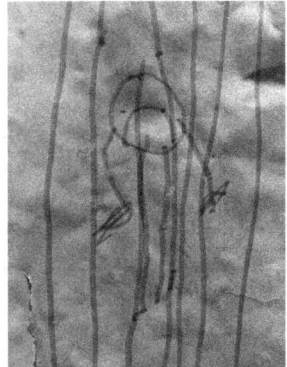

Figure 2.14 Drawing made by a six-year-old child placing himself behind bars to show how trapped he felt living with an abusive step-parent.

Figure 2.15 Close-up shows child's emotional response noted in forceful use of marker (dots) and paper rips.

Use of Drawing in the Context of Judiciary Aids

A representative sampling from various disciplines addresses the viability of the use of drawing in the context of judiciary aids and as a support to facilitate testimony (Burgess et al., 1987; Cohen-Liebman, 1995, 1999, 2003; Farley, 1987; Malchiodi, 1990;

Veltkamp & Miller, 1994). The function of drawing in the capacity of judiciary aids has been discussed by individuals both within and external to the field of art therapy (Burgess et al., 1981; Kelley, 1984; Landgarten, 1987; Miller et al., 1987). Drawing may help rule out alternative explanations and offer corroboration and clarification and contribute to verbalization and enhanced communication (Cohen-Liebman, 1999, 2003). In some states, statutes have been written that specifically provide for the use of drawing to assist a child witness at the discretion of the court (Haralambie, 1999). The child's identification of pictorial elements demarcates a drawing as a piece of evidence that is legally and clinically convincing and renders it admissible in court (Faller, 1993).

In the capacity of a judiciary aid, a drawing can evoke a response in the courtroom that can be profound. Drawing affords an objective and concrete statement that is reflective of the child's experience since it is client generated. Such a visual record serves not only to decipher the facts of the case and offer evidentiary material but also serves to convey the child's level of traumatization. Whether in isolation or combination, evidentiary material and emotional response can impact a legal proceeding and the courtroom.

Often children draw what they cannot say for whatever reason: fear, need to maintain secrecy, inability to verbally communicate what they experienced, lack of understanding and other factors that may inhibit disclosure. Drawing may promote verbal elaboration and add credence to what a child is expressing. Thus, reciprocity between drawing and verbal expression exists. A child may draw and then offer verbal explanation, or due to limitations or confines associated with the mode of verbal expression, a child may use art media to express what they wish to convey.

A child may depict developmentally incongruent knowledge in a manner that is congruent with developmental capacity, providing a means of assimilating disparate information (knowledge or experience). A child can show what happened and continue to articulate what happened through a pictorial narrative. This may illuminate a sequence of events, details and idiosyncratic elements. A drawing may contain a range of activities that were experienced whether in a singular event or over time. Discerning factors may be included that are consistent with evidence associated with the case. A child may, through a drawing, be able to clarify and communicate what they want to express even if they lack the skills or capability to do so in a different context. A drawing may contain the effects of the abuse; details of situational factors contributing to the abuse; the content of the abuse; related details (who, what, when, where, how); and also information regarding the setting, witnesses, victims and perpetrators.

If an investigative process moves forward into a judicial proceeding, the interviewer may be called into court to present evidentiary material as a witness. In this capacity, the interviewer may be asked to explain findings and conclusions that may be addressed in a report documenting the process, including artwork. As such, the interviewer brings the child into the court via the child's graphic productions. On the witness stand, the interviewer presents the evidence gathered through the fact-finding process. The findings derived from the drawing or drawings made by the child are discussed in relation to what the child communicated and expressed pictorially as well as verbally with regard to the allegations.

The child's associations, while creating the drawing as well as at any time during the process, merit attention. What the child says about and in conjunction to a drawing is significant. Verbal descriptions of depictions are to be sought from the child for clarification and understanding, thus alleviating an assumptive stance by the interviewer (Farley, 1987; Sorenson et al., 1997).

- process that involves many variables
- motivational factors
- charge enhancements
- consistency
  - core elements – a contributing factor
  - peripheral details may change
  - core components should remain constant
  - core vs. peripheral
  - must consider developmental application with regard to inconsistencies
- developmentally incongruent knowledge
- situational/contextual information
- multiple incidents over time
- progression of sexual activity
- continuum of behavior
- less intimate to more intimate activity
- alternative explanations
- idiosyncratic statements

Beneficial Considerations of Drawing

The benefits associated with the use of drawing are considerable for the child, the process and the system. Information derived from a drawing can assist in comprehensively understanding a child's experience as well as evaluating the child's skill level, coping mechanisms and level of trauma. The information is conveyed to the team and used in the determination of additional investigative measures as well as supportive interventions.

Advantages of Drawing Within the Interview Context

Intrinsic (Therapeutic) Value of the Integration of Drawing Within the Interview Process

- relate experiences through drawing pictures directly or indirectly
- may lack cognitive capability or verbal capacity to articulate verbally
- traumatic response may negate ability to verbalize
- once drawn, may elaborate verbally
- therapeutic distance
- picture is less threatening
- external object
- can stimulate conversation
- focus conversation
- provide structure to the process
- explore related topics and issues, both manifest and latent
- less threatening means of communication
- draw solutions to problems
- provide immediate gratification
- provide an opportunity to safely explore and alter feelings
- depict emotional reaction
- provide a sense of control
- can defend or protect self/others (something that a child may not have been able to do in reality)
- place self in control of situation
- gain mastery over the experience

(*Continued*)

(Continued)

Intrinsic (Therapeutic) Value of the Integration of Drawing Within the Interview Process

---

Therapeutic adjustments identified by Silver (1989) associated with the use of drawing by
   children factor into the interview process and are especially relevant.
Children, through drawing, may
- fulfill wishes vicariously
- experience unacceptable feelings in an acceptable way
- obtain relief from tension
- gain control over people and events
- transfer behavior
- personal involvement
   - Silver, 1989

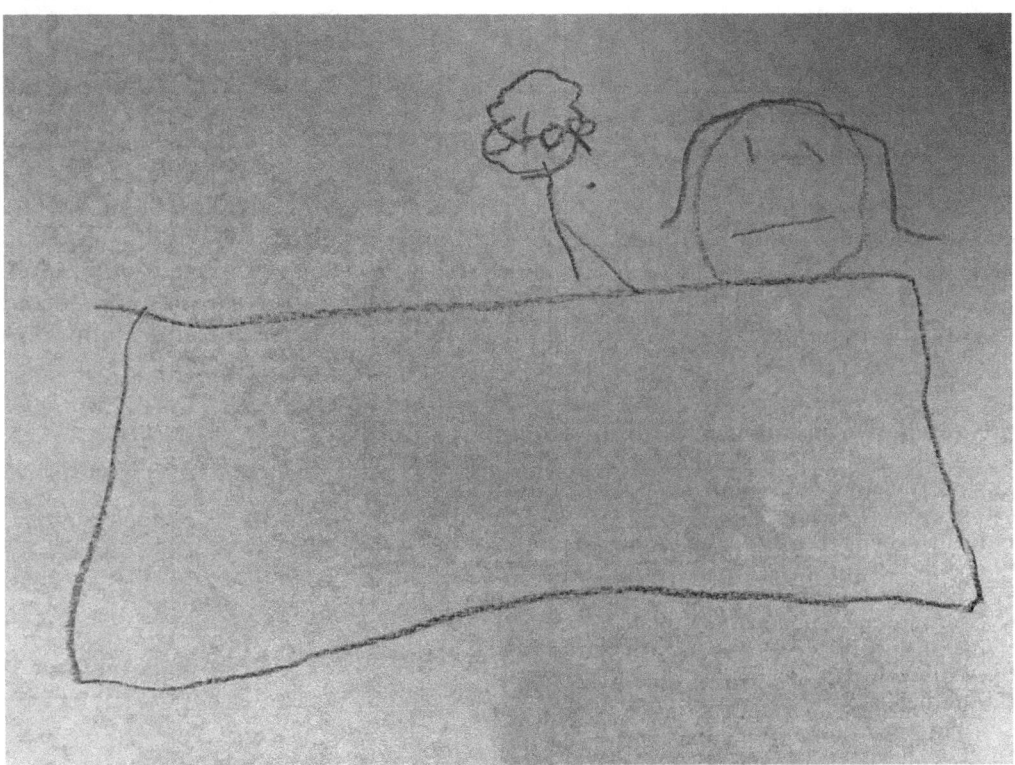

Figure 2.16 Drawing demonstrating empowerment and mastery, as the child was able to express
        what she had been unable to say when she was victimized in the bathtub.

Exemplar

A nine-year-old child who was abused in the bathroom by a relative drew a picture of herself sitting in a bathtub holding a sign that spelled out STOP (Figure 2.16). She explained
her drawing by saying that she wished that she had told the alleged perpetrator, an adult

male relative, to stop. The use of drawing within the interview context provided the means for her to express what she was unable to say during the assault. The drawing provided salient details, including corroboratory information; however, the drawing also provided a means for the child to integrate and process the experience. In addition, she was able to express and say what she had been unable to do at the time she was victimized in a manner that was ego syntonic.

The drawing served as a bridge to therapeutic intervention, as the child was prepared to discuss her thoughts and feelings surrounding her experience. The interview and the use of drawing enabled and empowered this child to give voice to what she had been unable to communicate prior to the interview. In essence, through the use of a stop sign, she was able to gain control over the situation and the perpetrator while obtaining relief from tension that permeated her need to master the situation.

In another drawing, the child was able to place the perpetrator behind bars, thus fulfilling wishes vicariously and owning her feelings that it was okay to want the perpetrator to be punished. The child was able to let go of her conflicted feelings and accept that her wish to have the perpetrator pay for his crime was positive; thus Silver's (1989) adjustment, *experience unacceptable feelings in an acceptable way*, was demonstrated through imagery and words. Although Silver may have intended these items as therapeutic adjustments, they are relevant for children within the context of investigative interviews, despite the emphasis on a nontherapeutic environment, and reflect the fusion of an interview process that integrates forensic and art therapy tenets.

The CIG is intended to support and safeguard the emotional well-being of the child within a forensic milieu. This hybrid configuration amalgamates investigation and support. This is demonstrated when a child draws scenarios related to an event that corresponds with the identified (therapeutic) adjustments. Sometimes, a drawing is the initial juncture wherein a child is able to reconcile something that may be difficult to articulate or express and process, thus initiating the commencement of recovery. The adjustments (listed earlier) correspond to the nature of the CIG, which is predicated upon the juxtaposition of art therapy principles and practices with judicial or legal tenets. Nonjudgmental support is embraced by the process, which promotes empowerment, which is often reflected in a drawing and/or a child's associations.

The investigative interview may precipitate the uncovering of information as well as associated thoughts related to the experienced event that may not have been acknowledged or understood, let alone integrated. Although the process is not intended to be a therapeutic process, the hybrid nature fosters a supportive context. Children may respond to the use of free drawing by expressing and/or depicting mastery of a situation or by placing themselves in control when disclosing what happened. Although the process is directed at fact-finding, a child may articulate verbally or nonverbally via drawing an alternative to what was experienced, or they may defend themselves or indicate punitive measures against the perpetrator. Drawing provides the opportunity to freely express what was personally experienced or endured. In addition, wishes and intentions, including what one may have been unable to say or do when victimized or abused, can be expressed without fear of retribution. The inability to defend one's self or protect a sibling is a sentiment frequently shared when allegations are disclosed and explored.

Interview Phases: Key Points

Rapport Building Key Points:

- engage
- empower
- encourage
- promote comfort
- address standard operating procedure
- emphasize accuracy
- assess suggestibility
- enhance resistance to suggestion
- promote trust
- activate participation
- address standard operating procedure (setting, task, expectations, documentation)
- choice
- challenge authority
- importance of accuracy
- acknowledge confusion rather than guess
- embolden child to disagree or correct
- clarify misperceptions
- ascertain who prepared child and what was said

Developmental Assessment Key Points:

- assess child's skills

    - cognitive, social, linguistic, artistic, psychosexual
    - memory
    - suggestibility
    - concept formation
    - expressive-receptive communication

- modify and adapt communication style
- critical, so interviewer is developmentally sensitive
- ascertain type of questions child can answer
- ability to interact and attend (attention and focus)
- does the child speak in a developmentally congruent manner
- are words used properly
- are words incongruous
- mirror sentence structure, choice of words
- responsive and reflective listening
- clarify and verify child's statements
- avoid interpretation or affixing meaning to a child's statements
- repeat back to child to reduce risk of misconstruing
- simple nonleading questions are recommended but not always plausible
- even if child is unclear with regard to qualification concepts, child can provide accurate information
- assess suggestibility

- assess congruency of concepts

  - truth versus lie, real versus pretend, right versus wrong
  - provide concrete examples rather than request a definition

- assess skill level

  - evaluate comprehension of prepositions
  - spatial relationships
  - developmentally congruent tasks

- practice and role play

  - issue of mistake

Anatomy Identification and Sensory Reference Key Points:

- identification of nonsexual and sexual body parts (within a developmental frame and as deemed applicable within the interview context)

  - location, function
  - sensory reference
  - see, smell, hear, taste, touch

- explore different types of touch

  - good/bad, comfortable/uncomfortable, safe/not safe

- serve as a demonstration tool

  - for externalization
  - provide distance
  - self-reference
  - concrete
  - objective

- assess suggestibility

Fact-Finding Key Points:

- fact-finding process
- assess and refute argument of suggestibility
- question continuum

  - free recall – narrative
  - open-ended, nonleading to more specific/focused
  - less focused and directed to more focused/directed
  - general to specific
  - step in and step out of question typology
  - vary question format
  - follow-up cues after less open-ended or more focused questions
  - reverse continuum of questioning – start open and focus/narrow as needed
  - use follow-up cues

- question types to avoid

  - double-barreled (two or more questions merged into a single question)
  - complex questions either grammatically or syntactically
  - negatively framed – insinuates the interviewer has an answer or response in mind

- continuum of question format
- contextual and situational information
- who, what, when, where, how
- corroboratory material

  - corroboration of verbal statements

- details and facts

  - collateral information, idiosyncratic details
  - multiple events versus isolated event
  - progression from less intimate to more intimate activity

- explore alternative hypothesis/explanations
- charge enhancements

  - pornography, media, sexual aids
  - coercion/threats/bribes/rewards/punishments/force/promises

Closure Key Points:

- ask if there is anything the interviewer forgot to ask
- thank child for participating/effort
- leave door open for possible reinterview
- address child's concerns/questions

  - respond truthfully but generally
  - avoid false hopes
  - address personal safety

- bridge to what happens next (transition)
- end positively rather than negatively
- allow child to regroup if child decompensated
- in certain circumstances – provide child with a means of contacting the interviewer
- very important piece of the interview

Credibility Assessment Key Points:

- process that involves many variables
- motivational factors
- charge enhancements
- consistency
- core versus peripheral details

  - peripheral details may change
  - core components should remain constant

- developmentally incongruent knowledge
- situational/contextual information
- multiple incidents over time

- progression of sexual activity
- continuum of behavior
- less intimate to more intimate behavior
- inconsistencies are addressed within a developmental application
- alternative explanations
- idiosyncratic statements

Interviewer Task and Observation Feedback Sheet

A sample feedback sheet with space for notes and observations is presented. This sheet allows team members to share impressions and offer constructive feedback when observing a process. It is a tool intended to enhance and acknowledge interviewing as well as observational skills that can be transferred into practice. It provides an opportunity to acknowledge strengths and identify areas that may need improvement. Names are omitted so that individuals share impressions openly and honestly. An interviewer is conducting a process on behalf of a team, so a willingness to take another point of view or perspective may inspire a different way of seeing or hearing that may be impactful for how an individual approaches and conducts a process.

Common Interview Guideline
Task and Observation Feedback Sheet

Task	Observations
RAPPORT BUILDING	
Engage	
Empower	
Encourage	
Promote Comfort	
Address Standard Operating Procedure	
Emphasize Accuracy	
Assess Suggestibility	
DEVELOPMENTAL ASSESSMENT	
Assess Skills	
Practice and Role Play	
Modify/Adapt Communication Style	
Spatial Relationships	
Congruency of Concepts	
Forensic Tasks	
Credibility Assessment	
Assess Competency	
Refute Suggestibility	
ANATOMY IDENTIFICATION	
Body Parts Inventory (in accordance with developmental level)	
Sensory Reference	
Explore Different Types of Touch	
FACT-FINDING	
Question Continuum	
Explore Details/Facts	

(Continued)

(Continued)

Task	Observations
Corroboration of Information	
Explore Alternative Hypothesis/Explanations	
Credibility Assessment	
Refute Suggestibility	
Charge Enhancements	
Gather Material Pertinent for Team	

CLOSURE

Thank Child for Participation	
Leave Door Open for Possible Reinterview	
Address Concerns/Questions	
Avoid False Hopes	
Address Personal Safety	
Bridge to Next Steps	
End Positively	
Transition	

INTERVIEWER BEHAVIOR

Developmentally and Culturally Sensitive	
Facilitative Utterances	
Nonverbal Behavior(s)	
Reinforcement Behaviors (negative/positive)	
Responsive Listening	
Affect	
Objectivity	
Neutrality	
Forensically Defensible Process	
Refrain From Interviewer Bias	

ADDITIONAL FEEDBACK/COMMENTS FOR INTERVIEWER

Use of Drawing Within the CIG

- integral component of multidisciplinary investigations
- incorporated in a supportive capacity
- assists in the investigative interview process
- complements the process
- can be used in a parallel manner to the guideline
- serves as a bridge to the respective phases as well as next steps
- serves as a stimulus for both the interviewer and the child to explore material, both manifest and latent

Integration of Drawing With the CIG

RAPPORT BUILDING

- ice breaker
- development of trust and rapport
- communication tool
- engagement on a nonverbal level

DEVELOPMENTAL ASSESSMENT

- quick/direct acquisition of information
- use of media and drawing assist in assessing

    - skill levels/ability to attend/focus
    - mastery of developmentally congruent tasks
    - adaptation of interviewer communication style

- artistic developmental level provides information pertaining to maturational spheres
- information assists interviewer in comprehending child's level of functioning

    - allows for modification and adaptation of language, communication, interactive patterns

ANATOMY IDENTIFICATION

- demonstration aid
- client-generated product
- externalization/distance
- evidentiary material
- screening tool
- body parts inventory
- follow verbal statement with demonstration/illustration
- concrete
- self-reference

FACT-FINDING

- evidentiary material
- situational, contextual details
- collateral information
- corroboration of facts
- confirmation of verbalizations
- imagery may promote enhanced verbalization
- stimulate free recall and narrative
- charge enhancements
- disclosure drawings
- judiciary aids
- objectification

CLOSURE

- review
- clarification
- revisit what was discussed/disclosed
- memory stimulus
- bridge
- regroup
- end positively
- transitional object

Benefits of the Integration of Drawing Within the Interview Process

Intrinsic (Therapeutic) Value

- children may relate experiences through drawing pictures directly or indirectly
- may lack cognitive capability or verbal capacity to articulate verbally
- interview process may negate ability to verbalize
- once drawn, may elaborate
- therapeutic distance
- picture is less threatening

  - external object
  - easier to talk about a picture of someone/something
  - self-referential

- can stimulate conversation
- focus conversation
- provide structure to the process
- explore related topics and issues, both manifest and latent
- less threatening means of communication
- draw solutions to problems
- provide immediate gratification
- provide an opportunity to safely explore and alter feelings
- depict emotional reaction
- emotional conflicts can be neutralized
- able to communicate what cannot say
- anxiety and stress are minimized
- process and use of art materials connotes child-friendly, child-focused process
- imaginal depiction may lead to enhanced verbalization
- provide a sense of control/mastery

Artistic Developmental Levels

In the mid-20th century, researchers and educators began to explore children's drawings and the phenomenon of graphic expression. Psychologist Rhoda Kellogg collected drawings from all over the world and discovered that children begin to draw at the same age and in the same manner (Kellogg, 1970). Kellogg focused on line formations and classified graphic production.

In 1952, art educator Victor Lowenfeld determined that artistic development occurs in combination with a child's emotional, physical and cognitive development. Lowenfeld placed artistic development into a stage theory. He is credited with recognizing and identifying sequential artistic development (Lowenfeld & Brittain, 1987). He determined that there is a correlation between intellectual, emotional and artistic development. Lowenfeld's work has been construed as analogous to Piaget's stage theory of cognitive or intellectual development (Malchiodi, 1998). The phase-specific developmental sequence associated with children's artistic development factors into the assessment of the graphic content and depictions created by children within an investigative interview.

Lowenfeld's stage theory of artistic development encompasses the developing child between the ages of 2 and 17 years. A child can be advanced or regressed within the phases, but development is sequential and contingent upon mastery of skills (Levick, 1998; Malchiodi, 1998). Although divided into different phases or stages, children's artistic development essentially encompasses three distinct sequences: scribbling, or the beginning of self-expression; schematic, or the child's perception of the environment including people, things and objects; and the naturalistic or realistic interpretation (Malchiodi, 1998). Graphic expectations are associated with each of the artistic developmental levels (Levick, 1998). Knowledge of "typical" (artistic) development is essential to understanding graphic productions created by children. Many factors and influences contribute to maturation or advancement in developmental spheres, including artistic. Just like with other developmental spheres, understanding what is considered to be typical helps in understanding and appreciating what is atypical.

Modifications of Lowenfeld's stage theory have evolved as the nuances associated with children's artistic development have been refined. Lowenfeld's work remains seminal to art therapy and provides a basis for understanding artistic development. Lowenfeld's stages are identified as scribbling, 2 to 4 years; preschematic, 4 to 7 years; schematic, 7 to 9 years; dawning realism, 9 to 11 years; pseudo-naturalistic, 12 to 14 years; and adolescent, 14 to 17 years. Specified elements and artistic features are associated with each stage of development. Drawing and representational characteristics commonly associated with the developmental phases articulated by Lowenfeld follow. The artistic characteristics typically associated with the various phases are highlighted. It must be reiterated that an individual may be advanced or regressed with respect to each phase. As such, the phases are guideposts and provide expectancies rather than norms associated with artistic development and progressive correlates. (Examples of graphic depictions associated with the developmental phases of artistic development were featured in a book chapter by Cohen-Liebman, 2002).

Cognitive, Psychosexual and Artistic Development

Myra Levick, a pioneer in art therapy education, went further in her exploration of graphic representation. She correlated the relationship between cognitive, psychosexual and artistic development (Levick, 1983). Levick's theoretical construct provides a foundation for the art therapist and a context for understanding drawing. The correlation between emotional development, intellectual development and creative expression is fundamental to art therapy (Levick, 1983). Levick also developed criteria for the identification of ego defense mechanisms and ascertained correspondence with graphic productions.

Defense mechanisms exist on a continuum and are indicative of a client's level of functioning. Levick proposed that conflictual and nonconflictual aspects of ego development and function are exposed through graphic expression. This knowledge aids in the identification of areas of fixation and issues that are central to the individual. These theoretical constructs in conjunction with the client's associations contribute to a foundation for understanding artwork as well as a framework for communicating this information.

- psychosexual and cognitive developmental levels relate to developmental sequences in children's drawings
- this knowledge assists in the identification of defense mechanisms in the artwork and areas of fixation, as well as conflicts and issues central to an individual

Rationale for Art Therapy and Art Therapists

Verbal associations in conjunction with graphic depictions foster an understanding of experience and are intrinsic to understanding client artwork. Art therapists are trained and skilled in a host of areas including the use of art media, the creative process and client response to the product generated. Coupled with knowledge of artistic developmental phases, rich foundational principles and teachings underlie art therapy as noted including the correlation with emotional and intellectual development as well as ego defense mechanisms and manifestation in graphic productions. A dynamic relationship, the creative process and the resulting artwork are intrinsic to art therapy. Drawings are not considered in isolation, nor do art therapists interpret for a client; rather, the art therapist assists the client with deriving understanding and making meaning from client-produced or client-created artwork within the context from which it emerges, thus demarcating a process-oriented approach. Not to be remiss, there is a dichotomy or perhaps a continuum that exists in the field that engulfs process versus product; art psychotherapy versus art as therapy which will be considered in Part V. For information about the profession itself, the reader is directed to visit www.arttherapy.org.

Proponents of multidisciplinary child sexual abuse investigations contend that drawing should not be overinterpreted by those not trained and skilled in the use of this technique (Farley, 1987; Hibbard et al., 1987). The supposition exists and is shared that care should be taken in the interpretation of drawings within clinical and forensic contexts (the American Academy of Child and Adolescent Psychiatry, 1990; Burgess & Hartman, 1993; Cohen-Liebman, 1995, 1999; Farley, 1987; Friedrich, 1990; Hibbard et al., 1987; Malchiodi, 1998; Schetky & Benedek, 1992; Sorenson et al., 1997). Reliance solely on a child's drawing as a means of confirmation of sexual abuse has not been established (Cohen-Liebman, 1995; Levick, 1986; Malchiodi, 1990, 1998).

Drawings created within the context of an investigative interview provide data for investigative and interventive purposes (Cohen-Liebman, 2003). When employed in combination with fact-finding processes, drawing may yield information which may contribute to additional or continual exploration, investigation and understanding of a child's experience. An investigative interview which includes drawing may provide insight into a child's coping skills, level of trauma, emotional reaction to the abuse and in many cases, abuse-specific information (Cohen-Liebman, 1999).

The use of art therapy and drawing within a forensic context extends the potentialities inherent in the modality beyond traditional application and signifies an interface within the realm of investigation and the judicial arena. Art therapy is process-oriented. It synthesizes the dynamic interplay that occurs within a relationship that includes the client, the art therapist and the creative process or the artwork, as well as the client's associations or the meaning attributed to the imagery by the client. Judy Rubin states that "whether art is creative or responsive, the therapeutic value is not limited to the clinic or hospital nor to deviant populations. It is a way of working with experiences which are difficult to understand or assimilate" (Rubin, 1979, p. 12).

Lowenfeld's Artistic Development Stage Theory (adapted from Lowenfeld & Brittain, 1987)

- Lowenfeld placed artistic development into a stage theory
- phase-specific developmental sequence associated with artistic development, which occurs in combination with a child's emotional, physical and cognitive development

Scribbling Stage (ages 2 to 4)

- composed of three stages/phases
  - disorganized scribble
    - child is not in control of movement
    - no eye/hand coordination
    - rely on kinesthetic feedback

- o controlled scribble
  - ▪ child realizes marks may be (self) controlled or generated
  - ▪ awareness of eye/hand connection – eye connected to hand
  - ▪ start and stop with the media (structured – crayon/marker)
- o naming of the scribble
  - ▪ progression from kinesthetic to imaginative
  - ▪ name marks
  - ▪ start and stop – control of marks
  - ▪ communication purposes

Transitional Stage (ages 4 to 5)

- • phase between scribbling stage and pre-schematic stage
  - o marks do not look like anything yet but they are more controlled than scribble stage
  - o design phase
  - o scribbles get organized
  - o geometric shapes and letters start to take form
  - o mandalas and tadpoles (head-body fusion) emerge

Pre-Schematic Phase (ages 4 to 7)

- • experiment with different ways of drawing something
  - o draw what they know, not what they see
  - o draw what is important to them
  - o importance is determined by size
  - o space looks haphazard but it is not
  - o space is related to self
  - o referred to as touch space
  - o not fixed forms
  - o children in this stage are egocentric
  - o will see exaggerations and omissions
  - o children leave this phase making a body including parts as relevant
  - o color is not realistic
  - o emotionally/socially children are in the phallic stage of psychosexual development
  - o conflict is oedipal

Schematic Phase (ages 7 to 9)

- o forms lose egocentricity and proportion becomes more real
- o can take another person's point of view
- o personification of sun
- o still see omissions and exaggerations
- o time sequences
- o story telling
- o detailing – use of detail to demarcate what is of interest and significance/importance
- o baseline and skyline
- o flip baselines
- o space becomes linear – horizontally and vertically
  - ▪ way of ordering things
- o use space subjectively
- o demonstrates that child can read – line elements up
- o color is realistic
- o schema is flexible
- o still see geometric shapes
- o tell a story
- o psychosexual stage – latency

(*Continued*)

(Continued)

Dawning Realism (ages 9 to 12)
  - children now draw what they see and how they see
  - schema no longer varies
  - rigid
  - realistic representation
  - no exaggerations and no omissions
  - use pencil and eraser
  - importance of elements is demarcated by details
  - multiple base lines
  - depth is implied – not perspective, but overlapping planes
  - color is more realistic/naturalistic

Pseudo-Naturalism (ages 12 to 14)
  - draw something the way it appears
  - shading, folds, shadows
  - perspective
  - foreshortening
  - natural action
  - three-dimensional tricks
  - secondary sexual characteristics
  - emphasis on details
  - exactness
  - stylizing
  - cartooning – if cannot draw something realistically or naturalistically

Adolescent (ages 14-17)
  - artistic elements
  - subjective interpretations
  - abstraction
  - naturalism
  - affect/mood
  - intentional distortions
  - exaggeration of details

Ethical and Legal Considerations Associated with Drawing

Graphic productions created as part of investigative interview processes are evidentiary material, and as such, confidentiality, ownership, display and disposition of artwork engender ethical concerns that vary from therapeutic processes. All information revealed or disclosed is documented, reported and shared with the investigative team. Intent is fact-finding. Records and process are not subjected to the same safeguarding as therapeutic processes given the emphasis on evidence gathering. Issues attributed to legal considerations are addressed at commencement of the process so that guardians or nonoffending caretakers, as well as children or adolescents, are aware of the nature of the process and the lack of confidentiality. Children are informed at the onset of the process that they are being observed and that information will be shared with the team, including pictorial renderings, to avoid surprises or deception. All parties are informed that information gathered will be shared with team members. Protecting the child's rights as well as the integrity of the process is essential.

Ownership

Artwork created for the purpose of fact-finding is evidence. Artwork relative to fact-finding is not typically shared with the family. The artwork may be retained along with the case file and maintained by the investigative team. It is typically housed where the interview was conducted (this is contingent upon agreements and may extend to jurisdictional oversight). In this way, the evidence is accessible and retrievable in the event it is needed for a judicial procedure or to prepare a child for court.

Confidentiality

* Confidentiality is overridden due to forensic standards
* Everything is "discoverable"
* Not extended to client/interviewer relationship
* Issue must be addressed at commencement of the process (child and nonoffending caretaker)
* Extends to the artwork

References

American Academy of Child and Adolescent Psychiatry. (1990). *Guidelines for the evaluation of child and adolescent sexual abuse.* Author.

American Professional Society on the Abuse of Children. (2002). *Practical guidelines: Investigative interviewing in cases of alleged child abuse.* Author.

Barlow, C. M., Jolley, R. P., & Hallam, J. L. (2011). Drawings as memory aids: Optimising the drawing method to facilitate young children's recall. *Applied Cognitive Psychology, 25,* 480–487.

Burgess, A. W., & Hartman, C. R. (1993). Children's drawings. *Child Abuse and Neglect,* 17, 161–168.

Burgess, A. W., Hartman, C. R., Wolbert, W. A., & Grant, C. A. (1987). Child molestation: Assessing impact in multiple victims (Part I). *Archives of Psychiatric Nursing, 1*(1), 33.

Burgess, A. W., McCausland, M. P., & Wolbert, W. A. (1981). Children's drawings as indicators of sexual trauma. *Perspectives in Psychiatric Care, 19*(2), 50–57.

Butler, S., Gross, J., & Hayne, H. (1995). The effect of drawing on memory performance in young children. *Developmental Psychology, 31,* 597–608.

Cheung, K. F. M. (1997). Developing the interview protocol for video-recorded child sexual abuse investigations: A training experience with police officers, social workers, and clinical psychologists in Hong Kong. *Child Abuse and Neglect, 21*(3), 273–284.

Cohen-Liebman, M. S. (1995). Drawings as judiciary aids in child sexual abuse litigation: A composite list of indicators, *The Arts in Psychotherapy,* special issue on sexual abuse, *22*(5), 475–483.

Cohen-Liebman, M. S. (1999). Draw and tell: Drawings within the context of child sexual abuse investigations. *The Arts in Psychotherapy, 26*(3), 185–194. https://doi.org/10.1016/S0197-4556(99)00013-1

Cohen-Liebman, M. S. (2002). Intro to art therapy. In A. P. Giardino & E. R. Giardino (Eds.), *Recognition of child abuse for the mandated reporter* (3rd ed.). G.W. Medical Publishing.

Cohen-Liebman, M. S. (2003). Drawings in forensic investigations of child sexual abuse. In C. Malchiodi (Ed.), *Handbook of art therapy* (pp. 167–179). Guilford Press.

Cohen-Liebman, M. S. (2007). Parent support group: A non-traditional use of art therapy. In D. Spring (Ed.), *Art in treatment: Transatlantic dialogue* (pp. 68–85). Charles C. Thomas.

Cohen-Liebman, M. S. (2016). Forensic art therapy. In D. Gussak & M. Rosal (Eds.), *The Wiley Blackwell handbook of art therapy* (pp. 469–477). Wiley-Blackwell.

Cohen-Liebman, M. S. (2017). *Drawing and disclosure of experienced events in an art therapy investigative interview process with school aged children: A qualitative comparative analogue study* (Doctoral dissertation). Retrieved from ProQuest Dissertations and Theses database.

Cohen-Liebman, M. S. (2020). Drawing to disclose: Empowering child victims and witnesses in investigative interviews. In M. Berberian & B. Davis (Eds.), *Art therapy practices for resilient youth* (pp. 285–312). Routledge.

Cohen-Liebman, M. S. (2021). Drawing to disclose: Findings from an art therapy-based investigative interview process. In V. Huet & L. Kapitan (Eds.), *The art of practice & research: Art therapy international practice research conference proceedings* (pp. 77–85). Cambridge Scholars Publishing.

Falk, J. D. (1981). Understanding children's art: An analysis of the literature. *Journal of Personality Assessment, 45*(5), 465–472.

Faller, K. C. (1993). *Child sexual abuse: Assessment and intervention issues.* U.S. Department of Health and Human Services, National Center on Child Abuse and Neglect.

Faller, K. C. (2005). Anatomical dolls: Their use in assessment of children who may have been sexually abused. *Journal of Child Sexual Abuse, 14*(3), 1–21.

Faller, K. C. (2014). Forty years of forensic interviewing of children suspected of sexual abuse, 1974–2014: Historical benchmarks. *Social Sciences, 4*(1), 34–65.

Farley, R. H. (1987). Drawing interviews: An alternative technique. *The Police Chief, 54*(4), 37–38.

Friedrich, W. N. (1990). *Psychotherapy of sexually abused children and their families.* Norton.

Gee, S., & Pipe, M. E. (1995). Helping children to remember: The influence of object cues on children's accounts of real events. *Developmental Psychology, 31,* 746–758.

Gross, J., & Hayne, H. (1998). Drawing facilitates children's verbal reports of emotionally laden events. *Journal of Experimental Psychology: Applied, 14,* 163–179.

Gross, J., & Hayne, H. (1999). Drawing facilitates children's verbal reports after long delays. *Journal of Experimental Psychology: Applied, 5,* 265–283.

Gussak, D. (2013). *Art on trial: Art therapy in capital murder cases.* Columbia University Press.

Gussak, D., & Cohen-Liebman, M. S. (2001). Investigation vs. intervention: Forensic art therapy and art therapy in forensic settings. *American Journal of Art Therapy, 40,* 123–135.

Haralambie, A. M. (1999). *Child sexual abuse in civil cases: A guide to custody and tort actions.* American Bar Association.

Hewett, S. (1999). *Assessing allegations of sexual abuse in preschool children: Understanding small voices.* Sage.

Hibbard, R. A., Roghmann, K., & Hoekelman, R. A. (1987). Genitalia in children's drawings: An association with sexual abuse. *Pediatrics, 79*(1), 129–137.

Hoorwitz, A. N. (1992). *The clinical detective: Techniques in the evaluation of sexual abuse.* W.W. Norton.

Jolley, R. P. (2010). *Children and pictures: Drawing and understanding.* Wiley-Blackwell.

Katz, C., & Hershkowitz, I. (2010). The effects of drawing on children's accounts of sexual abuse. *Child Maltreatment, 15*(2), 171–179.

Katz, C., & Hershkowitz, I. (2013). Repeated interviews with children who are the alleged victims of sexual abuse. *Research on Social Work Practice, 23*(2), 210–218.

Kelley, S. J. (1984). The use of art therapy with sexually abused children. *Journal of Psychosocial Nursing, 22*(12), 12–18.

Kellogg, R. (1970). *Analyzing children's art.* Mayfield Publishing Company.

Kendall-Tackett, K. A. (1992). Beyond anatomical dolls: Professionals' use of other play therapy techniques. *Child Abuse & Neglect, 16*(1), 139–142.

Lamb, M. E., & Brown, D. A. (2006). Conversational apprentices: Helping children become competent informants about their own experiences. *British Journal of Developmental Psychology, 24*(1), 215–234.

Lamb, M. E., Orbach, Y., Hershkowitz, I., Esplin, P. W., & Horowitz, D. (2007). A structured forensic interview protocol improves the quality and informativeness of investigative interviews with children: A review of research using the NICHD investigative interview protocol. *Child Abuse & Neglect, 31*(11), 1201–1231.

Landgarten, H. (1987). *Family art psychotherapy.* Brunner/Mazel.

Levick, M. F. (1983). *They could not talk and so they drew.* Charles C. Thomas.

Levick, M. F. (1986). *Mommy daddy look what I'm saying.* M. Evans.

Levick, M. F. (1998). *See what I'm saying: What children tell us through their art.* Islewest Publishing.

Lippmann, J. (2002). Psychological issues. In M. Finkel & A. Giardino (Eds.), *Medical evaluation of child sexual abuse: A practical guide* (2nd ed., pp. 193–211). Sage Publications Inc.

Lowenfeld, V., & Brittain, W. L. (1987). *Creative and mental growth.* MacMillan Publishing Company.

Lyon, T. D., & Ahern, E. C. (2011). Disclosure of child sexual abuse. In J. E. B. Myers (Ed.), *The APSAC handbook on child maltreatment* (3rd ed., pp. 233–252). Sage Publications, Inc.

Malchiodi, C. A. (1990). *Breaking the silence: Art therapy with children from violent homes.* Brunner/Mazel.

Malchiodi, C. A. (1998). *Understanding children's drawings.* The Guilford Press.

Miller, T. W., Veltkamp, L. J., & Janson, D. (1987). Projective measures in the clinical evaluation of sexually abused children. *Child Psychiatry and Human Development, 18*(1), 47–57.

Myers, J. E. B. (1992). *Legal issues in child abuse and neglect.* Sage Publications, Inc.

Patterson, T., & Hayne, H. (2011). Does drawing facilitate older children's reports of emotionally laden events? *Applied Cognitive Psychology, 25*, 119–126.

Poole, D. A. (2016). *Interviewing children: The science of conversation in forensic contexts.* American Psychological Association.

Poole, D. A., & Bruck, M. (2012). Divining testimony? The impact of interviewing props on children's reports of touching. *Developmental Review, 32*(3), 165–180.

Poole, D. A., & Lamb, M. E. (1998). *Investigative interviews of children: A guide for helping professionals.* American Psychological Association.

Poole, D. A., & Lamb, M. E. (2009). *Investigative interviews of Children: A guide for helping professions.* American Psychological Association.

Powell, L., & Faherty, S. L. (1990). Treating sexually abused latency age girls: A 20 session treatment plan utilizing group process and the creative arts therapies. *The Arts in Psychotherapy, 17,* 35–47.

Rubin, J. (1979). Art therapy: An introduction. In *Conference on creative arts therapies [Monograph]* (pp. 12–14). American Psychiatric Association.

Salmon, K. (2006). Toys in clinical interviews with children: Review and implications for practice. *Clinical Psychologist, 10*(2), 54–59.

Salmon, K., Roncolato, W., & Gleitzman, M. (2003). Children's report of emotionally laden events: Adapting the interview to the child. *Applied Cognitive Psychology, 17*(1), 65–79.

Saywitz, K., Lyon, T., & Goodman, G. (2011). Interviewing children. In J. Myers (Ed.), *The APSAC handbook of child maltreatment* (3rd ed., pp. 337–360). Sage Publications, Inc.

Saywitz, K., Lyon, T., & Goodman, G. (2018). When interviewing children: A review and update. In B. Klika & J. Conte (Eds.), *The APSAC handbook on child maltreatment* (pp. 310–329). Sage Publications, Inc.

Schetky, D. H., & Benedek, E. (1992). *Clinical handbook of child psychiatry and the law.* Williams & Wilkins.

Shepherd, J., Dworin, B., Farley, R., Russ, B., Tressler, P., & National Center for Missing and Exploited Children. (1995, April). *Child abuse and exploitation investigative techniques* (2nd ed.). Office of Juvenile Justice and Delinquency Prevention.

Silver, R. A. (1989). *Developing cognitive and creative skills through art: Programs for children with communication disorders or learning disabilities.* Ablin Press.

Smart, M. (1986). Expanded work settings for art therapy. *Art Therapy, 3*, 21–26.

Sorenson, E., Bottoms, B., & Perona, A. (1997). *Handbook on intake and forensic interviewing in the children's advocacy center setting.* Office of Juvenile Justice and Delinquency Prevention.

Steele, L. C. (2012). The forensic interview: A challenging conversation. In P. Goodyear-Brown (Ed.), *Handbook of child sexual abuse; Identification, assessment and treatment* (pp. 99–119). Wiley-Blackwell.

Veltkamp, L. J., & Miller, T. W. (1994). *Clinical handbook of child abuse and neglect.* International Universities Press.

Wadeson, H. (2010). *Art psychotherapy* (2nd ed.). John Wiley & Sons.

Wakefield, H., & Underwager, R. (1998). The application of images in child abuse investigations. In J. Prosser (Ed.), *Image-based research: A sourcebook for qualitative researchers* (pp. 176–194). Falmer Press.

Wesson, M., & Salmon, K. (2001). Drawing and showing: Helping children to report emotionally laden events. *Applied Cognitive Psychology, 15*, 301–320.

Part III   The Art of Testifying

Legal, Forensic and Judicial Tenets

Modern use of expert testimony developed in the 18th century. Witnesses provided a trier of fact, meaning a judge or jury, with knowledge rather than opinion. The adversary system of justice was founded on the belief that the most effective way to arrive at just results was predicated upon each side presenting evidence which encompassed knowledge and facts. The belief was that from the presentation of evidence by each side of an issue, the trier of fact would be able to decipher the truth. As such, the determination of truth was relegated to the judge or jury, which had sole province on deciding the issue before the court. The trier of fact was tasked with concluding from the evidence the facts of the case. Exercising opinions and conclusions to determine a verdict became the domain of the jury.

This practice necessitated that the trier of fact was provided with informed and unbiased material, including opinions proffered by experts. Ultimately, the goal of the adversary system was the acquisition of the truth. The procedural method established that truth would emerge through courtroom confrontation of adversaries (Myers, 1992). To obtain credence in the courtroom and in accordance with proceedings and to thwart bias, the process of cross examination, an antibiased device, was conceived to establish and confirm competency and credibility of witnesses in the courtroom. Cross examination is utilized as a means to assist the court in the evaluation of a witness's reliability and credibility, as well as the accuracy of the evidence the witness presents. The primary focus of cross examination of an expert witness "[m]ay be to challenge the expert's qualifications or impartiality, as well as the factual and theoretical basis of his opinions" (Barsky & Gould, 2002, p. 178).

Adversary System of Justice

- modern use of expert testimony developed in the 18th century
- witnesses provided the trier of fact with knowledge rather than opinion
- exercising opinions and conclusions to determine a verdict became the sole province of the jury
- founded on the belief that the most effective way to arrive at just results is for each side to present evidence and let the judge/jury decide where the truth lies
- ensures informed, unbiased expert opinion
- antibiased device which tests competency and credibility

    - cross examination

The Court System

In the United States, a two-court system exists. This system is composed of state and federal courts. State courts mediate and lobby jurisdiction over state laws, while federal

DOI: 10.4324/9781003225041-4

courts provide guidance and governance over federal laws. In some cases, the notion of dual sovereignty exists in which a case may be tried in both state and federal court. The Supreme Court is the final authority for the court system.

Legal Proceedings

In the United States there are two types of legal proceedings: civil and criminal. Each has a respective burden of proof that is distinct and distinguishes the type of proceeding. The goals and objectives differ depending upon the nature of the court. In family or civil court, the aim is protection and resolution, whereas in a criminal process the emphasis is directed toward punitive measures, restitution and even rehabilitation. It is incumbent upon the individual (expert) working within the court system to know the jurisdictional proclivities of the community, county and state where the individual practices and serves clients.

Juvenile Court

Juvenile court is considered by some jurisdictions as a partner with child protective services (CPS); however, different goals and allegiances exist. Although juvenile court has the authority to intervene to protect children, the court also has a duty to protect everyone within the court, which means the family, which encompasses the child or children (who may be present due to allegations of abuse) as well as the parents and the government (which is represented by CPS). Myers (2011a) explains that CPS workers "are the gatekeepers to juvenile court", yet the responsibility initially is to the law, despite an emphasis on protection of youth, as CPS determines "when and whether to invoke the authority of the juvenile court" (p. 57). CPS also must take into consideration protection of all rights and the welfare of the parties involved; however, "CPS workers are primarily concerned with "protecting children from maltreatment" (Myers, 2011a, p. 56).

> [T]he different perspectives of social work and law engender beneficial checks and balances that temper the tendency toward extremes that are inevitable in complex human endeavors – particularly endeavors involving intense emotion and the exercise of state power over individuals. (Myers, 2011a, p. 57)

A formal proceeding begins with the filing of a petition, which is applicable to all lawsuits both civil and criminal (Myers, 2011a). In juvenile court, where the burden of proof is with child protection, abuse or maltreatment must be proved by CPS such that a preponderance of evidence exists.

Civil

Civil proceedings encompass many types of litigation, including cases that may be associated with family court or juvenile court where child welfare is a primary focus. In a civil case, the burden to be met to establish guilt is a "preponderance of evidence". Depending upon the jurisdiction, courts may organize and assign cases differently. In a civil proceeding there is more leeway regarding process and procedure. These proceedings are less formal than criminal proceedings, and the environment may be referred to as relaxed in some settings. The fact-finder role is ascribed to the judge because typically there are no juries.

Through time and experience, an individual will develop understanding and skills and form relationships with key personalities that subsist and interface in this court context. The flexibility and less strident ambiance that pervade civil court are congruent with the permissibility of experts testifying. The rationale is that without the presence of a jury (usually just a judge), acquiescence to the expertise communicated either due to presentation or status is not an issue. The proceedings are focused on the child rather than the guilt or innocence of an individual. It is believed that the judge will weigh the facts and evidence in assessing the truth and not be unduly influenced by an expert witness.

Criminal

The burden in criminal proceedings is definitive: "beyond reasonable doubt". As such, the defendant (offender) must be found to have committed a crime with unlawful intent. The focus is directed at offender accountability. The defendant must be found to be guilty or not guilty beyond a reasonable doubt (95%). The fact-finder may be either a judge or a jury. Strict adherence to rules of evidence pervades criminal proceedings. If a defendant is found not guilty, that finding does not necessarily mean the trier of fact did not believe the person committed the crime they are on trial for. Rather, it means that the evidence to establish and meet the burden of proof was not met and, as such, the defendant is determined to be not guilty in accordance with the law.

Legal Proceedings

- **Criminal**
    - burden – beyond reasonable doubt
        - committed crime with unlawful intent
        - guilty or not guilty
        - strict adherence to rules of evidence
- **Civil**
    - burden – preponderance of evidence
        - encompasses many types of litigation
        - in family court – aim is to protect child or children and resolution

Testimonial Capability

In the court system a witness may testify in one of two capacities: a lay witness or an expert witness. Litigation often involves technical, clinical or scientific issues that are beyond the understanding of the average juror. Assistance is provided by individuals with specialized knowledge that serve in the capacity of an expert witness.

Lay Witness

The concept of a lay witness is expansive in that anyone can present at court and testify in this capacity. A lay witness is also considered a fact witness. An individual who presents as a lay witness is called to testify about knowledge or facts pertaining to a topic or a subject that the witness has experience with, meaning that the lay witness provides information about something they have observed or, in the case of a person, interacted with or engaged with in some manner. Lay witnesses speak about relevant facts related to the matter in which they have personal information. The testimony provided by a lay witness is based on personal knowledge rather than opinion or inference. Lay witnesses are limited to discussing personal observations. A lay or fact witness does not garner special status like an expert who is awarded certain privileges. Fact or lay witnesses may not testify as to matters of opinion. In a case related to sexual abuse, a lay witness might repeat what a child disclosed (depending upon admissibility rules), while an expert may offer interpretation.

Lay Witness

There are guiding principles that are aligned with what a lay witness may and may not offer in court. Lay witnesses are not allowed to offer an opinion as to the issue that is before the court, for example, if a child was sexually abused. A lay witness is constricted to providing factual information, meaning they may speak to personal knowledge that they possess such as facts, observations or knowledge gathered from their experience with an individual or related to the issue before the court.

- direct observations
- cannot give an opinion in court
- speak to knowledge, facts, observations

Expert Witness

An individual presenting in court as an expert witness presents differently than a lay witness. Certain expectations accompany this status and are associated with the presentation offered by an expert on the witness stand. As such, expert witness status garners special privileges in court because the expert must demonstrate and meet certain qualifications to be considered an expert. The judge, through a special process (if deemed applicable or necessary), will determine if an individual is qualified to present as an expert through a procedure known as voir dire.

Voir dire provides the calling counsel (the attorney who asks for the individual to be qualified as an expert) with an opportunity to establish a foundation for the expertise of the proposed expert. This method takes precedence to admittance of an expert stating an opinion. Once qualified as an expert in a particular subject, topic or area, the expert may provide an opinion as well as respond to hypothetical questions. An expert does not have to be the foremost authority on a particular topic; however, expertise must be established in order for the individual to be recognized as someone that is qualified to provide expert testimony on a given subject.

Expert witness testimony is deemed prudent when specialized knowledge will help the trier of fact. An issue need not be completely beyond the understanding of the trier of fact (judge or, in criminal cases, jury) in order for an expert witness to be retained. Expert testimony can add depth to understanding. Expert testimony can also be used to disabuse commonly held misperceptions about relatively common topics. The judge will determine if an individual offered by either side, meaning the prosecution or the defense, has the expertise to assist the jury to understand the evidence or to determine a fact in issue. Again, an expert does not have to be the ultimate authority on a specific topic.

Experts speak about topics familiar to them and in which they have experience such as child abuse. An expert is brought into court to help inform the judge or jury about topics that may not be common or familiar to the average juror or to offer assistance, as noted earlier. Jurors are citizens who are randomly selected from a pool of individuals requested to come to court and serve as jurors. Jurors may fill out a questionnaire and be subjected to questioning by attorneys as well as the judge assigned to a case to determine if an individual satisfies the criteria to serve as a juror for the case that a jury is being seated for. If chosen by the lawyers assigned to a case, these individuals remain in the courtroom, listen to the facts of the case as presented by both sides and deliberate before rendering a determination on the matter before the court.

Expert testimony has different manifestations within a courtroom. An expert may offer an opinion about the issue that is before the court. The opinion is based upon a reasonable degree of certainty about a subject. Myers (2002) explains this concept in the following manner: Certainty "lies somewhere between guesswork and complete certainty" (p. 248). Experts may provide information about a topic, and they can speak to questions not posed to lay witnesses. Expert witnesses are expected to be unbiased and credible. The information proffered by an expert witness is utilized to either support or defend an opinion.

> Whenever the trier of fact is confronted with issues which cannot be determined intelligently based on ordinary judgement and practical experience gained through the usual affairs of life, the benefit of scientific or specialized knowledge or experience may be provided by use of expert testimony. The expert provides an opinion "that is a reasonable probability rather than conjecture or speculation".
>
> (Ladd, 1952, p. 419)

Forms of Expert Testimony

Expert testimony may take one of three forms: an opinion, a response to a hypothetical question and providing education about a topic (Myers, 2011c). An expert is not limited to one form when testifying. An expert may combine the different forms of testimony.

- an opinion
  - must be reasonably confident (Myers, 2011b)
- answer to a hypothetical question
- dissertation providing background information on a relevant topic

Experts do not need to know all of the rules associated with expert testimony (that is for the attorney to know and to prepare the expert accordingly), but an expert should know enough to avoid mistakes when presenting testimony. Experts are not allowed to testify that a child told the truth. Judges grant more latitude to experts in noncriminal cases. For example, a judge might allow an expert to give an opinion in juvenile or family court that would not otherwise be sanctioned in criminal court. In certain circumstances, a judge may limit or disallow expert testimony due to concern that the jury will defer to the expert and abdicate the role assigned to the jury.

Opinion Testimony

Opinion testimony is offered based upon reliable certainty. Experts are not supposed to speculate or guess. They do not, however, have to be completely certain before offering opinions. Degrees of certainty as noted range between guesswork and absolute certainty

(Myers, 1996). The judge or jury considers how much confidence can be placed in the facts underlying the expert's opinion. The important question is "whether the expert's opinion is logical, consistent, explainable, objective and defensible" (Myers, 1996, p. 322).

Examples of questions to consider with regard to opinion testimony are provided by John Myers (Myers, 1996):

- Does the expert have adequate understanding of pertinent clinical and scientific principles?
- Have the principles been subjected to rigorous testing?
- Have the principles the expert is relying on been published in peer-reviewed journals?

    - Are they accepted as reliable by experts in the field?

- Did the expert employ appropriate methods of assessment?
- Are the inferences and conclusions defensible?
- Is the expert reasonably objective?

Experts draw upon many sources of information to reach a conclusion. Generally, experts are allowed to base their testimony on the same sources of information they rely on in their daily work. Experts typically do not address credibility or truthfulness of others, as that is for the trier of fact to determine.

Combination Testimony

Another form of expert testimony that is utilized in child sexual abuse cases consists of a combination of lay and expert testimony. As such, behaviors observed in sexually abused children as a class are discussed by the expert in combination with lay testimony (by a fact witness), establishing that the child or complainant demonstrates such behaviors. This type of expert testimony does not focus specifically on the child involved in the case; rather, it speaks to sexually abused children as a class. Expert testimony that a child demonstrates behaviors commonly associated with sexually abused children is distinct from expert testimony that a particular child was sexually abused. In this capacity, the expert is not offering an opinion on the ultimate question of whether abuse of a particular child occurred (Myers, 1996).

Experts do not need personal knowledge of a case or a particular child (for example, in a child sexual abuse case). In certain cases, an expert who is not personally involved with a particular case or client may be brought into the court to discuss a group of individuals or behaviors associated with a genre such as sexually abused children and speak to the genre as a whole. This type of testimony is used to clarify or explain why a particular child may have acted in a particular way or exhibited a type of behavior that is consistent with sexually abused children. In some cases, an expert can testify as both lay and expert witness, depending upon whether the individual was involved in the case personally and if the witness also has expertise about the topic beyond a lay witness, which may be useful in court.

Exemplar

Perhaps a young child disclosed to an adult that something happened to the child. The adult to whom the child made the disclosure may be brought into court to testify as a lay witness and provide knowledge about what the child said. The adult may speak about the context and explain the circumstances in which the disclosure was made by the child. If later the child denies making the allegations and recants or takes back what was originally shared, an expert who may not know the child but is someone identified as a specialist in sexual abuse may be asked to testify about sexually abused children and recantation. The expert will ideally possess knowledge about the dynamics and mechanics of child sexual abuse and the process of disclosure. This individual will be asked to clarify and educate the trier of fact as to why a child might recant allegations of sexual abuse. This is done when information is beyond the scope of the lay witness, who may not possess expertise in the dynamics and mechanics of sexual abuse, including the process of disclosure, thus necessitating the introduction of an expert to testify about why a child who made allegations of sexual abuse may recant.

The goal of integrating lay witness and expert testimony is to educate the jury or the judge about why a particular child may be doing something that is consistent with a given population. In this case, explaining the behavior that the child is exhibiting in relation to what is commonly associated with child sexual abuse by the expert is offered to assist the trier of fact in understanding what may be compatible or consistent with this class or group of people (sexually abused children). The expert will also most likely demonstrate general acceptance of the issue which will be addressed later.

Experts Testify

- on subjects which are familiar
- to help explain subjects beyond the ken of the average juror
- to clarify commonly held misconceptions about common events/subjects
- testimony should be relevant, helpful and reliable
- the issue is whether the expert can assist the jury to understand the evidence or to determine a fact in issue
- an expert supports and defends an opinion
- are expected to be unbiased and credible

Mental Health Expert Witnesses and Child Sexual Abuse

To serve as an expert mental health witness, an individual must qualify under the rules of evidence and belong to a legally recognized mental health profession (Bolocofsky, 1989). These requirements in and of themselves do not ensure that an individual is a competent witness. Discretion resides with the court in determining the competency of a mental health professional to present as an expert.

Three critical factors relate to the qualification of an expert in child sexual abuse: extensive firsthand experience with sexually and nonsexually abused children, a thorough and up-to-date knowledge of the professional literature on child sexual abuse and objectivity and neutrality about individual cases (Myers et al., 1989). Techniques and skills employed by the expert are important to consider, as is admissibility. The party or the attorney (prosecution or defense) that offers the testimony has the responsibility of establishing the witness's qualifications. The experience through which an expert has gained specialized knowledge is important to the weight of the testimony as well as for admissibility of the testimony.

Witnesses establishing expert qualification are questioned on the witness stand regarding education, specialized training and relevant experience. Advanced degrees, membership in professional organizations and publications regarding child sexual abuse are additional areas that are explored. Previous expert status in prior cases of child sexual abuse litigation is another consideration in the qualification process, as is current employment status and past professional experience. Experience working with sexually abused children will be questioned as well. Expert witnesses need not be knowledgeable about all aspects of an issue.

Testimonial Privileges

Privileges exist within legal proceedings that involve testifying or when an individual is requested to provide testimony such as during a deposition. This means that some confidential communications may not be disclosed if a privilege is determined. Myers (2011a) states, "A privilege gives protection that is greater than the protection afforded by the ethical duty to protect confidential information" (p. 365). A witness is advised to discuss what constitutes privileged communications when contacted to testify by an attorney in a particular case. If a witness is court-appointed, that witness acts in a quasi-judicial capacity and is entitled to protection of absolute immunity, so the expert presents objectively (Schetky & Benedek, 1992).

Testimonial Capability

Lay Witness	Expert Witness
• provides personal knowledge • cannot offer opinion • reports direct observations • speaks about knowledge, facts or observations	• may testify in the form of an opinion • judge determines who qualifies as an expert • does not need to be foremost authority on a particular topic • may answer hypothetical questions • provides information about individuals he or she may not have had contact with • can apply group data to individual cases • can aggregate information or data and relate it to an individual

Federal Rules That Govern Expert Testimony:

Rule 702

Federal Rule 702 is the basic principle governing admission of expert testimony in a court of law. The rule states:

> If scientific, technical or other specialized knowledge will assist the trier of fact to understand the evidence or to determine a fact in issue, a witness qualified as an expert by knowledge, skill, experience, training or education may testify thereto in the form of an opinion or otherwise.
>
> (Myers et al., 1989, p. 6)

The rule establishes that testimony must be relevant to a matter that is in dispute. It must be reliable; thus, it must have a scientific or some other basis. Finally, it must be not otherwise available to the average juror. In essence, the probative value must be greater than the prejudicial effect (Smith, 1989).

Update Regarding Rule 702 (adaped from)

American Prosecutors Research Institute National Center for Prosecution of Child Abuse (Brown, 2001)

In 2000, Federal Rule of Evidence 702 was updated by Congress and included a clause at the end of the definition that reads: if (1) the testimony is based upon sufficient facts or data (2) the testimony is the product of reliable principles and methods, and (3) the witness has applied the principles and methods reliably to the facts of the case (Brown, 2001).

Essentially the inclusion of this addition means that the Federal Rule is applicable to all experts from all disciplines, not just scientific experts. Moreover, the language "defines the role of the court as gatekeeper based on criteria of reliable methodology" (Brown, 2001), which means that reliability of the information must be proven prior to testifying. The methodology of the expert's basis for testimony, rather than the content of the testimony, is for the court to determine. This provides courts with the ability to determine what information is reliable versus what is unreliable. "When conclusions are examined, it is always in the context of what process was used to reach them" (Brown, 2001). This refers not to the expert's conclusions or opinion, but rather the method(s) "applied to form those conclusions".

In total, the new language "merely serves as a way to perform a gatekeeping function to ensure that all testifying experts used reliable methods when reaching conclusions" (Brown, 2001). "A court's ruling on an expert's testimony is based on the reliability of the methodology used, not on the content of the testimony" (Brown, 2001). Reliable means "as determined by the standards of the Field". The rule still encompasses the standards utilized to assess reliability that are articulated in Daubert (to be explained).

Finally, Brown (2001) states that "prosecutors should also consider the new Rule 702 a valuable tool when using experts for their own cases. Because the new language explicitly sets the same standard of scrutiny for all experts, prosecutors should aggressively use testimony from soft science experts in their cases". As such, experts on "interviewing techniques, memory and suggestibility or other psychological topics should be seriously considered because now there is a demonstrable, definite standard against which to demonstrate to the courts that their testimony is reliable and beneficial".

Federal Rules of Evidence 703, 704 and 705 permit experts to base an opinion on information that would not ordinarily be admissible as evidence, to testify to ultimate issues and to express opinions without first having disclosed the underlying facts that gave rise to the opinion, respectively (Myers et al., 1989). With regard to the ultimate issue, many scholars believe that mental health experts should not be allowed to provide an opinion regarding ultimate legal issues. This is based on the belief that it is not within the jurisdiction of the expert to speak to the ultimate issue that is before the court in the manner of an opinion. The limitation on opinion testimony is known as the ultimate issue rule.

An opinion that a child has been sexually abused mirrors the legal issue that is before the court in such cases. An expert can testify through alternative means about the sexual abuse of the child without resorting to an opinion. For instance, in child sexual abuse litigation, an expert can discuss inappropriate sexual knowledge possessed by the child. The ultimate issue is whether the abuse has occurred. In most states experts are allowed to state their opinions as being of "reasonable certainty" due to the belief that the jurors will be able to weigh appropriately the opinions and information entered as evidence.

It is the jurisdiction of the trial judge to determine if the proffered testimony meets the requirements of Rule 702. Admissibility of the testimony is determined with regard to whether the testimony will assist the trier of fact. In cases without a jury, the judge is the trier of fact. In a jury trial, the jury assumes the role of the trier of fact. It bears repeating that a jury is composed of a body of ordinary people, necessitating the dissemination of information in a manner that allows the jury to exercise sound judgement in determining the ultimate issue. Testimony that is applicable for one case may not be admissible in others.

The federal rules allow that expert testimony need not be limited to subject matter that is beyond the understanding of the average juror. Experts can offer depth and insight to subjects of familiarity, and their testimony can be admitted to disabuse misconceptions about commonly held subjects. Testimony should be relevant, helpful and reliable (Myers, 2011a). The issue is whether the expert can assist the jury to understand the evidence or to determine a fact in issue. As such, the expert provides testimony that is unbiased while providing opinions, which the expert must support and perhaps defend, for instance, when being cross examined.

Voir Dire

In order for a judge to confer expert witness status, especially if the expert is being offered to the court in the guise of an expert for the first time, a judge may conduct a separate hearing known as voir dire. This process is intended to establish an individual's credentials. Voir dire, which means "to speak the truth", is a preliminary examination of a potential witness's qualifications. The proceeding is directed at establishing the qualifications of the witness in order for the witness to present testimony in the manner designated, such as in the guise of an expert. In alignment with Federal Rule 702 as noted earlier, the judge conducts the process to establish the proffered expert's knowledge, skill, experience, training and/or education on the issue or related issue before the court. Voir dire is essentially a hearing within a hearing to establish a foundation of expertise. Expertise must be established before the expert's opinion is admissible. Opposing counsel will have the opportunity to conduct a "mini" cross examination of the expert after the expert's qualifications have been presented.

Voir dire is a three-part process designed to establish expertise. Questions will focus on three areas:

1. The witness's credentials, including background and training, in an attempt to establish and showcase why this individual should be considered an expert on a particular topic (which is designated in relation to the case).
2. The nature of the witness's expertise; the field and type of practice that make the individual a witness.
3. The specific case.

It is the responsibility of the party offering the expert testimony to establish the expert's qualifications. As such, the expert will be asked questions directed at the credentials, including background, experience and expertise regarding a particular subject. Educational accomplishments, specialized training and relevant experience may be assessed in an effort for the judge to render an opinion as to whether or not an individual may be qualified as an expert witness as opposed to a lay witness. The expert is granted special privileges.

The expert witness should have a court-ready curriculum vitae (CV) listing information pertinent to the material to be asked on the witness stand. The CV is designed for court and may not be inclusive of information that may be presented in the same manner as if the individual were applying for a job or an academic position. For the most part, the information is essentially the same, as it details the individual's background and training and reflects the strengths of the witness with regard to specialization. It is designed to be informative for the qualification process and highlight the information that will be concentrated on by the presenting counsel. (CV prep and scripting will be addressed later and sample material will be provided).

Novel Scientific Evidence

Expert testimony based on scientific principles or techniques may require a special rule of admissibility. This rule governs techniques that are of novel or dubious reliability. The purpose of the rule is to exclude expert testimony based on unreliable scientific principles or techniques. This type of evidence comes into play when expert testimony is based on scientific principles or techniques of questionable reliability, including machines, devices and techniques (Myers, 2019). Such evidence may garner a special admissibility hearing to thwart the presentation of unreliable scientific principles or techniques in court. Novel scientific evidence may be considered in one of two forms. Different tests that can be used to determine reliability are Frye (general acceptance) and Daubert (relevance analysis).

Novel Scientific Evidence Rule, Two Forms

1. **FRYE RULE – General Acceptance Rule**
2. **DAUBERT – Relevance Analysis**

Frye Rule

The Frye rule, which was the standard for many years before Daubert was recognized, means that the trier of fact must be convinced that the (novel) principle is generally accepted as reliable in the relevant professional community. Frye used to be the dominant rule, but in recent years it has been challenged or rejected since it sometimes excludes scientific and clinical information that may help the jury (Myers, 1992). Four sources of evidence can be used to establish general acceptance in accordance with the Frye rule: informed testimony (testify to general acceptance), relevant literature, guidelines from professional organizations and prior court decisions.

Novel Scientific Evidence

Novel scientific evidence is subjected to a special admissibility test. Reliability is the issue of concern. It is the court's jurisdiction to decide if evidence is reliable or not. When expert testimony is based on scientific principles or techniques of dubious or questionable reliability, such evidence may be subjected to a special admissibility hearing so that the presentation of unreliable scientific principles or techniques is prevented in court.

With regard to Frye and Daubert, not everything is subjected to either principle, as courts limit the use of these principles "to expert testimony based on novel scientific principles, machines, devices and techniques" (Myers, 2019, p. 91). Essentially Myers states, "If the primary concern is protecting juries from 'junk science' the best approach is to apply Frye or Daubert to any expert testimony of dubious validity or reliability, whether in the form of opinion or a little black box" (Myers, 2019, p. 92).

- special rule of admissibility
- purpose is to exclude unreliable scientific principles or techniques
- subjected to a special admissibility test
- applicable when expert testimony is based upon scientific principles of questionable, dubious or ambiguous reliability
- it is the court's jurisdiction to decide if evidence is reliable or not
- issue of concern is reliability
- different tests can be used to determine reliability, Frye or Daubert

Daubert

In 1993 the U.S. Supreme Court adopted Daubert for federal courts, rejecting the Frye rule and general acceptance. The Daubert rule stems from the case *Daubert v. Merrell Dow Pharmaceuticals, Inc.* Daubert is not binding on state courts; however, it tends to influence judges. Daubert consists of a process referred to as relevance analysis. This two-step process involves a judge conducting an inquiry to assess the reliability of scientific principles supporting the expert testimony. In assessing reliability, the judge considers whether "the rule can be and has been tested to determine its reliability and validity" (Myers, 1992, p. 324).

Daubert, in essence, incorporates the Frye rule, which is predicated upon general acceptance. The standards governing the use of the principle address whether peer-reviewed literature incorporates discussion of the principle, as well as the standards governing the use of it and how often the results are accurate. Daubert entails subjective analysis versus objective analysis. With relevance analysis, the judge conducts an inquiry into the reliability of scientific principles supporting the expert testimony.

Daubert involves (Myers, 1992)

- how often the principle yields accurate results
- the existence of standards governing use of the principle to ensure accurate results
- degrees to which expert testimony is based on subjective analysis as opposed to objective analysis
- publication in the peer-reviewed literature – publication is but one element of peer review
- whether the scientific or clinical practice is generally accepted by experts in the field
  - Frye rule – widespread acceptance can be important in determining admissible evidence
- whether the principle or technique is consistent with established and proven modes of analysis
- when the special rule governing scientific evidence applies;
  not every time and when an expert's testimony is based in whole or in part on scientific principles
- many scientific principles are well established; thus, a judge takes judicial notice of the reliability of the principles

---

Frye – General Acceptance Rule

- must convince trier of fact that the principle is generally accepted as reliable in the relevant professional community
- four sources of evidence can be used to establish general acceptance through informed testimony

  - general acceptance
  - relevant literature
  - guidelines from professional organizations
  - prior court decisions

Daubert – Relevance Analysis

- adopted in 1993 for federal courts rejecting Frye (general acceptance)
- relevance analysis – two-step process
- judge conducts an inquiry to assess the reliability of scientific principles supporting the expert testimony

- in assessing reliability, the judge considers whether the principle can be and has been tested to determine its reliability and validity
- how often accurate results are yielded
- standards governing use
- subjective analysis versus objective
- publication in peer-reviewed literature
- general acceptance (Frye)

Myers (2019), states:

It is the court's jurisdiction to decide if evidence is novel or scientific. The issue of concern is reliability. The different tests are used by the court to determine reliability with regard to novel scientific evidence. With regard to Frye and Daubert, Myers (2019) states that "in the vast majority of cases involving expert testimony, there is no Frye or Daubert hearing". Rather, "the expert gets on the witness stand, is qualified, testifies, is cross-examined, and that is the end of it. Frye or Daubert only arise in exceptional cases" (Myers, 2019, p. 90).

Drawings as Novel Scientific Evidence

Drawings are considered novel scientific evidence in the court system. In order to be admitted as evidence, the admissibility of drawings is determined through specific principles. Novel scientific evidence is subjected to a special admissibility test if proffered expert testimony is believed to be based upon novel scientific principles. A hearing may be conducted to evaluate the admissibility of the evidence. The special admissibility test is applicable when expert testimony is judged by the court to be less accessible to lay analysis than other types of evidence. The special admissibility test is applicable when expert testimony is based on scientific principles of questionable reliability (Myers et al., 1989).

If the Frye rule is invoked, four sources of evidence can be used to establish general acceptance. Witnesses may be called to testify regarding general acceptance. The quality of the testimony, rather than the number of witnesses, aids in the establishment of acceptance. Witnesses should possess significant expertise regarding the scientific principle at issue and demonstrate this through informed testimony. Knowledge about the status of the principle among other qualified professionals is important information for the witness to present. An informed witness will have comprehensive knowledge of published literature on the topic as well as materials presented at professional conferences and unpublished data. The informed witness will also be aware of the views of leading authorities in the field. The witness should not present as an advocate for the principle; rather, the witness should be neutral and provide information assessing the position of the scientific community with regard to the principle.

The other three sources of evidence used in the establishment of general acceptance include the introduction of relevant literature, guidelines from professional organizations and prior court decisions. Guidelines from professional organizations provide the court with a consensus of the members of an organization. Moreover, the status of the sponsoring organization may be a prominent factor in establishing general acceptance.

Wilkerson v. Pearson

Wilkerson v. Pearson was a landmark case that established the credibility of art therapists as expert witnesses and the validity of drawings as judiciary aids. Art therapy was presented as novel scientific evidence, and the Frye rule was invoked. General acceptance of art therapy and its reliability within the scientific community were established through the presentation of the four types of evidence needed to assert general acceptance within the larger scientific community. Dr. Myra Levick, a pioneer in the field of art therapy, provided testimony in the hearing, which was hailed as a precedent-setting case.

The following discussion of the case provides a lens into how the Frye rule may be invoked when scientific evidence is novel, construed as ambiguous and subsists outside of mainstream consciousness or the professional community from which it originates. Specifically, the case presented surrounds art therapy; however, the manner in which the Frye rule is applied is applicable and illustrative to practitioners and professionals outside of art therapy who may be presenting scientific evidence in which general acceptance and reliability may need to be established in court. This information is relevant for art therapists as well as other professionals who present as expert witnesses, as the documentation showcases how an expert is qualified, how novel scientific evidence is subjected to a special admissibility test and the four types of evidence invoked to establish general acceptance are highlighted.

The case is indicative of how general acceptance is established and thus provides a snapshot into the judicial process. The case involves art therapy; however, the use of evidence in compliance with meeting the Frye test to substantiate novel scientific evidence transfers to other professions and professionals who bring novel scientific evidence into court and must defend the use of it.

Wilkerson v. Pearson

- landmark case (1985)
- established the credibility of art therapists as expert witnesses
- the validity of drawings as judiciary aids was acknowledged
- Frye rule was invoked
- general acceptance of art therapy and its reliability within the scientific community was established

---

Wilkerson v. Pearson was a court proceeding that was tried in New Jersey in 1985. The credibility of art therapists as expert witnesses, as well as the validity of drawings as judiciary aids, was brought up on appeal. In order to establish the validity of art therapy, experts in the fields of art therapy and psychiatry provided expert testimony. The case involved a mother trying to stop supervised visitation between her former husband and their daughter because of allegations of sexual abuse involving the father and daughter.

A registered art therapist, who was working with the child, was asked by the mother to testify in support of the allegations. The art therapist was qualified as an expert; however, her testimony was challenged on the basis that it did not meet the standards and criteria established in *State v. Cavallo* (1982) and *State v. Kelley* (1984). The standards and criteria established in *State v. Cavallo* (1982) involve the relevance of the proffered expert testimony. Once the proper foundation is established, expert opinion testimony is admissible. New Jersey Rules of Evidence were consulted and adhered to since the case was tried in Bergen County, New Jersey. Aspects of the trial that included the testimony provided by the art therapist as well as the qualification of expert status were appealed by the defendant. The points of contention were examined individually with respect to the aforementioned court case.

In order to validate the acceptance of art therapy as recognized and accepted within the larger scientific community, it was determined that relevant evidence, defined as "evidence having any tendency in reason to prove any material fact" (*State v. Cavallo*, 1982) had to be established. New Jersey case law defines the test to be whether the evidence "renders the desired inference more probable than it would be without the evidence" (*State v. Cavallo*, 1982). The general standard of admissibility is whether the proffered evidence will be an aid to the court or jury in determining the question in issue. Under New Jersey Rule 56(2)(b) expert testimony is admissible only if the expert has sufficient expertise to offer the intended testimony and the testimony itself is sufficiently reliable (*State v. Cavallo*, 1982).

New Jersey's standard of acceptability for scientific evidence was an important issue in *Wilkerson v. Pearson*. Scientific evidence is admissible if the proposed technique or mode of analysis has "sufficient scientific basis to produce uniform and reasonably reliable results and will contribute materially to the ascertainment of the truth" (*State v. Cavallo*, 1982, p. 517). An expert opinion is not helpful if it is based upon unreliable premises. What constitutes reasonable reliability depends in part on the context of the proceedings.

Although a judge may not necessarily determine the inherent reliability of expert evidence, the judge can decide whether the proffered evidence has gained "general acceptance" in the scientific community. The proponent of scientific evidence can prove its "general acceptance" and thereby its reliability by the three methods of proof that have been recognized by the courts: expert testimony, scientific and legal writings and judicial opinions (*State v. Cavallo*, 1982, p. 521).

General acceptance of art therapy within the scientific community and its reliability were established in *Wilkerson v. Pearson* through the utilization of the three methods of proof. The prosecution introduced duly qualified experts in the fields of child psychiatry and art therapy. Dr. Allwyn Levine, a child psychiatrist, (substantial support for the general acceptance of psychiatric witnesses was established in 1972) was proffered as was Dr. Myra Levick, as an art therapist and a psychologist. These two individuals were presented as experts in their respective fields and were presented to the court to aid in the qualification of art therapy. Both of these experts referred to relevant literature in their associated field(s), and another form of evidence, judicial opinions (from prior court cases), were consulted during the proceedings.

Dr. Levine was introduced by the prosecution in order to provide evidence of the acceptance of art therapy by professionals in different disciplines. Dr. Levine testified as to his understanding of the modality as well as the general acceptance of art therapy in the field of psychiatry. He also discussed the use and value of art therapy. He provided testimony regarding the acceptance of art therapy by a professional organization, the American Psychiatric Association.

During cross examination, the defense questioned the reliability and validity of psychological tests, including the house-tree-person drawing. Levine replied with a unique and appropriate analogy. He discussed the "tranquilizer as an example of an accepted modality of treatment, even though there are no statistical studies to validate it" (Levick, Safran, & Levine, 1990, p. 50). The court ruled that the witness was not being asked to establish the validity of the tests; rather, he was speaking to general acceptance in the field.

Dr. Levick was presented to the court by the prosecution and introduced in the following manner:

> Dr. Levick is the person who can describe to this court the very nature of Art Therapy, its history and the fact that it is a reliable and, in fact, in some cases a valid scientific tool for use in diagnosis and therapy.
>
> (Levick et al., 1990, p. 51)

Dr. Levick then presented her credentials to the court. She explained that she coordinated the first graduate training program in art therapy and the first graduate program of creative arts in therapy in the United States at Hahnemann University (which is now Drexel University) in Philadelphia. Dr. Levick informed the court that she is a licensed psychologist and a registered art therapist. She also stated her professional affiliations as well as her previous tenure as the first president of the American Art Therapy Association (a nationally recognized professional membership organization).

Levick's testimony included the definition of art therapy and a historical overview of the modality, as well as the development of the American Art Therapy Association. She expounded upon the professional and educational membership organization and addressed the educational standards and the programs that meet the criteria established by the American Art Therapy Association for approval. Levick also spoke about pioneers in the field and their respective contributions and backgrounds in relation to the development of the profession of art therapy. Questions regarding the current state of the profession with regard to training programs was another topic.

Dr. Levick's qualifications were examined and accepted on the basis that the witness (Levick) was the director of a graduate training program for art, music and dance therapists; all three programs had been approved by their respective national associations; and the witness had served as the education chair for the American Art Therapy Association and as the first president of the association (Levick et al., 1990, p. 51).

Much of the testimony centered around the issue of scientific evidence. Levick was asked to distinguish between empirical data and experimental studies. She testified that empirical data are available and acceptable in psychoanalysis and psychiatry as well as in art therapy (Levick et al., 1990). An example utilized by Levick included the way in which a psychologist uses the house-tree-person drawing and the manner in which an art therapist "draws inferences from the same objects used in these tests" (Levick et al., 1990, p. 51). Levick explained that a qualified art therapist does not make interpretations from a drawing just as the psychoanalyst does not make interpretations from a dream; rather, both elicit associations from dream and drawing. This point needed to be underscored repeatedly during Levick's testimony (Levick et al., 1990).

Levick was asked to identify previous cases in which she was qualified as an expert witness. Dr. Levick's previous experience as an expert witness was considered, including the use of drawings as part of her testimony. She recounted two custody cases and one criminal case. A detailed description of one of the custody cases was provided, including a discussion of the artwork that was presented as evidence in the proceeding. This information was requested in order to explore "in depth the conclusions that are made from drawings" (Levick et al., 1990, p. 52). Additionally, Levick provided information about the use of art therapy in evaluating, diagnosing and treating children and adults by referencing professional literature and speaking about her personal experience.

The presentation of evidence provided by both Levine and Levick contributed to the presiding judge, the Honorable Harvey R. Sorkow's, opinion in which he accepted the testimony supplied by the art therapist that was originally challenged. The judge designated that this individual qualified as an expert in the field of art therapy. The opinion written by the judge set a precedent in the state of New Jersey, making it a landmark case (Levick et al., 1990). In deciding his opinion, the judge followed the three basic requirements for the admission of expert testimony as established by Chief

Justice Robert Wilentz in *State v. Kelley* (1984). The judge found the art therapist's testimony to meet the three criteria as follows:

> The interpretation of an individual's drawings as an expression of nonverbal communication of thoughts stimulated by internal psychological conflicts and external pressure is, indeed, beyond the understanding of this court or the average juror if this were a trial by jury. The second criteria was met because recognized proofs of scientific basis for producing uniform and reasonable reliable results were given by other expert testimony. As to the third requirement, it is noted again that the expert's qualifications were stipulated.
>
> (Levick et al., 1990, p. 52)

In defining art therapy, Judge Sorkow combined the testimony supplied by the original art therapist and Dr. Levick. He wrote:

> Art therapy is defined as a form of nonverbal expression and communication. It is a means of expression that synthesizes internal and external stimuli of an individual, so that feelings and thoughts stimulated by internal conflicts and external pressures can be synthesized into the nonverbal form of art communication or art expression. It is a tool used to diagnose and interpret. It can be bridge between the conscious and unconscious.
>
> (Levick et al., 1990, p. 52)

Judge Sorkow discussed the acceptance of art therapy and its reliability in his opinion in the following manner:

> This court is satisfied that Art Therapy has a sufficient scientific acceptance and basis. It is not a test such as a breathalyzer that establishes a result given certain facts. Rather Art Therapy is a modality of treatment that is subjective in nature but has within its discipline fundamental criteria that if found to exist lead to certain inferences and conclusions. To this extent such evidence is reliable.
>
> (Wilkerson versus Pearson, 1985, p. 338)

In order to allow the testimony of the art therapist (who was working with the child in the case), Judge Sorkow had to determine general acceptance of the profession of art therapy and qualify the art therapist as an expert witness. Levick et al. (1990) state, "We reinforce our integrity and credibility by identifying the capabilities and limitations of our profession" (p. 53). Judge Sorkow's opinion was summarized as follows:

> With his decision, Judge Sorkow has added another expert viewpoint to the already recognized disciplines of psychiatry and psychology to aid the courts in these difficult decisions. Art Therapy adds the component of nonverbal communication of thoughts and feelings and thus is an important addition.
>
> (Levick et al., 1990, p. 53)

Qualification of Art Therapists as Expert Witnesses
The following material is adapted and excerpted from publications written by the author
   regarding the *Art Therapist as Expert Witness in Child Sexual Abuse Litigation* including a Master's
   thesis (Cohen-Liebman, 1991), an article that appeared in the *American Journal of Art Therapy*

(Cohen-Liebman, 1994) and a book chapter in 2002. The thesis (1991) and article from 1994 were written prior to the establishment of the Art Therapy Credentials Board (ATCB, www.atcb.org) and board certification process, which is integral information to include/ discuss when testifying. The explanations and words as quoted (from the article) highlight the acceptance of art therapy by the American Psychiatric Association and contribute to recognition of the profession within the larger scientific community.

Although the information may seem dated, the material contained is nevertheless enduring and immutable. The recognition and acceptance of art therapy, which has existed since the latter half of the 20th century by other professions, is relevant and, as articulated, timeless and abiding.

A review of the standards and criteria for the education, training and registration of art therapists indicates that art therapists meet the standards and criteria for expert status as stipulated in the Federal Rules of Evidence (Cohen-Liebman, 1991, 1994). The Federal Rules state that in order to testify as an expert witness, it is necessary to qualify under the rules of evidence and belong to a recognized, national mental health profession. An individual qualifies as an expert by knowledge, skill, experience, training and education. The field of Art Therapy is considered to be a recognized, national mental health profession.

The American Art Therapy Association, (AATA) is a national membership organization for Art Therapy. It is dedicated to "the growth and development" of the profession of Art Therapy (https://arttherapy.org). The Art Therapy Credentials Board, Inc., ATCB, (www.atcb.org) is the governing board that manages credentialing (registration) and certification of art therapists (Cohen-Liebman, 2002). AATA is a separate entity and has no influence or oversight with regard to the credentialing process. AATA is recognized by the American Psychiatric Association. AATA has developed guidelines for the training, membership and practice of art therapists (AATA, 1999). AATA designates and establishes professional standards and criteria for its membership. Specific goals govern the organization, including "the progressive development of the therapeutic use of art, the advancement of research, the improvement of standards of practice, the development of criteria for training art therapists, and the exchange of information and experience through publications, meetings and seminars" (Rubin, 1979, p. 14).

Professional qualification for entry into the field requires a master's degree from an accredited academic institution or a certificate of completion from an accredited institute or clinical program (Levick, 1983; Lusebrink, 1989). Graduate training programs are required to include practicum experience in addition to didactic training.

Dr. Michael Vaccaro, an assistant professor at Hahnemann University (now Drexel University) in Philadelphia, proposed soon after the establishment of the American Art Therapy Association (in 1969) that art therapy be understood as a branch of psychiatry (1973). He wrote, "Art therapy is steeped in theoretical principles and therapeutic practices" (Vaccaro, 1973, p. 253). He acknowledged that The American Art Therapy Association "has recognized and accepted its role of formulating guidelines for accredited education and training; validating research; and promulgating an ethical code of professional conduct for its members" (Vaccaro, 1973, p. 253). Vaccaro (1973) defines the education and training of the art therapist in the following manner:

The art therapist undergoes a specialized training graduate program affiliated with a medical college or a university where he is offered sound theoretical principles and therapeutic techniques which have been tested by time and scientific experiment. Concomitant with his academic training he is gradually exposed to the vicissitudes of a supervised clinical experience (Vaccaro, 1973, p. 255).

Child Sexual Abuse Litigation and Mental Health Expert Testimony

The degree of expertise depends on the type of testimony. To qualify as an expert in child sexual abuse or a related designation, some of the questions posed to an individual during voir dire might include:

- education, including advanced degrees and postgraduate training
- credentials specific to sexual abuse

- specialization in a particular area of practice
- specialized training in child sexual abuse
- extent of experience with sexually abused children
- familiarity with relevant literature
- membership in related professional associations
- publications/presentations regarding child sexual abuse
- prior qualification as an expert on child sexual abuse

The last point is important because once an expert is qualified as such, especially outside of a criminal court (typically but not always), the individual's credentials are stipulated to (meaning accepted by both parties) and the individual is not subjected to voir dire in a later proceeding. Rather, both parties typically will agree to the previous voir dire designation and qualification of the individual as an expert. The status is acceptable, given the previous confirmation.

To be fair, in my experience, depending upon the semantics of a particular case, expert witness status was aligned with the agenda of the presenting attorney and in deference to case considerations. Thus, the nature of the expert witness status was determined in relation to what the attorney deemed was in the best interest of the case. As such, the specification of my expert status varied from expert in art therapy to child sexual abuse, child abuse, sexually abused children and their drawings, the use of drawing and other designations in accordance with the proceedings that correlated with how the calling attorney wanted to present my expertise (which was contingent upon the subtleties of each case).

My status remained as an expert, but the specifics of my expertise depended on how the presenting party (the prosecution) qualified me. The presenting attorney requested the designation in relation to the dynamics of the case, my involvement and my role. Sometimes, this was determined as a result of the attorney's preparedness for the case, prior preparation with me and/or the attorney's familiarity with my background and expertise (if we had worked together previously on a case).

Ethical Issues for Mental Health Expert Witnesses

There are a host of practice and procedural concerns that an expert mental health witness should be cognizant of when preparing for courtroom participation and testimony. Foremost is the responsibility to remain within the limits and boundaries of one's identified area of expertise. As such, an expert should not attempt to speak to issues that are beyond the expert's realm of expertise. This is not a negative, but rather being forthright about what is within one's purview versus what is not will help avert potential pitfalls on the stand, including diminished credibility. An expert should prepare above and beyond as well so that one is able to demonstrate one's competence in a professional and reliable manner. A suggestion is to be well read in one's area of expertise so when explaining or discussing a particular issue, the literature is cited in a relevant and impressive manner. This entails being current on scientific literature, and if an issue is controversial, it is best to be familiar with both sides of an argument or issue in anticipation of cross examination which is impacted by the knowledge and preparation that opposing counsel conducts. For example, with regard to child sexual abuse, if asked about recantation and dynamics of child sexual abuse, it is important to know what the arguments are as to why children might or might not recant disclosure.

The expert mental health expert should admit limitations and weaknesses and address such on direct examination in anticipation of cross examination. By doing so, one may avoid potential issues that may manifest on cross examination. (Different forms of testimony and how to prepare and present will be considered shortly.) If an expert provides an opinion, the expert should be able to articulate the scientific basis that supports the opinion. The expert is advised to answer as unequivocally as possible and not let opposing counsel mar or diminish the expert's integrity (tips on how to do this will be shared as well).

Ethical Considerations

- maintain expertise
- be current on scientific literature, including controversial points of view so one can address both sides of an issue/argument
- know biases
- testimony should be the same regardless of which side testifying for
- should be an active practitioner rather than a full-time expert witness
- be aware of compromising objectivity
- stick to ethical standards (professional and personal)
- avoid manipulation of beliefs
- do not be cajoled into supporting a position that may be counter to the expert's belief/opinion

As an expert mental health witness, privileges extend. In this capacity, the expert may offer information about individuals they may not have had direct contact with; they can aggregate information or data and relate this information to an individual.

Mental Health Fact/Lay Witness Versus Expert Witness

- a treating clinician typically is presented as a lay witness and speaks to the particulars of a case
- as an expert, can provide information about individuals one has not treated
- expert can apply group data to individual cases

  - aggregate data and relate to an individual

Issues may arise pertaining to the role of a treating provider. Can a provider be an expert witness? There is concern with regard to a treating clinician versus forensic evaluator versus both roles. The question is: Can a provider be an objective evaluator? Typically, roles should be separate. Distinctions need to be clear regarding the role of a treating clinician in court versus a forensic evaluator because this impacts how one presents and testifies. The treating clinical is typically sworn in as a lay witness if speaking (testifying) to the particulars of a case.

Within the role of a clinician, an individual is presenting as a provider of treatment rather than as a fact-finder. Confidentiality extends to a certain degree, with exceptions depending upon circumstances. The provider is supportive of the client and concerned with the welfare of the client. Most importantly, the mental health provider is not able to argue the case or to assume the role of trier of fact, but is brought in to provide information meaning personal knowledge or firsthand information which is consistent with a lay witness.

The issue of a forensic versus a clinical role is relevant to the function of a mental health provider serving in the capacity of an expert witness. Within a forensic role the purpose is to form an opinion about the matter before the court. As a forensic evaluator corroboration is important and confidentiality is not protected or extended. The forensic evaluator may be working for the court. Neutrality is important, as is objectivity. Distinctions that are associated with forensic evaluators and mental health providers encourage that each retain the role ascribed. Providers actively treating a client should most likely not conduct the forensic evaluation, just as the evaluator should maintain a forensic role rather than conduct therapy after the evaluation. Clearly stated:

> The forensic evaluator's task is to gather data and information for investigative purposes . . . while the therapist's role is that of a helping agent who provides emotional support, education and appropriate treatment (Mannarino & Cohen, 1992, p. 3).

Presentation in court will differ depending upon the role assumed and contribute to witness status. Typically, the forensic evaluator presents as an expert and may provide opinions and speak to credibility. The mental health provider most likely will present in the capacity of a lay witness and speak to information or knowledge stemming from personal association with the case. The latter is precluded from offering an opinion or speaking to credibility.

Forensic Role	*Clinical Role (mental health provider)*
• fact-finder	• treatment provider rather than fact-finder
• role to gather information	• role to provide support and validation as well
• purpose to form an opinion	as intervention
• address likelihood of abuse	• confidentiality except in certain
• may offer an opinion (expert witness)	circumstances
• need for corroboration	• client is the client
• confidentiality not protected (anything	• client welfare is addressed
may be used in court)	• sessions are informal/supportive
• nature of client – may include court or	• not the role of the mental health provider to
other parties	argue the case
• neutrality	• not the trier of fact
• objectivity	• if testify – fact/lay witness

Confidence in an Expert's Opinion

Confidence in an expert's opinion typically increases as the amount and quality of evidence increase. Confidence in expert opinion declines as the amount and quality of evidence supporting the opinion decrease. An expert's opinion has a higher degree of confidence that a child was sexually abused when an expert's opinion is based upon a combination of data that may include but is not limited to a child's disclosure and corroborating information. Myers (1996) cautions that one should not conclude that the quantity of evidence is a satisfactory basis for judging expert opinion; rather, sound decision making rests on careful assessment of the quantity, quality and context of the evidence.

Evidence in the Context of Testifying

Evidence, like testimony, is characterized as substantive or rehabilitative. Substantive evidence is offered to prove a matter or an issue. This type of evidence is associated with a high level of expertise and may be directed at an opinion – perhaps that a particular child was a victim of sexual abuse. Expert testimony plays an important role according to Myers (1996) in describing medical evidence, psychological effects of abuse and developmental differences between children and adults. Myers (1996) states that the degree of expertise required to testify as an expert depends on whether the testimony is offered as substantive or rehabilitative. A high level of expertise is needed to give substantive testimony, whereas with rehabilitative evidence, an expert only needs limited expertise.

Expert testimony in child sexual abuse litigation falls into two categories:

substantive – proof that a child was sexually abused (opinion that a particular child was abused)
rehabilitative – a child's impeached credibility merits explanation (for example, a delay in reporting)

Rehabilitative Versus Substantive

Rehabilitative evidence does not necessarily rise to the same level of expertise as substantive evidence, meaning that the information presented by the expert is offered to dispel misconceptions and to educate the judge or jury about a topic. The expert provides information to assist the trier of fact in rendering a decision. This type of evidence also consists of an expert explaining the fundamentals associated with child sexual abuse such as why children delay in reporting or recant disclosure. Rather than provide an opinion as to whether a particular child was abused, this type of evidence is designed to inform or assist the judge and/or jury to understand a fact or matter. An expert, for example, may provide testimony to explain why a child might recant disclosure, or the expert might speak to why sexually abused children may delay in reporting. The expert does not need to defer to the child that is the subject of the proceeding, but instead the expert may speak to sexually abused children as a whole or a class and provide information based on relevant literature or research.

Rehabilitative evidence is not offered as substantive evidence but may be presented to rehabilitate a child's credibility after the defense has attacked it (the child's credibility) on cross examination. Rehabilitative testimony is not subjected to the special rule governing scientific principles, but there are guidelines that govern the use of it. When presenting such testimony, the expert usually speaks about a group of children rather than a specific child. The expert's testimony is directed at what is being rehabilitated, and an opinion about whether the specific child was abused is not offered. This kind of testimony is straightforward and simple. The expert demonstrates knowledge of relevant literature, research or study to support the testimony.

Expert testimony is not allowed with regard to credibility of children either singularly or as a group. An expert cannot say the child in a particular case told the truth or was believable because assessment of credibility is the determination of the trier of fact and not the mental health expert. This is considered the province of the jury and as such the expert cannot usurp the trier of fact. As such, experts may not testify that a particular person perpetrated abuse. There is no single symptom or behavior, whether sexual or nonsexual, that is significant or remarkable for sexual abuse (Myers, 1996). Courts take three positions regarding expert mental health substantive testimony in child sexual abuse: mental health professionals are properly qualified to offer some forms of substantive evidence, some or all forms of substantive evidence from mental health professionals is sanctioned and it can provide a form of scientific evidence and be subjected to the special rule applied to such evidence.

Corroborative or Substantive Testimony	Rehabilitative Testimony
<ul><li>opinion</li><li>high level of expertise</li><li>offered to prove</li></ul>	<ul><li>expert needs little experience/training</li><li>speak to child sexual abuse issues such as recantation or delay in reporting</li><li>expert does not venture an opinion that the child in the case was abused</li><li>expert need not refer to a specific child</li><li>straightforward and simple testimony</li><li>need knowledge of relevant literature</li><li>not substantive</li><li>need not be the foremost expert on a topic</li></ul>

References

American Art Therapy Association, Inc. (AATA). American Art Therapy Association, Inc. (1999). Art therapy: *The profession.* Mundelein, IL: Author. www.arttherapy.org

Art Therapy Credentials Board, Inc. (ATCB). www.atcb.org

Barsky, A., & Gould, J. (2002). *Clinicians in court: A guide to subpoenas, depositions, testifying, and everything else you need to know.* The Guilford Press.

Bolocofsky, D. (1989). Use and abuse of mental health experts in child custody determinations. *Behavioral Sciences and the Law, 7,* 197–213.

Brown, D. (2001). The new 702: How it affects the use of experts. In *National center for prosecution of child abuse update* (Vol. 14, No. 3). American Prosecutors Research Institute. APRI.

Cohen-Liebman, M. S. (1991). *The art therapist as expert witness in child sexual abuse litigation.* Master's Thesis, Hahnemann University.

Cohen-Liebman, M. S. (1994). The art therapist as expert witness in child sexual abuse litigation, *Journal of the American Art Therapy Association, 11*(4), 260–265.

Cohen-Liebman, M. S. (2002). Intro to art therapy. In A. P. Giardino & E. R. Giardino (Eds.), *Recognition of child abuse for the mandated reporter* (3rd ed., pp. 227–257). G.W. Medical Publishing.

Ladd, M. (1952). Expert testimony. *Vanderbilt Law Review, 5,* 414–431.

Levick, M. F. (1983), *They could not talk and so they drew.* Charles C. Thomas.

Levick, M. F., Safran, D., & Levine, A. (1990). Art therapists as expert witnesses: A judge delivers a precedent-setting decision. *The Arts in Psychotherapy, 17,* 49–53.

Lusebrink, V. B. (1989). Education in creative arts therapies: Accomplishments and challenges. *The Arts in Psychotherapy, 16,* 5–10.

Mannarino, A. P., & Cohen, J. A. (1992). Forensic versus treatment roles in cases of child sexual abuse. *Protective Services Quarterly, 7,* 1–6.

Myers, J. E. B. (1992). *Legal issues in child abuse and neglect.* Sage Publications Inc.

Myers, J. E. B. (1996). Expert testimony. In C. Jenny, J. Briere, J. Bulkley, L. Berliner, & T. Reid (Eds.), *The APSAC handbook on child maltreatment* (1st ed., pp. 319–326). Sage Publications, Inc.

Myers, J. E. B. (2002). Legal issues in the medical evaluation of child sexual abuse. In M. Finkel & A. Giardino (Eds.), *Medical evaluation of child sexual abuse: A practical guide* (2nd ed., pp. 233–250). Sage Publications Inc.

Myers, J. E. B. (2011a). Juvenile court. In J. E. B. Myers (Ed.), *The APSAC handbook on child maltreatment* (3rd ed., pp. 53–66). Sage Publications, Inc.

Myers, J. E. B. (2011b). Legal issues in child abuse and neglect practice. In J. E. B. Myers (Ed.), *The APSAC handbook on child maltreatment* (3rd ed., pp. 361–376). Sage Publications, Inc.

Myers, J. E. B. (Ed.). (2011c). *The APSAC handbook on child maltreatment* (3rd ed.). Sage Publications, Inc.

Myers, J. E. B. (2019). *Mental health law in a nutshell.* West Academic Publishing.

Myers, J. E. B., Bays, J., Becker, J., Berliner, L., Corwin, D. L., & Saywitz, K. J. (1989). Expert testimony in child sexual abuse litigation. *Nebraska Law Review, 68*(1–2), 1–145.

Rubin, J. (1979). Art therapy: An introduction. In *Conference on creative arts therapies [monograph]* (pp. 12–14). American Psychiatric Association.

Schetky, D. H., & Benedek, E. (1992). *Clinical handbook of child psychiatry and the law.* Williams & Wilkins.

Smith, S. (1989). Mental health expert witnesses: Of science and crystal balls. *Behavioral Sciences and the Law, 7,* 145–180.

State v. Cavallo, 88 New Jersey, 508 (1982).

State v. Kelley, 97 New Jersey, 178 (1984).

Vaccaro, M. (1973). The responsibility of the art therapist. *Philadelphia Medicine, 69,* 253–256.

Wilkerson v. Pearson, 210 New Jersey, Super. 333, 335. Chancery Division. (1985).

Part IV   The Art of Mock Court

Effective Witnessing and Evidentiary Presentation

A unique feature of my course on forensic art therapy included a mock court forum, which I presented through the years as a workshop for art therapists and other professionals. Standard courtroom procedure, judicial hearings and a foundation for testifying were topics presented through didactic teaching coupled with experiential exercises. The workshop was designed to address practical strategies for effective witnessing. Conceived as a venue for skill building, the material was designed to promote the development of analytic and communication skills to enhance courtroom engagement. Litigation tactics were explored to prepare participants with an understanding of courtroom strategy through the unique and dynamic format.

Modeled after mock court competitions, the program provided interactive and simulated exercises surrounding courtroom engagement that exposed participants to techniques, tactics and strategies to understand and manage direct and cross examination. A compendium of resource information was provided surrounding judicial proceedings, legal terminology, testifying or witnessing and evidentiary presentation. Finally, tip sheets that addressed preparation, presentation, practice, behavior and scripting were disseminated to provide participants with information in the event they received a subpoena to appear in court.

The first half of the workshop presented information pertinent to legal proceedings, testimonial capability and evidentiary material to establish a foundation for eventual participation in a hypothetical case scenario. Participants assumed designated roles, including courtroom personnel, attorneys and witnesses. The premise was directed at practicing and augmenting testimonial capability. Application of learned knowledge culminated in a mock courtroom exercise wherein participants assumed roles and enacted a judicial proceeding predicated upon a child abuse investigation. The premise was to provide participants with the opportunity to experience and apply skills acquired with respect to investigation, litigation and judicial presentation of evidence. At the culmination of a course/workshop, students were able to integrate material from the modules in the form of testimony and evidentiary material; the latter included the use of drawing within the context of judiciary aids.

The use of drawing as related to each facet was also practiced: investigation, litigation and evidentiary presentation. Students were allotted time to craft role plays pertaining to the objectives of the course, and the final project was the enactment, which demonstrated learned skills and application within a child sexual abuse investigation. The case scenario centered around a child forensic interview process promoting interaction and engagement pertinent to process, procedure and presentation within a judicial realm.

DOI: 10.4324/9781003225041-5

Role plays also included voir dire and scripting exercises to help with preparation and to give authenticity to the portrayal. A prosecution side and a defense team were designated so that witnesses had to prepare and present as either lay or expert witnesses and manage direct and cross examination. Skills and strategies were intended to be transferred to real-world situations should one be engaged in an eventual court proceeding. The forum provided participants with the opportunity to apply and integrate learned concepts through an experiential format.

Participants were divided into a prosecution team and a defense team. Additional participants were designated as court officers and assorted personnel as related to the role play and improvised scenario. Teams drafted scripts in anticipation and considered strategies for managing direct, cross examination and rehabilitation or rebuttal testimony stemming from a mock case. Often, investigative interviews, including the use of the Common Interview Guideline (CIG), were enacted prior to the strategizing sessions for participants to fully engage with the process and to be able to present authentically. The forum was designed to familiarize and acquaint participants with courtroom procedure and protocol.

The mock court, whether offered as part of a full course or in a separate workshop, coalesced around the material presented on legal proceedings, courtroom protocol and effective techniques for presenting on the witness stand regardless of capacity (lay witness, expert witness, mental health expert). As such, participants were given the opportunity to engage in a simulated interview process prior to the courtroom enactment, which entailed melding the course material surrounding investigating, interviewing and testifying.

In concert with the material shared during the entirety of the program, role plays centered on the use of the CIG, the investigative interview guideline that was elucidated during the didactic portion of the program, which also included a hands-on component for demonstration purposes. Although workshops were limited to specific time frames, participants were able to construct brief encounters to address unscripted vignettes centered around the development, practice and enactment of judicial engagement, testimonial capability and evidentiary presentation.

Students enrolled in a forensic art therapy course were provided with an extended time frame to prepare, practice and implement a simulated experience that integrated and merged the course components. In some mock settings, participants truly were immersed in the process and utilized props, modified costumes and made mock drawings to present on the witness stand in the guise of expert witnesses or related capacities. The "attorneys" were prepared to challenge, and witnesses were prepped to defend the interview process as well as the use of an art therapy–based investigative interview process on the witness stand.

Within the mock court scenario, litigation tactics were explored to prepare participants with an understanding of courtroom strategy to enhance performance. Tips for testifying were shared in this novel format. Participants learned how to handle and identify motivations, methods of attack and strategies employed by defense attorneys to anticipate and prepare for cross examination. Practice tips addressed preparation, presentation, qualification, courtroom protocol, ethical considerations and effective witnessing.

Another aspect incorporated into the unique format was the use of a peer review worksheet. Participants/students were asked to provide and relate feedback in a written format. Identifying information was omitted. The purpose is two-fold: to offer commentary that is constructive and helpful to the enactor, while providing an opportunity for reflection and education for the person providing feedback/commentary. One learns by doing and through experiencing. As such, the person sharing thoughts is broadening personal perspective and understanding while also offering constructive feedback. It is a reciprocal process that has proven to be very successful as an educational and teaching tool, at least for this conceptual process and format.

Sample Peer Review Worksheet for Mock Court Scenario		
	Observations	*Reflections*
Qualification/Voir Dire		
On Direct Examination		
On Cross Examination		
On Redirect Examination		
General Thoughts		

A worksheet was provided for teams to utilize in strategizing for the mock court role play. Teams were instructed to work together and formulate ideas while planning and strategizing how to effectively present the team's side. Presentation of witnesses and the incorporation of strategies (akin to real-world application) of courtroom engagement are to be addressed and demonstrated. Ideas to consider are noted.

Team	*Strategy Worksheet for Mock Court Case Scenario* Goal: Consider courtroom strategy as it pertains to team assignment	
	Prosecution or Plaintiff	*Defendant or Defense*
	plan and strategize identify objectives for witnesses themes and line of questioning anticipate cross prepare for redirect	plan and strategize formulate objectives and lines of questioning consider cross examination techniques for prosecution witnesses anticipate how to use plaintiff witnesses to support team's position
	opening statements	closing statements

strengths		
weaknesses		
strategies		

	direct	cross	redirect
strengths			
weaknesses			
strategies			

The objectives of the course and abbreviated workshop were the same:

- identify standard courtroom procedure
- comprehend practical strategies for effective witnessing
- understand how to qualify as an expert witness
- practice cogent witnessing
- enhance skill as expert witness
- develop an understanding for courtroom tactics to enhance courtroom performance
- apply learned knowledge in the areas of preparation, presentation, qualification, articulation
- identify ethical considerations associated with testifying in the capacity of an expert witness

---

Expert Witness Forum Outline

---

preparation
ethical concerns
practice tips

   preparation
   presentation
   behavior
   general
   testifying

direct examination
cross examination
rebuttal or redirect examination

   effective versus not effective witnessing

practice exercises

   scripting
   voir dire
   courtroom strategy

litigation tactics
cross examination
motivations and methods of attack
peer review
mock court

   explanation
   distribution of role play
   enactment
   debrief

review and processing
summation

Impetus for Mock Court Exercise

The lack of preparation and education regarding effective witnessing in tandem with presenting evidentiary material in court contributed to the creation of a mock court exercise/component. Originally intended for art therapy students and professionals, content is applicable and transferable for anyone who works with related populations and may potentially be called into court. In a survey conducted as part of my doctoral program, creative arts therapists were asked a series of questions pertaining to the paucity of curricula surrounding judicial interaction, specifically understanding of legal proceedings and issues affiliated with testifying. Respondents conveyed the lack of as well as the need for education in these areas. Several respondents expressed the need for preparation for possible and (as I always stress, most likely at some point in one's career depending upon the nature of one's work and the setting where one conducts his/her practice) potential courtroom involvement.

Preparatory knowledge in anticipation of a command (subpoena) from the court to present either oneself or one's records will obviate misunderstanding with regard to legalities and noncompliance with formal requests. Knowledge and experience will effectively (or hopefully) minimize angst, although anxiety and court do go together. In truth, one should be concerned because it is difficult to anticipate what one will encounter within a judicial realm; however, preparation and cognizance of fundamental precepts will assuage apprehension and temper fear.

Nothing prepares one for the first time they are called into court. Despite meeting with a deputy solicitor and extensive preparatory work, it was difficult to quell my nerves prior to my first foray as an expert witness, yet it was imperative not to show dread or worry. In fact, my mindset shifted from nervous to impassioned readiness when the defense attorney sauntered into court (looking like he had just rolled out of bed with his hair askew and his suit astray), approached the judge and handed him a piece of paper. The attorney had a sheepish grin on his face, thinking that whatever was on the piece of paper he had presented to the judge (this was civil court) was going to literally be his get out of jail card and the case was going to be dismissed. Well, much to his dismay and eventually my chagrin (because he decided to target me given his lack of preparation and no defense strategy), the attorney was blasted by the judge and told whatever he had displayed was outdated and invalid and the proceeding was moving forward that day, that morning, in just a few short minutes, and the judge instructed the attorney that he had better be prepared. Well, of course, the man was not ready to present a case of any sort. So, at a loss since he was not prepared for the case, the attorney looked around at everyone assembled in the courtroom and his gaze landed on me.

Thinking he had found his mark, he proceeded to walk by me and made a few remarks under his breath. Since the judge was willing to give the man a bit of time to get himself and his case together, we were in a holding pattern of sorts. I went to make a phone call from the phone booth that was inside of the lobby (yes, again dating myself – pre–cell phones and an old-fashioned phone booth with a glass door that had to be pushed). As I was standing inside of the booth, having not yet closed the door, the attorney, who had followed me, made remarks insinuating he was going to attack me (meaning my credentials) as well as my report, which I doubt he had even read given that he thought he had the golden ticket that would preclude forward movement in the case.

Trying to intimidate me, his threats escalated until I realized that I could not let him be in control of me or the situation. I politely told him I could not speak to him outside of the courtroom and I had a call to make. I then shut the door and turned my back to him. (I have to thank the old-fashioned door of the phone booth, which necessitated force to shut it.) The attorney stomped off. He had no ammunition outside or inside of the courtroom after that encounter. The judge let him know that, and I have to say my anxiety evaporated. I was ready to do what I was there to do.

I have to thank this person for his behavior that day because had I not had to contend with his behavior and his lack of preparedness, as well as the verbal exchange (as noted), I might have let my nerves get the best of me. Instead, I was so annoyed and truly angry at this person that I was determined to show who he was dealing with and present as effectively as possible in a professional and commanding manner. Frankly, I had no choice but to master my emotions and discuss the case and present evidence in a cogent manner. Negative situations do have positive benefits, but more than that, one has to be prepared for anything when called into court. Predictability is not guaranteed in a court of law. Expectations may very well require adjustments.

The best advice is to be prepared for anything when testifying. I would be remiss if I did not acknowledge directly the work of John Myers, legal scholar extraordinaire. I have referenced his work throughout this text and I thank him for his work, including his emphasis on preparation. I highly recommend his publications as resource material for anyone engaged in forensic or legal work especially professionals in the multidisciplinary field of child abuse.

Preparation is definitely key. The best way to manage courtroom machinations is to understand process and protocol and not to personalize anything that occurs within this context. This is imperative and merits understanding and acceptance by anyone enmeshed in legal, judicial and forensic work. Everyone in the courtroom has a job to do, be it good or bad, positive or negative. Both sides, prosecution/plaintiff and defense, will engage in dual roles, offensive and defensive, depending upon the nature of the case and the objectives.

Sometimes upon leaving a courtroom after a relatively robust and lively exchange on the witness stand, opposing counsel would comment on "performance" and the use of strategies as an expert witness. Adversarial prowess inside the courtroom did not necessarily extend outside. I witnessed opposing attorneys engage in friendly banter outside of the courtroom setting after intense drama had unfolded or been enacted. Compliments were frequently exchanged on the deftness invoked or exhibited whether by attorneys or witnesses. Kudos and praise were mutually shared. Relationships might have been suspended inside the courtroom but were evident outside in the corridors. Truly a remarkable and enlightening experience given some of the exchanges that took place when everyone was enmeshed in their respective roles/positions. It was always an education to be privy to what goes on inside as well as outside of the courtroom and the dynamics.

Typical art therapy graduate curriculum does not include a module or a course designed to familiarize, acquaint and prepare art therapists for possible and oftentimes likely courtroom encounters. I trust this is true in other fields and professions, including creative and expressive arts therapies. This aspect of my teaching and work was intended to remedy this paucity not only for art therapists but for a range of individuals who might find themselves subpoenaed to appear in court and potentially testify, whether in child abuse cases or other legal matters.

Unfamiliarity with the expectations, process, procedures and protocol and a lack of actual experience with courtroom involvement promotes consternation, anxiety and stress. Trying to rectify this paucity, I developed an expert witness forum and workshop to provide a platform for interactive and experiential opportunities. The concept was designed to provide introduction and explanation of courtroom proceedings and judicial practices in a way that was engaging and informative. Pragmatically, the concept was intended to provide a way to orient individuals and provide them with an arsenal of information that would be useful in the event of actual courtroom participation. Anyone engaged in the realm of child maltreatment (previously defined as an umbrella term that encompasses an array of disciplines and practitioners as well as professionals and students) may at some point in their career encounter the need to present information in a court of law, including mental health practitioners and members of multidisciplinary investigative teams, as well as others committed to investigation and intervention.

Too often, acquisition of information and exposure is garnered through on-the-job training which originates due to participation in a case that, for whatever reason, may merit legal or judicial engagement. The expert witness forum presented basic information pertaining to courtroom participation and inculcated mechanisms for preparation in the event one is to appear in court either physically or by virtue of reports and/or records relative to a particular case. Even if one is not specifically requested to appear for a proceeding, the possibility exists that records may be subpoenaed or requested and that extends to contacts, conversations and memorialization of any kind.

As technology has evolved, so too has the wording on subpoenas that may list every conceivable type of product that falls under record keeping such as emails, text messages and, back in the day, faxes. As such, it behooves practitioners from whatever background to have preparatory knowledge about the legal system as well as testifying, record-keeping, documentation and presentation of evidentiary material. It is also essential to understand what constitutes evidence in a court of law.

Myers (2011a) identifies two types of subpoenas issued by a court, usually at the request of an attorney

Subpoena ad testificandum	Subpoena duces tecum
Requires an individual to testify	Requires a person to produce documents or records

---

Courtroom Materials

For many years I presented expert witnessing workshops and generated packets and notebooks full of resources. Participants were told they need not memorize what was in the packet/notebook but to keep the resource material in a location that was accessible for reference in the event a courtroom request should manifest. The mock court module followed introduction to courtroom procedure, protocol and process. As such, an introduction and explanation of the adversary system of justice was followed by information pertaining to the judicial system, including legal proceedings and expectations associated with witnessing. Particular attention was directed at effective witnessing, including qualification and testimonial capability. Evidentiary material and presentation of such was explained, and basic courtroom procedure was demonstrated to provide exposure to the legal system and allow for practice opportunities through a mock court or simulated judicial experience.

Prior to engaging in this aspect of the program, participants and students were advised not to take anything personally within the scope of courtroom interaction. One must master their emotions and understand not to take to heart or personalize anything that may be said or directed at one's presentation on the witness stand. Everyone in the courtroom has a specific purpose and intention. Everyone has a job to do whether as an officer of the court, an attorney on either side of the matter and each witness as well. Court is a theater of sorts. One must always rise above the dynamic interplay and present in the best possible manner with respect to presence in the courtroom and one's designated as well as perceived role.

Therefore, it is critical to be prepared for the proposition of having to provide testimony and appear for a judicial matter. Preparation may be time consuming and challenging; however, without proper and adequate preparation, one should not attempt to provide testimony. Basic information regarding courtroom procedure and judicial proceedings should be incorporated as standard graduate curricula for creative arts therapists, mental health providers and evaluators, forensic interviewers and multidisciplinary team members, since many will, whether purposefully or inadvertently, end up in court at some point. Knowing process, procedure, rules and protocol will help one to prepare and effectively present information.

This section is devoted to providing an overview and identifying resource material for interest in acquiring basic information that may be of use for eventual and possible courtroom participation. Preparation extends to the following arenas:

- presentation
- behavior
- general information about legal proceedings and courtroom etiquette
- testifying/testimony
- cross examination/strategies/principles

Mock Court Exercise

Mock court is based on the simulation and enactment of a trial (judicial proceeding). A trial is a judicial procedure conducted to determine if the rights of a person or entity have been violated. Typical mock court exercises are competitive and team based and as such scored on identified criteria, including how well everyone performs in designated roles as well as overall team performance. Individuals portray lawyers, court officers and witnesses and enact a judicial proceeding based on a dedicated scenario. Specific rules apply and pertain to procedure and format as well as process and courtroom protocol. Scoring in a mock court considers the performance of lawyers, witnesses and "the team" in concert with the rules and procedures of the process. Within the context of the course or workshop, scoring and competition were not the intended objectives rather the point of the exercise was for teaching and instructional purposes.

Mock court provides an experience that is relevant to understanding and interacting in a court of law and offers an experiential component to acquire knowledge about courtroom participation. The three major elements associated with effective trial advocacy, whether in real life or in a mock presentation, are *planning, preparation and presentation*. Rules govern how a trial is to be conducted whether in real life or in a mock scenario.

Mock court exercises proved to be rewarding and exciting for professionals as well as students in a workshop format or as the culmination of a graduate-level course. Teams strategize how to present their side of the trial and showcase strengths predicated upon preparation, investment and engagement. Mock court scenarios invoke an aura of performance, which is akin to how courtroom engagement may be understood and appreciated. For some, the interactions and encounters that occur within the guise of courtroom combat often reflect theater or performance. Often improvisation seemingly comes to mind when observing and critiquing how examiners conduct themselves and "perform" their "roles". This sentiment is not meant to be negative or flippant, but rather is conveyed to help neutralize the emotions that accompany courtroom engagement. If one thinks in terms of enactment and considers dance as a metaphor for court, one will appreciate how to incorporate the pressure and fear that may be generated. Rather than allow process and procedure to manipulate and minimize one's ability to cope with the myriad of elements and strategies that are invoked, crafted and even dare I say performed, an analogy of movement, rhythm and syncopation is prudent. Truly, courtroom participation, whether voluntary or commanded, is a dance of sorts and once one understands the tempo, rhythm and the cadence as well as the routine, one will be better equipped to mirror and move in sync and respond within this domain. One truly has to experience the process as it unfolds and engulfs, yet one can learn how to regulate, modulate and assimilate.

The following material is structured to introduce and familiarize participants with basic awareness surrounding judicial processes, legal proceedings and courtroom conventions. Typically, teams are determined and roles assigned that correspond with the personnel associated with the case: attorneys, witnesses and support figures such as judge, jury (if there are enough participants to include this body), court reporter and bailiff. Similarly, each side, prosecution and defense, will have attorneys and witnesses. Depending upon the nature of the case, civil or criminal, the prosecution side is referred to differently. In a civil case, the litigant or the complainant is referred to as the plaintiff (prosecution side). On the defense side, a defendant is the accused in a criminal proceeding. Nomenclature may vary depending upon the jurisdiction.

The mock trial follows the sequence of a regular proceeding with both sides presenting opening statements starting with the prosecution. After, direct examination is conducted to introduce witnesses and present evidence. The opposing side conducts cross examination of a witness if it so chooses after direct examination of the witness. If additional testimony is desired or there is a need to rehabilitate a witness or their testimony, redirect examination may follow cross examination.

After all witnesses have concluded testimony and the evidence has been presented by each side, the attorneys will deliver closing arguments directly to the trier of fact. Closing arguments provide the attorneys with the opportunity to appeal to the judge or jury (if there is one) to find in favor of their client. In closing, attorneys will provide a summary of the evidence within the context in which it was presented during the trial. They may reaffirm the credibility of their witnesses and perhaps try to diminish opposing counsel's presentation through pointing out problems such as inconsistencies in witnesses' statements or they may try to malign the credibility or evidentiary material that was presented. This is an effort to implore the judge or jury to find in favor of the case they presented and side with their client. Essentially, the attorneys review the facts of the case (as they interpret them in accordance with the agenda they have presented and the response they wish to invoke). Essentially, each side reviews what evidentiary material they presented and recapitulate the basis for a favorable ruling.

Trial Terminology

What follows is a listing of terms and processes that are considered pertinent to the enactment of a mock court and that relate to courts in general. Terms that are fundamental to courtroom process and procedure are listed, although scoring, which is directly associated with the mock court exercise, is included here for reference only. The terms are concomitant with a mock court scenario as well as real-world involvement, given that mock court is derivative of courtroom practice. Familiarity with presentation, tactics and strategies with regard to direct examination and cross examination will be of use in preparing for court, and as such this information is presented here to provide an overview and appreciation of what is entailed when court beckons. The information is presented in an effort to identify, introduce and explain the roles and the processes within a mock court scenario, which are reflective of actual courtroom encounters (minus scoring, yet scoring points in the mind of jurors or others in the courtroom is applicable).

Lawyers

These individuals are scored on opening statements, direct examination and cross examination. In addition, they are scored on how they demonstrate and exhibit knowledge and trial skills as well as understanding of procedures including laws, rules and objections. The ability to display knowledge and demonstrate trial skills is considered. The more convincing and believable an individual is in their presentation and interactions with other attorneys, witnesses and jury are additional factors that garner points.

Trial Lawyers

Trial lawyers typically are prepared to perform in a sense. As such, the way they conduct themselves embraces all aspects of comportment, including attitude, demeanor, posture, presentation and behavior. They present themselves in a stylistic manner such that they have presence. They know that everyone in the courtroom is observing and hopefully listening and following their presentation, and they use their talents and skills to make an impression, which extends to how they address and engage with witnesses and evidence. Through the years, as cameras have been permitted inside courtrooms, sensationalized cases have acquainted us with skills and talents by trial attorneys in an effort to be persuasive.

Opening Statements

The opening statements will begin with the prosecution. The prosecutor will introduce and present the allegations or the charges against the defendant. As such, the prosecution presents and sets the stage or the groundwork of the case. The prosecutor will explain to the trier of fact what will be proved and how that will happen through presentation of witnesses and evidence. The attorneys will engage with the jury in a conversational manner to engage them and enable them to understand and appreciate what the attorney is going to do over the course of the trial with respect to their client. Essentially, a road map is provided through verbal statements to enlist the support of the jury to find in favor of their client via the information to be offered, including real and demonstrative evidence.

The entirety of the case is summarized in advance to provide the jury with an overview of what is going to be discussed and presented and the order in which the process will be unveiled. Establishing the path to the platform for where the attorney hopes to conclude is primary to opening statements. Final remarks are reserved for a summation as to why the jury should support a particular outcome. The material presented during opening statements will be revisited upon closing arguments. The attorney will repeat information that was presented at the beginning of the trial to the jury to demonstrate how everything that was promised to happen did, meaning that the attorney will indicate that everything that was to be presented and proved during the trial was achieved and the objectives as initially outlined or stated were met, leading to an appeal from the attorneys for the verdict they have strived to convince the jury is the only desirable outcome.

The opening statements consist of four parts:

- a synopsis of what happened in relation to the client or via the client's viewpoint
- relating such to a wrong or loss suffered by the client
- introduction of the principal facts and who will testify to them
- the prosecutor will seek a favorable decision in support of the plaintiff through direct appeal to the jury and will reiterate this during closing arguments

Synopsis: The prosecutor will explain to the jury in a conversational manner who the client is and why the client and, by extension the jury, is in the courtroom. In other words, the lawyer will explain the circumstances that gave rise to the proceeding. The lawyer will inform the jury what will be presented and who will be providing information or evidence to help the jury understand the facts of the case (the witnesses to be called).

The lawyer will also explain what must have occurred and ask the jury to render a verdict in concert with the presentation of the facts essentially to find in favor of the plaintiff (civil) or the prosecution (criminal). The plaintiff may also be referred to as the complainant. It is the job of the prosecution, meaning the attorney who represents the state or the entity pursuing justice (so to speak), to meet the burden of proof.

If the case is a criminal proceeding, the prosecutor will present opening statements first. The defendant's attorney follows. Each side provides the trier of fact with information about what evidence will be presented. Each side explains what the lawyers will prove and what they hope the outcome will be.

The defendant's side will explain the evidence to be presented and what the defense hopes to prove on behalf of the client. Witnesses are subjected to direct and cross examination by the opposing counsel or side.

Witnesses

Witnesses are scored on character portrayal. They are assessed on preparation and how it relates to character presentation as well as their testimony on direct and cross examination. Testimony by a witness is admitted into evidence via procedure. This entails identification of the witness for the court, swearing under oath about the truthfulness of the testimony to be given and direct and cross examination in the presence of the trier of fact. The presentation of evidence is central to trial. Rules of evidence govern the procedure and process so that evidence is offered in a fair and just manner such that the facts are presented accurately.

Team Performance

Team performance is scored on overall performance, preparation and understanding of judicial process and procedure.

The following terms are associated with judicial proceedings and are relevant, whether in a mock scenario or a real-world setting.

Burden of Proof

A judge will explain to a jury the charges at the conclusion of the trial and describe what standard(s) are to be met in order to meet the specified burden of proof, which depends upon the nature of the court proceeding.

Myers (2011b) outlines that American courts subscribe to three burdens of proof depending upon the nature of the proceeding and the type of litigation.

Proof beyond a reasonable doubt – is the most difficult to meet 95% certainty. "To satisfy the standard, "evidence does not have to eliminate all doubt. Yet, the evidence must be so strong that the judge or jury is nearly certain that the evidence is right" (Myers, 2011b, p. 61).

Preponderance of evidence is, according to Myers (2011b), the least demanding of the burdens, meaning it is the easiest to meet (p. 61) with 51% certainty associated with it. This is satisfied "when the evidence in favor of a proposition is even slightly greater than the evidence against the proposition" (p. 61).

Clear and convincing evidence lies between the two burdens described earlier. Myers attributes 75% of certainty to this standard.

In a civil matter, the burden of proof is "a preponderance of evidence", whereas if the matter is a criminal case, then the accused must be found "guilty or not guilty". As stated earlier, if a defendant is found not guilty, that does not mean that the judge or jury believes the defendant is innocent; rather, it means that the circumstances as determined by the trier of fact did not meet the standard or the burden of proof to render a guilty verdict.

In deciding if a burden has been met, the jury will apply the judge's instructions to the evidence that has been introduced during the trial and in regard to how it relates to the law. The judge's instructions follow closing arguments and precede jury deliberation.

Preliminary Hearing

Although this is not necessarily a part of a mock court scenario, for explanatory purposes it is included here in the event one might encounter such a proceeding. This is a matter wherein a judge determines if enough evidence has been rendered by the prosecution to justify a defendant to stand trial. As such, this proceeding preempts what comes next. Preliminary hearings do not happen in every matter. Children may be asked to testify and provide evidence in support of the prosecution's case that a defendant should go to trial on a crime. Essentially the prosecutor is charged with the task of meeting the criteria of the judge to accept that a crime was committed and/or that the defendant is the person responsible (Myers, 2011c).

In reality, only a small number or percentages of cases actually proceed to trial. Some forms of child maltreatment are considered to be a crime; however, according to Myers (2011b), most "child maltreatment is not criminal" (p. 99). As Myers explains, to protect children in some cases, the intervention and juvenile court, in conjunction with the intervention of child protective services, is sufficient to protect children and assist families and parents. In some cases, no court involvement is necessary. However, Myers expresses that in other situations when abuse or neglect is great, criminal law is warranted (Myers, 2011b).

Trial

A trial is a judicial procedure conducted to determine if the rights of a person or entity have been violated. A trial is a method of procedure to determine the guilt or innocence of a person with respect to the violation of rights. In a civil case, an individual must establish that his or her rights have been infringed upon. In criminal court, a trial is conducted to determine if someone has violated laws that pertain to society as a whole or an individual. Laws are associated with a governing body which will prosecute, such as the state. One must be cognizant of the law as it pertains to the jurisdiction where the trial is being held.

In a trial, rules exist that pertain to procedure, conduct of participants and the submission of evidence. To ensure a fair process, objections may be raised in response to the areas where rules are applied, meaning objections may be directed at procedure, conduct and evidence. Discussion of objections follows.

Plaintiff

The plaintiff is the person who is bringing some sort of legal action, and in some instances, the prosecution is responsible for bringing action on behalf of an individual.

Defendant

The defendant is the person or perhaps a body such as an institution that is being brought up on charges of some sort in court. The defendant is the accused.

Jury

The jury is composed of individuals from the community. To serve as a juror, one must be a U.S. citizen, be 18 years old and live in the jurisdiction of the court. Jury selection is necessary because the individuals selected are invested with the power to render a verdict or a decision based upon the evidence presented in a trial. They are charged with deliberating and determining a just and proper finding in accordance with the adversarial system of justice. Jury duty is considered an obligation.

Alternates are selected as well. Alternates are present during the trial to hear the case; however, they do not participate in deliberations unless selected to take the place of a juror should a need arise to remove someone. A jury is selected via a process which may involve responding to questions and inquiries through voir dire, which means "to speak the truth". Questions are asked by the various attorneys involved in a particular case. The process is intended to weed out individuals who may have a connection to someone involved in the case, including the attorneys, or if someone is unable to participate in an unbiased or nonprejudicial way. For example, if the case involves someone who was hurt because they fell outside of a store while walking on an icy sidewalk, someone may have had a similar experience and may be unable to separate their situation from the case being presented (an actual case where a potential juror was dismissed).

The lawyers and the judge have the opportunity to explore how potential jurors think and feel, and they make determinations as to which individuals they think are acceptable to serve given the particulars of a case. Jurors may request to be excused when called to jury duty; however, the judge will decide if such is granted. Excuses are offered depending upon an individual's needs and life situation and whether or not, if selected, jury duty might create a hardship either personally (young child at home and no one else is available to babysit) or financially (self-employed).

Sometimes an individual may be dismissed after responding to questions because they are viewed as not able to be impartial for whatever reason or an attorney does not think the individual is the best person for a particular case. There is latitude with regard to arguing for or against a potential individual to be seated as a juror; however, the judge is the final arbitrator. An attorney may request that a potential juror be dismissed "for cause", perhaps because an attorney believes the individual presented information that indicates preference for the other side for whatever reason. There is no set number of these requests that attorneys may seek; however, there are also "preemptory challenges" where an attorney does not have to specify why they wish for the potential juror to be dismissed. These types of challenges do have a finite number depending upon the type of proceeding (American Bar Association, n.d.).

Jury Instructions

Follow closing arguments and preceding deliberations, the judge will instruct the jury about the rules of law. The instructions inform the jury about weighing the evidence in concert with the applicable law as denoted by the judge.

Objections

There are three broad types of objections: procedure and rules, admission and use of testimony and evidence and conduct of a participant with regard to procedure or evidence (American Mock Trial Association, 1985).

- three broad types
    - procedure and rules
    - admission and use of testimony and evidence
    - conduct of a participant: procedurally or evidentiarily

Attorneys for the opposing side can object to something the other side's attorney questions or asks as well as object to a witness as noted earlier. The judge may ask for the reason why the objection should be overruled.

If overruled, the witness is allowed to answer the question because the judge disagrees with the reason offered by the objecting attorney.

If sustained, the witness may not answer the question because the judge agrees with the objecting attorney that the question is improper under the rules of evidence.

It is the responsibility of the attorneys to identify points of law involved in the issue to support the objection and to know when to object, and it is up to the judge to determine how to rule and in support of which side given the law and the objection made. The witness must be alert to the judge's ruling so as not to respond when directed not to.

If the judge stipulates overruled, then the witness should answer the question. If, however, the judge sustains the objection, then the witness must not answer. It is important to understand the process and the meaning of objections and how this impacts a witness when testifying on the stand. The witness does not want to be admonished for giving a response when directed not to or for not replying when told to do so.

Standard Objections

A judge may rule once an attorney has objected to something said or presented by a witness. Standard objections include:

Irrelevant Evidence

Lack of personal knowledge, improper character testimony, irrelevant to the facts of the case or beyond the scope of direct examination, for example, when information is not presented on direct examination.

Opinion

When the witness is not qualified to give an answer, for instance, if not qualified as an expert

Leading Question

Objectionable only when done on direct examination

Hearsay

Hearsay is a statement made to the witness by someone not in the court. Hearsay has been defined as "an out of court assertion that is required in court to prove the truth of the matter asserted" (Myers, 2011d, p. 378). When this objection is made, an attorney asks for a statement to be stricken from the record (of course, once something is said, it has been heard by the jury and even though it may not be reflected in the official record or transcript, it still has the potential to influence). Hearsay is offered to prove the truth of the fact and may be admissible in certain circumstances. According to the American Mock Trial Association (1985), "If testimony is offered for the sole purpose of proving that the statement was made, it is not hearsay".
Objection examples follow and include examples drawn from personal and first-hand exposure/experience.

Objection Examples:

Leading Question

Objection: Counsel is trying to get a witness to contradict previous testimony
Response: Counsel is leading the witness to substantiate a claim by the attorney
Objection: Badgering the witness
Response: Counsel is attacking the witness and not letting the witness answer questions
Objection: Asked and answered
Response: Counsel has already asked the question and the witness has responded

Irrelevant Evidence

Objection: Irrelevant evidence; witness is discussing a different client to make a point
Response: The information exceeds the scope of information needed for a fair hearing
Objection: Character of the witness is being challenged
Response: Such information cannot be introduced unless it is an issue in the case
Objection: Witness offers an opinion when not asked to do so or when a lay witness
Response: Witness is testifying to an opinion on the ultimate issue, which is the jurisdiction of the trier of fact, or the witness is not an expert

Hearsay

Objection: Hearsay
Response: Immaterial, as the information is not from the witness

Objection: Counsel has not laid the proper foundation for evidentiary material
Response: Not presented on direct examination

Opinion

Objection: Lack of foundation to qualify as an as expert
Response: The witness is a lay witness and as such cannot offer an opinion about the issue
Objection: Witness is giving an opinion they are not qualified to give
Response: Speculation to a hypothetical question or testimony is not factual
Objection: Stating a conclusion
Response: Witness is going beyond material introduced on direct examination

Closing Arguments

Attorneys for each side will provide a summation of the evidence they presented. Their presentation is essentially a plea for the trier of fact to find in favor of the arguments they have presented and to find in favor of their client. Each side will indicate what they proved and what the other side failed to prove. They will do this by addressing the credibility and presentation (performance) of the opposing side's witnesses and even counsel (lawyers).

Closing is a last-ditch appeal for the jury to hear from the defense as to what the defense did that was advantageous versus what the prosecution did that was not propitious. The goal is to summarize for the jury the facts (as they see it) of the case. The defense will try to make the case for why the jury should believe the facts as they presented them, including the evidence they presented to contradict the other side. The defense will call into question what they feel has holes in it with regard to witness testimony or evidentiary material in an effort to make a strong and convincing case for why the jury should find in favor of their side or for the defendant. The defense will highlight what is helpful for the case from what was presented and may summarize or repeat what was presented during opening statements, including witnesses and their testimony. The defense will take apart the other side's presentation and try to identify weaknesses in the case, the prosecution witnesses and their testimony on direct and cross examination and attack credibility as well as the presented evidence. This will culminate in a final appeal to the jury for a verdict in favor of the defense.

In sum, the closing argument is an opportunity for each side to say what they proved, what the other side failed to prove, what was favorable and what supported their version of the facts and why they deserve to have the jury find in their favor.

Hired Gun

This person is an expert hired by one side to present an opinion favorable to that side. Compensation is customary, and as such the expert is brought into court to support a position or an agenda (usually). This witness's testimony is contracted as such and may imply or suggest a lack of impartiality and partisanship. Monetary compensation and other expenses vary according to the expert witness's experience and notoriety. Sometimes just the presence of this individual in the courtroom or waiting to be called has a resultant impact on the other side's presentation and may lead to a change in strategy (which may be the intent by counsel).

An expert witness, including a hired gun, should in reality not be swayed or pressured to follow a particular agenda. Experts are brought in to assist the court. Even hired guns presenting as forensic experts have an ethical responsibility to present information in a reliable and accurate manner. "A forensic specialist hired by one side will provide an honest appraisal of the facts and, if permitted to testify, will provide an honest accounting of the accumulated data and its derived interpretations". Moreover, "[t]he best interests of the court are served when the expert witness performs in an objective, impartial manner regardless of who hires him" (Barsky & Gould, 2002, p. 149).

Subpoena

Court participation is often initiated through a subpoena. A subpoena has an official court seal and is signed by a court clerk, judge or attorney. It is a command by the court and merits a response. It is delivered by a process server. Lack of response can be punishable, and a person may be considered in contempt. There are two types of subpoenas: one that designates a certain time and day to be present to testify, while the other requests specified documents be brought at a certain time and day to court.

Once a subpoena is served, contact should be made with the individual or entity that sent the document. Myers (2002) eloquently states, "Understanding where the lawyer is coming from helps the expert set proper boundaries and maintain objectivity" (p. 244). A discussion may reveal that the potential witness may not be the best person to provide testimony. Documentation of contact is recommended in the event a subpoena is voided so that one is not held in contempt if this information is not communicated to the court.

Legal Representation

Individuals should be cognizant of the policies and practices associated with one's legal obligations related to their workplace. Individuals are advised to speak directly with in-house counsel or agency affiliated legal representation upon receiving a subpoena to discuss one's responsibilities about courtroom participation and direct response (to a subpoena). If legal counsel is not a function of one's work environment, then seeking outside counsel to address concerns, queries or one's participation related to a specific case is recommended.

A subpoena is a command that is normally issued by a court at the request of an attorney (Myers, 1992). It mandates that the professional go to court; however, it does not mean that the individual has to disclose privileged information (Myers, 1992). It is prudent and wise to contact the attorney who signed the subpoena to ascertain the reason and rationale for being asked to appear.

Deposition

A deposition is a proceeding that is used by attorneys to ascertain the content of the testimony of an opposing witness. It is part of the discovery process (collection or exchange of information/evidence) conducted during pretrial proceedings. Depositions consist of sworn testimony taken in the presence of a recorder (stenographer) and are certified by the witness as correct. No trier of fact is present. Normally the attorney who requested the deposition asks the questions, but the witness has counsel present to object or advise not to answer.

A transcript of a deposition may be requested by the witness and reviewed prior to trial. It is strongly recommended that a witness review a deposition transcript in anticipation of what defense will ask on cross examination and to make sure sworn testimony is consistent on the witness stand with what was deposed. The transcript should be logical and organized, as it is reflective of the testimony provided during the proceeding, which is typically an indication of how the witness will appear on the witness stand. If the written testimony does not appear coherent, the need to prepare accordingly is highly recommended.

A deposition is a tactic that provides insight for opposing counsel regarding what the expert intends to say during the trial. This allows for the opinions of the expert to be shared, as well as the basis for them. Counsel also can assess how witnesses handle questioning through this process.

If the testimony of a witness differs substantially during trial, which it should not, the witness may need to explain discrepancies on the stand. The purpose of the deposition is to gather sworn statements for discovery purposes and to use the information to impeach during cross examination.

Evidence

Evidence encompasses a wealth of forms. Evidence can include testimony by witnesses, and it is also defined as written documents or objects. Evidence is admissible unless some rule exists to exclude the evidence. Evidence is defined as "any matter, verbal or physical that can be used to support the existence of a factual proposition" (Lilly, 1996, p. 2). Moreover, Lilly (1996) asserts that "this definition is useful because it emphasizes the perspective of the legal profession, which associates evidence with the facts of a case" (p. 2). As such, evidence may include testimony which is admitted into evidence via procedure in which the witness is identified, testifies under oath and is subjected to questioning by both plaintiff and defense. The manner in which and how evidence is offered and delivered may impact a trial and is critical for accomplishing the goals of each side. Thus, evidence may be presented as a mechanism for proving or disproving (facts).

Admissibility of evidence is governed by complex rules administered by a judge. Evidence may be substantive or rehabilitative. In child sexual abuse cases evidence is used to accomplish different objectives. Substantive evidence is evidence offered in court to prove that the child was sexually abused such as a medical exam or a disclosure statement. Substantive evidence is based on many factors, including a child's statements, behavior and symptoms. Demonstrative evidence can be used to clarify or illuminate or explain oral testimony, such as a chart or a photograph. The jury can take this evidentiary material when deliberating to recall what the witness's position was about a particular matter. Evidence enhances the effectiveness of witness testimony.

Questions

The rules of trial prohibit leading questions. A leading question is one that suggests the answer. Typically, on direct examination, narrative testimony is elicited via open-ended questions.

Three types of questions may be used and combined: open, closed and leading questions.

Open is associated with a narrative response.

Closed is associated with a specific response such as a yes or no answer.

Leading questions contain the intended response, or they may be restrictive such that a response is limited in scope. Leading questions are not to be asked on either direct or redirect questioning; however, leading and closed questions are used to orchestrate what an attorney wants a witness to say. Closed questions limit what a response may be, whereas a leading question suggests what response is desired.

A Line of Questioning

A line of questioning refers to a single question or a series of related questions asked by the examining attorney. Questions are grouped such that they assist counsel in achieving objectives or an agenda. Lines of questioning are essential to consider when preparing for testifying.

Theme

A theme is given to identify each particular line of questioning.

Direct Testimony

The basic points that will be covered on direct questions are designed to elicit the facts in the most effective manner possible and to give the witness the chance to affirm or deny. Testifying is a verbal process predicated upon language; however, nonverbal communications may impact or affect the outcome. A record of verbal transactions is recorded so witnesses must speak and not respond nonverbally or risk being admonished to say an answer rather than nod. The court reporter is not watching, but rather listening, so it is important to use words rather than provide an answer that is not heard and may not be recorded.

Topics addressed on direct testimony include:

- the expert's qualifications
- the expert's knowledge of the facts of the case
- the steps that the expert has taken in formulating an opinion
- if the expert has formed an opinion to a reasonable degree of professional certainty on the question at issue
- the expert's opinion
- the reasons and basis for the expert's opinion

Direct examination consists of a three-part structure that includes an introduction wherein the witness is introduced to the trier of fact and testimony is proffered to establish credibility. Direct examination affords an opportunity for the witness to offer information pertaining to the facts, and it allows for a narrative. Typically, the exchange between the attorney and the witness is a question-and-answer pattern with opportunities for narration. The body of testimony consists of information to prove the elements of the case and to refute the opposing case and rationale. This is done through evidence presented, including details relevant to the matter. To avoid the witness being effectively impeached, on direct examination, negatives that might impact or be used to impeach the witness on cross examination are brought to light. Admission of weakness such as lack of experience, or recent employment with a specialized population or whatever is deemed to be an issue is acknowledged to preempt cross examination, which will try to establish incompetence and undermine credibility by honing in on perceived areas of weakness.

Cross Examination

Cross examiners will seek to undermine the credibility of a witness and look for weakness in preparation and presentation as well as testimony. Cross examination is known as an antibiased device (Myers, 1992). Objectives and strategies associated with this judicial process are designed to impeach the testimony and ultimately the credibility of a witness and their testimony. The cross examiner will attempt to minimize an expert's qualifications, highlight perceived bias and dismiss evidentiary material including negating a written report. All witnesses are subjected to cross examination, and preparing for the possibility and likely interaction is paramount to managing one's ability to tolerate this process and remain professional.

Courtroom strategy considers witness order, and an experienced witness is typically presented first. If the witness is familiar with the dynamics and strategies of cross examination and able to contend with the questions, this will be a positive first impression. If, on the other hand, the witness is unable to handle the cross examiner, the witness's presentation may negatively impact the case. Of course, the cross examiner may also be seen in a hostile way by the jury. Cross examination is all about strategy, tactics and technique. The more one is versed in these elements, typically through exposure and previous experience as well as preparation, the better equipped one may be to handle cross strategies and devices and present effectively.

Understanding the objectives and studying the strategies that are employed are key to surviving cross examination. There is no standard structure for cross examination. Cross examiners will utilize every skill and technique that is permissible to undermine a witness (Myers, 1992). Witnesses must be attentive to how they present and the language they use. Devoting time to understanding cross examination, its objectives and strategies through practice and role play is recommended.

Myers (1996) has described techniques on cross examination as negative and positive. Cross examiners may try to engage a witness in a positive and friendly manner only to later employ strategies to discredit through negative tactics that undermine the testimony that was elicited to confirm or support the cross-examiner's case (Myers, 2011c). Cross examination strategies do not necessarily subscribe to negative engagement, which is a ploy in and of itself and at times is used to snare unsuspecting witnesses.

During cross, it is the role of the direct examiner to protect the witness. As such, the attorney has to be vigilant and appeal to the judge if the witness is being manipulated, or badgered. The attorney representing the witness can object if, for example, the witness is not being given adequate time to respond to cross inquiries, etc. The goals associated with cross are multifaceted and the direct examiner has to be mindful of the tactics as they unfold and intervene accordingly. Cross is an attempt to discredit the witness and help the defense. The cross examiner will use the witness's presentation to advance the defense agenda, if possible, by discrediting testimony and integrity.

Objectives on Cross Examination

- impeach the accuracy and truth of the testimony
- discredit the testimony through identifying omissions and commissions
- downplay the significance of the witness's testimony to cast doubt

- undermine the facts on which the expert bases an opinion
- point out how an opinion would differ if certain assumed facts were changed

Strategies/Approaches

- cross examiners try to lead the witness through tone of voice and pace of speech
- use of leading questions
- examiners do not ask a question on cross examination unless they know the answer
- on cross examination the attorney will make it clear that they are in charge
- the lawyer may present aggressively
- the lawyer will provoke the witness into responding
- compound and hypothetical questions will be utilized
- the witness will be baited to venture beyond their expertise
- weakness will be preyed upon: personality, character, presentation and be used to the advantage of defense
- be mindful of traps and being boxed into a corner (Vieth, 2000)

Myers (1992) lists the following strategies invoked during cross examination:

- Defense avoids a full-frontal attack because it makes the cross examiner look bad and rarely works.
- The jury's discontent with the attack by the attorney may be generalized to the client.
- Cross examiners may use more subtle techniques that use indirect methods to undermine an expert's testimony.
- Cross examiners try to raise questions and doubts about the expert's testimony that can be used against the expert during closing arguments.

Challenges on cross examination may be directed at:

- expert's credentials
- certainty of the expert's opinion
- witness's interest in a case or the outcome – impartiality
- perceived bias

Myers (1992) describes three cross examination strategies that are predicated upon controlling the witness.

Cross examiners will ask leading questions. Leading questions suggest the answer and permit only short responses, usually yes or no. They do not afford an opportunity to clarify or explain a response in a narrative fashion.

The second way a witness is controlled is by limiting the opportunity to explain answers. As such, Myers (1992) states that a witness needs to find a way to express the answer without resorting to a yes or no response. At times, the witness may need to directly appeal to the judge to be allowed to respond accordingly.

The third strategy the witness may encounter while being cross examined is "hiding the ball" (Myers, 1992). Myers (1992) explains that an attorney will ask questions that seem innocuous but ultimately lead the witness into a predetermined position through hiding the objective.

Myers (1996) describes strategies and principles associated with cross examination

---

Cross examiners will seek to undermine a witness by employing various strategies and
techniques, including:
- inconsistencies in prior statements
- leading questions
- questions that foster a desired response
- provoking a negative response
- minimizing qualifications
- cornering into yes/no questions without a way to expound

Barsky and Gould (2002) in their text provide information for the clinician in the
courtroom. They caution not to take cross examination out of context. They state, "the
vast majority of cases are won or lost on the facts rather than one witness's performance
on the stand" (p. 119). They offer that "consistency is key to whether your evidence will
be believed" (Barsky & Gould, 2002, p. 120). Discrepancies in a witness's testimony and
thus the evidence they offer may be challenged.

Barsky and Gould (2002) discuss strategies they refer to as ten tactics or methods
associated with cross examination. Some are consistent with the strategies outlined by
Myers (1992, 1996) as noted. I include Barsky and Gould (2002) for additional reference. They offer supportive information pertaining to coping with as well as preparing
for cross examination. The text is another valuable resource to delve deeper into the
complexities associated with cross examination of witnesses (in addition to the material
referenced by Myers).

Tactics for Cross Examination adapted from Barsky and Gould (2002)

- **Tactic 1: Challenging Credibility**
- **Tactic 2: Establishing Doubt**
- **Tactic 3: Logic Funnel** – Ask a series of questions intended to nudge the witness in
  a particular direction. Similar to Myers's hiding the ball, whereby answering earlier
  questions in a certain direction means one may not be able to avoid an answer
  that appears contradictory or that is in opposition to something that was asked
  previously.
- **Tactic 4: Leading Questions**
- **Tactic 5: Feigned Ignorance** – Typically an attorney does not ask a question unless
  the answer is already known or possessed by them. This is a tactic used when the
  attorney may be fishing for something or intends to direct the witness into a hidden
  area (strategy – like Myers's hiding the ball).
- **Tactic 6: The Cutoff** – This occurs when the attorney does not want the witness to
  provide information that may not be helpful for that side.
- **Tactic 7: Rapid Fire** – Asking questions in a "machine-gun-like fashion" (p. 123). The
  witness will need to be aware of the strategy, which is to unbalance the responses of
  the witness, so remaining calm and responding as if the questions were being asked
  in a nonrapid manner is the best way to handle this tactic.
- **Tactic 8: Intentional Ambiguity** – The authors state that this tactic is meant to confuse the witness and say something that was unintentional (p. 124).

- **Tactic 9: Implying Impropriety** – This tactic tries to make the witness look bad on the stand in a dishonest or immoral way. Barsky and Gould provide an example surrounding a witness's compensation. The witness, they say, should not be embarrassed to admit accepting payment and instead should instruct the attorney and the court if asked about such that they are being paid for time, not testimony. "A direct and non-defensive response is the best way to respond to a question that attacks your integrity" (p. 126).
- **Tactic 10: Rattling the Witness** – Whereby an attorney engages in intimidating and even offensive behavior to try to provoke an untoward response. Remain calm and carry on, as has been explained in the tips for cross examination.

Redirect Examination

This type of testimony allows for rehabilitation of a witness. For example, if opposing counsel tries to discredit something about the witness's testimony or credentials that may have been brought out during cross examination, redirect examination gives the presenting counsel an opportunity to try and correct or clarify a misnomer identified on cross examination. It also affords the opportunity to explain mishaps or miscommunications that may have occurred during cross examination and that were intended to discredit the witness and their statements. This type of testimony is not always easy to prepare or script because it is conducted after direct and cross examination and is used to address something that may have occurred on the witness stand that may not have been anticipated, such as a witness's words being taken out of context. Hopefully, on cross examination, the direct examiner is wise to the cross-examiner's tactics and is making objections when appropriate and if the witness is being beleaguered, pressured or harassed in some way. Questions should not go beyond what was discussed/asked in cross examination unless truthfulness of the witness is raised.

Objectives

- rehabilitating the witness
- re-emphasizing what was presented on direct examination
- remedying oversights from direct examination
- correcting mistakes
- opportunity to clarify and remediate something that went awry during cross examination
- giving the witness an opportunity to explain answers from cross examination
- examining issues raised by cross examination not previously addressed

Witnesses

Witnesses are integral to the trial system and provide various roles within the court. They educate, inform, disabuse commonly held misperceptions and provide opinions as experts. They are necessary to present information and knowledge as well as evidence. Witness testimony is evidentiary material.

The order in which witnesses are called is a factor in planning case presentation. Although a strong and favorable witness is desired to open the trial, the order of witnesses may be determined upon the foundation that the calling attorney is attempting to establish. The witness lineup may be cumulative such that there is a motive behind introducing witnesses in relation to one another and in the presentation of evidence that each will offer with respect to the facts of the case. Witnesses are brought in to testify, as well as to establish or corroborate facts that are salient to the case.

In some instances, certain witnesses such as an external expert (someone not involved in the particular case) may be asked to participate and speak to a class of individuals or provide consultation and not testify on the witness stand and may not be needed depending upon how the case develops. Sometimes these witnesses are held in abeyance in an annex or waiting area until such time that they may be needed to offer testimony. These witnesses may be held in reserve in the event that there is a need to have an effective witness to offset something that may have occurred on cross examination with a different witness. As such, this witness may be brought in for rebuttal purposes and may not be extended a lengthy preparatory period given the need to respond to a tactic or strategy that was utilized on cross examination. Seemingly, this type of a witness is someone who has experience and expertise presenting in such situations where elongated preparation is not feasible.

At times, some individuals may be construed as hired guns, brought in to support an agenda. They may have well-known names or reputations in a particular area. Sometimes just having such individuals in the building is a strategy in that the other side may not wish to have this individual present on the stand for a myriad of reasons. These types of witnesses may receive payment for their presence without stepping inside the courtroom or presenting testimony. They may also be in reserve in the event that the case is in need of extra help or support from having this individual participate or be present. This is not always advantageous, as an expert's time constraints and fees may be implausible with regard to how a case is unfolding in real time. When an outside expert is brought in, they will be presented in order such that the evidence and facts have already been presented by prior witnesses about the individual case. The external witness may offer an opinion and speak to a class of individuals in some fashion.

The fact-finder (judge or jury) wants three pieces of information from a witness: who is the witness, what does the witness know about the case and is the witness testifying honestly and accurately. With regard to an expert testifying, the witness may be placed in the witness lineup after the facts and information that the witness will base his or her opinion on has been presented and entered into evidence so that the opinion offered is most effective.

The last person on the witness stand is ideally a strong witness for the calling side. The first witness sets the stage for the information or evidence to be offered. The last witness is positioned to reaffirm the main points presented in relation to the case and the evidence presented. In some instances, this person may be sought in response to a cross examination attack on a witness, and this person may not have a great deal of time to prepare. Witness scheduling is a part of strategizing how the case will be presented and the manner in which evidentiary material will unfold.

Considerations addressed in preparing witnesses encompass presentation as well as content of information. Questions to be considered include whether the witness can refute or contradict evidence offered by the opposing party and whether the witness will offer evidence that may bolster the case. Witnesses may also be used to corroborate evidence in alignment with the facts being offered, and conversely a witness may purposefully be asked to testify to cast doubt on testimony or credibility by a witness offered by the opposing counsel.

In preparation, attorneys will balance the probative (positive) value against the prejudicial (negative) effect of presenting a particular witness to testify. Another consideration for the attorney to consider pertains to the witness's innate presentation. The attorney may need to balance if a witness's inherent personality traits might be offensive or not conducive to a positive outcome against what the witness may be able to offer in support of the case.

There is some juggling that must be considered in strategically planning the witness list. Consideration must be directed at understanding whether a witness may be used by opposing counsel in a manner that refutes the purpose of the testimony and instead ends up helping the opposing side. An expert may also be utilized in the role of an advisor wherein testimony is not warranted, but rather emphasis is placed on how the expert can assist the attorneys with the case dynamics.

Finally, effective witnesses are familiar with procedures and the dynamics of testifying. Effective witnesses anticipate responses and shape the feel as well as the substance of the exchange with the calling and/or defense attorney. If the witness is in control, testimony will conform to what the witness knows rather than the intimations of the attorney.

Witness Planning and Preparation Tips

- know the attorney's expectations regarding your testimony
- have the attorney be direct in stating and outlining the purpose of your testimony
- clarify what you are/can be an expert on
- identify matters you will not discuss
- educate the attorney about your field/area of specialization
- explain your training and related experience
- provide resource materials to educate the attorney about your profession and type of work
- review the report that you will be testifying about, which may be entered into evidence
- the effectiveness of witnesses has an impact on a case and may influence the outcome
- have the attorney read back notes during prep to identify and clarify misperceptions
- anticipate possible questions to be asked on cross examination
- ask the attorney for a list of prepared questions that will be asked and script expected answers
- request a list of the facts to be examined when on the witness stand
- prepared questions can help the lawyer get a desired response or help to modify questions
- prep participation with calling counsel can increase the effectiveness of the testimony
- develop and review strategies with presenting counsel for direct examination and possible redirect examination
- consider what might be a potential target for cross examination and prepare accordingly
- identify weaknesses in the curriculum vitae (CV) and testimony and develop strategies to combat on cross examination

Witness Presentation Tips

- everything in the courtroom is open to scrutiny
- witnesses' physical presentation, posture, attitude and demeanor are scrutinized
- be mindful of nonverbal behaviors such as fidgeting or nervous habits

- affect will be observed
- be aware of communication patterns, how to relay information and speak
- talk in a manner that is confident
- if you do not know something, say, "I do not know" or "I do not have an answer for the question"
- be honest and sincere in response and delivery
- direct testimony to everyone in the courtroom, including judge, jury and counsel
- speak clearly
- vary answers in length and tone, and be mindful of inflection and how it may contribute to testimony
- ensure everyone in the courtroom can hear you and is receptive to what you are saying
- how you say something matters
- do not let counsel control you or "flip the script" – stay in control of counsel and testimony
- do not volunteer additional information, especially on direct examination
- only answer the question asked
- anything you provide on direct examination is subject to cross examination
- make sure you understand the question before responding
- pay attention and stay engaged
- remember you are being observed at all times
- be objective
- avoid professional jargon
- master your emotions
- maintain a professional demeanor
- do not argue or become defensive
- never make a statement or give an opinion you cannot support
- be respectful
- be deferential
- provide observations, not conclusions, unless an expert
- if technical terms are required, then use a lay definition
- as much as possible answers should be short, direct and to the point
- express findings and opinions in understandable but memorable terms
- present opinions with persuasive and compelling language
- communicate clearly and effectively
- know the goals of your testimony and the limits
- prepare ahead of time
- be aware of nonverbal behavior
- do not memorize testimony – may sound stilted
- let the presenting attorney develop your testimony

Tips for Cross Examination

- be mindful of cross examination strategies and potential traps
- as a witness, you have more power than you think
- do not succumb to intimidation
- maintain a professional posture
- resist being controlled
- do not fall into innuendos that the cross examiner may be making

- if the cross examiner has the witness under control, the cross examiner will direct the flow of the testimony
- anticipate responses and shape the feel and the substance of the exchange
- learn to control cross examination through speech techniques
- listen with care to the nature of the questions and use to your advantage
- disagree with cross examination when possible
- be aware of the use of positive and negative ploys
- do not hide on the stand; command personal space – it denotes power
- sit tall, do not fidget or show nerves
- listen to what is being asked and answer only what is asked
- do not volunteer information beyond what is asked
- answer compound questions by breaking up the question so you avoid giving an answer that may only be responsive to part of the long-winded question
- remain impartial
- do not be reactive – maintain a professional demeanor
- maintain objectivity
- exhibit neutrality

Tips for Testifying and Techniques

- do not answer when an objection has been made until the judge rules on the objection
- be loud – audible – do not rely on the microphone and do not lean into it
- speak in a clear and controlled voice
- include the judge and jury in responses – speak directly to them
- take time to think about where the cross examination is going and give an appropriate response
- do not allow yourself to be pressured to answer
- if things go sour, do not show frustration – redirect examination will follow
- present the same as if on direct examination
- do not engage with cross examiner in a way that invalidates previous testimony
- stay strong willed and remain vigilant to cross examination tactics
- know and respect the limits of your expertise

I recommend Brodsky's (2004, 2013) texts as pertinent resources for understanding testifying and handling cross examination. He identifies and discusses common issues expert witnesses confront on the stand. He highlights these dilemmas with useful resolutions summed up in a maxim (a concisely expressed principle or rule of conduct). Brodsky's maxims or adages are intended to help prepare witnesses to manage courtroom scenarios and master the adversarial process with aplomb. In a recent text that expands upon his work in collaboration with a co-author they write, "Unlike the majority of our peers, we find testifying to be personally fascinating, intellectually challenging, and emotionally satisfying (usually)" (Brodsky & Gutheil, 2016, p. xii). Their strategies combine useful and pragmatic information to assist with comprehending, addressing and effectively managing the nature of the process, as well as responding cogently to the various strategies invoked. Brodsky (2004) as well as others have described characteristics associated with witnesses, both persuasive and not persuasive. These descriptors are fundamental to presenting as an expert witness and can be attested to by having had reason to present in the guise of an expert witness.

Throughout the years, via personal experience coupled with interactive, didactic and experiential training opportunities, as well as attention to the literature and scholarship on effective and ineffective methods of witness comportment, demeanor and presentation, these tips and tenets have been inculcated and merit continued propagation. (Information is presented as an amalgamation as described earlier and emanates from collective and personal integration and experience). The references provide resourceful material, yet the literature in this area continues to evolve.

Witnesses That Are Not Overly Effective, Convincing, Persuasive or Compelling *Some material attributed to Brodsky (1991, 2004, 2013); Brodsky and Gutheil (2016); Myers (1992, 2011c)*	*Witnesses That Are Effective, Convincing, Persuasive or Compelling* *Some material attributed to Brodsky (1991, 2004, 2013); Brodsky and Gutheil (2016); Myers (1992, 2011c)*
• talk too much • exaggerate • appear angry, defensive or antagonistic • overdramatic and appear superficial • take too long to respond • over qualify what say • use unfamiliar words • use conventional analogies • do not appear authentic and genuine	• do not talk too much or too little • calm and poised, professional demeanor • not too quick or too slow in answering • use narrative, smoothly flowing statements • use original analogies • personalize testimony • vary format of answers • humanize statements • personalize testimony • respectful, honest, genuine, authentic, confident not arrogant
Additional Descriptors for Not Overly Effective or Influential Witnesses	*Additional Descriptors for Effective or Influential Witnesses*
• lack of preparation • reactionary • labile affect on the stand • lack of professionalism • disrespectful/combative • argumentative • not prepared for cross examination • lack of awareness of relevant literature • not answering questions • talking in jargon	• appear reasonable and knowledgeable • do not overstate facts/opinions • demonstrate lack of bias • remain calm and attentive • do not argue with opposing counsel • concede when appropriate • support opinions with current literature • avoid anecdotal references • know literature that demonstrates awareness of controversies so can offer both sides of an issue • have case material organized • identify weaknesses in CV and present on direct examination in anticipation of cross examination • testimony should appear cogent and organized when transcribed • truthfulness and candor • look for opportunities to give long narrative answers during cross examination • use pronouns in a purposeful manner – 'we' connotes general acceptance

Testifying – Process/Procedure

1. swearing in
2. identification
3. qualification

4.   direct questioning
5.   cross examination
6.   redirect examination

Tips on Ethical Issues

- competence – limit testimony to areas of expertise
- maintain expertise – be current on relevant research, publications, developments in the field
- know scientific basis for opinions
- know courtroom basics
- familiarity with Frye and Daubert in the event special admissibility tests are invoked (not necessary but helpful to be informed – attorneys will address)
- know personal biases
- know consequences of an opinion – be able to support via testimony
- do not compromise one's ethics to meet an agenda
- if not qualified to speak to a particular subject, own it
- do not exceed scope of expertise
- admit when purview is beyond expertise
- be clear with attorney as to expectations, limits, boundaries
- maintain integrity
- authenticity factors into professional representation

Voir Dire: Qualification Process

- establish credentials as related to case
- questioning surrounding CV
- may be waived if testified in the same court system previously and if all parties stipulate to witness's qualifications
- typical to be qualified as an expert in predominate area of specialty
- will usually be asked location of training
- education, degrees, internships
- specialized training
- area of board certification or licensure
- membership in professional organizations
- experience with the population (length of time served, how many children worked with, etc.)
- publications/presentations
- prior court involvement (as expert)
- academic affiliations

Direct Testimony

- attorney usually asks questions intended to develop a logical and cohesive train of thought that leads to a conclusion
- role for the witness is to educate the trier of fact about specialized knowledge – parallels a teaching process – consider how to instruct students by building upon prior knowledge and experience
- use common sense

Cross Examination

- it is fundamental to the adversarial process, which is dedicated to finding the truth, yet the nature of it leads one to believe otherwise (Myers, 1992)
- the goal is to negate the testimony offered on direct examination
- the task is for opposing attorney to impeach the expert using whatever legal means are available, and there are plenty (Myers, 1992)
- cross examination may focus on inconsistencies in prior statements, or leading questions may be used in an attempt to structure responses so they are tailored in the way the attorney wants

Rebuttal/Redirect Examination

- contradicts testimony given by a previous expert for the other side
- defense can usually find someone who will testify to whatever position is needed
- rebuttal evidence often provided by expert witnesses and is designed to inform jurors
- may encounter redirect and recross examination, which allow for an opportunity for elaboration and witness challenge
- new material cannot be introduced during redirect examination

Testifying in Court as an Expert Witness Case Preparation

- review documentation of interview
- pay attention to details in report – location, time of day, who was present, child's affect
- note tools used in the interview
- length of interview
- note observations – physical, behavioral, emotional
- be able to speak to and defend the interview process, highlight main elements
- explain if interview process has been accepted in court – may need to explain and define the process, including who subscribes to it (multidisciplinary team) and where it is accepted (jurisdiction)

Memorialization of Documents (Reports)

- document during interview and review after
- make sure salient information is detailed
- describe observations
- identify source of information
- write clearly
- avoid vague statements
- do not use subjective or judgmental terms (for example – obviously or clearly)
- quote the child – direct quotes
- discuss nonverbal behaviors
- avoid mixing opinion with fact
- provide basis for conclusions, which should be clear from observations
- clarify contradictory information
- impressions and recommendations should be supported by data in the report
- keep report professional

- handwritten notes can be subpoenaed – make sure notes are clean – no doodles or subjective comments

Courtroom Procedure Preparation

- know courtroom policy and procedure
- be familiar with courtroom process and judicial procedure
- observe a similar process in anticipation
- objection – let the attorneys argue the merits of the objection and wait for the judge to rule and instruct you on whether to respond
- an objection is not a personal attack; it is based on legal precedent

Expert Witness Preparation

- know what is expected of you
- know why you are being called
- relevance of testimony
- find out agenda of attorney who executed the subpoena
- educate counsel about background, experience and training
- inform attorney about professional practice and area of specialization
- find out what is acceptable to discuss and what is not
- discuss hearsay issues – evidence that has been excluded
- be familiar with factual material about the case
- attorney will not necessarily want you to repeat contents of report
- find out the agenda of the attorney and the role of your testimony
- try to ascertain a hidden agenda
- identify and discuss problem areas in your testimony ahead of time
- be direct with calling attorney about what you will and will not say on the witness stand
- be mindful of compromising integrity and ethics
- let attorney know in advance the limits of your expertise – what you will and can speak to versus what you will not comment about when testifying
- do not compromise ethical boundaries to meet someone's agenda
- it is okay to disagree if the attorney mistakenly poses erroneous information (maybe wires were crossed during prep) or presents information that is incorrect about qualifications when on the stand
- the attorney will often tell the expert witness what is expected and what the attorney wants the expert witness to say
- clarify and agree to disagree and let the attorney know that if something is brought up or asked that will compromise integrity, you are not going to agree and you will indicate as such on the stand
- need to educate the attorney about information on CV and instruct how to rehabilitate
- before discussing a case with anyone, know the affiliation of the person seeking information
- professionals are under no legal obligation to communicate with the defense whether by phone, in person or by letter as well as digital communication
- preparing with calling counsel will effectively enhance testimony through developing strategies

- identify potential areas of conflict or weakness in anticipation of cross examination and promote strategizing

Cogitations

Prior to my first foray into court, I met with the deputy city solicitor to be instructed and informed as to how my presentation as a witness and testifying should be handled. It was an interesting discussion, especially with the words imparted prior to the conclusion of our meeting. This person stated unequivocally that how I presented the first time, meaning my presentation and my presence on the witness stand, would establish my reputation and seal my fate regarding my ability and competence in court as an expert witness in the community. Prosecutors and defense attorneys will be aware of what kind of witness I am and will address me and perceive me as such in future proceedings. What follows is a synopsis of the conversation with the city solicitor.

The solicitor (city attorney that represented the department of human services) said that I need to educate the attorney about my background and my area of specialization. She was very enamored with my thesis, *The Art Therapist as Expert Witness in Child Sexual Abuse Litigation*. Essentially, the material was parceled into segments; art therapy/art therapists; expert witnessing and evidentiary material in the form of drawings, child sexual abuse and children as witnesses. The solicitor felt the material was very important, especially for my initial qualification in the court and her comment about the thesis, "It's kind of overwhelming which is fun" set the tone for our meeting. She instructed me to always bring my CV and to include in it research and papers I have presented or published. She said to bring several copies of the CV for the defense and prosecution. She proceeded to describe the three judges that I would most likely encounter including their personalities and individual style on the bench. Her advice after providing the detailed descriptions was to "play to your judge" including directing my responses to the judge when speaking rather than the attorneys (this process was configured around dependency court or civil matters rather than criminal court). I learned which judge was hard of hearing and which one was new and how each was perceived and what their reputations were at that time. The solicitor also stated at the beginning of our conversation not to take anything personally, especially something conveyed by a judge. She also related that dependency court is in the business of reunifying families. She informed me that where I was working was very well respected and being an unknown professional was a good thing because "I can set the tone for how I'll be perceived". She explained that my job was to state clearly my recommendations based on my process; what I identified and how I support the recommendations from my findings. She told me to "be self-assured and confident" which she said was "the bottom line without being cocky". She also said to be firm with what I say. "If you hedge on answers, you'll get torn up and you'll lose credibility so say my recommendation is. . .". She also instructed me to give solid answers. She explained how to respond to inquiries or if my recommendations were questioned. She gave the following example, "I would never choose to do that but if the court chooses to do that the ramifications will be. . .". She offered, "They will look for my recommendations and findings". I can testify as to what a child said to me. For example, say "I interview a child to obtain information to reach my recommendations or say, in the course of interviewing the child . . .". She said to state that the information (based upon the interview) is used to make recommendations that will include what is in the best interest of the child and give specifics as to the nature of what I am recommending (investigative, therapeutic or supportive measures) and to explain what was determined and what the recommendation was based upon. She discussed that in this court, the judges are more lenient and they will push the rules of evidence.

The solicitor continued to describe what I would need to do on the stand; establish a chronology, explain how and what I record (behavior and observations, associations, media behavior, time factor) and my bottom line, what did I determine. She also said, I would need to explain what does an art therapy evaluation entail and what does one expect to learn as my role is to educate the judge. She told me to say this is what I am trained to do. She reiterated that my role is to provide recommendations based upon my process – not to identify a specific treatment intervention or program. She was adamant and instructed me to, "Tie it all back into the drawings and tie the recommendations in to the drawings". She said that the defense would ask about my expertise. I would need to state the basis for my conclusions based on the interview, the child's behavior, and the art work. I would need to clarify the investigative interview process and explain that it combines art therapy and forensic tenets. I was told by the solicitor as well to give a "textbook answer" for example with regard to what a typical child for a particular age might draw.

She said unequivocally to respond to the questions asked and "don't hide the fact that you're knowledgeable. Impress us with your knowledge". She indicated that it would increase my credibility and she offered, "explain it but don't preach". She related that there are 30–40 lawyers in the court and "word will spread". She instructed me to give complete answers and not to leave the door open for the attorney to challenge or question (or interpret) what I mean. She told me to say what I mean. The solicitor stated that prep is designed so that a witness can answer questions exactly as "they've been asked"; questions are very specific. She was direct when she expressed, "answer and don't offer anything more". She firmly reiterated, "Only answer what has been asked". She conveyed her hope that the attorney would stipulate that I am an expert in art therapy with sexually abused children. She said once qualified as such; they will build on that. She discussed that as far as qualification, I would be asked about educational history, employment history and what have I done in the field including internships and direct practice work. She provided, "This is your time to boast" and she told me to speak about anything that I have written that is related to art therapy, sexual abuse, use of drawings with the population and related materials (essentially anything that would support/reflect my expertise). She discussed proposals (abstracts) that I had submitted to speak/present to indicate how the community at large might be impacted by my work. She advised me that I would need to talk about the interview process; what does it include, how many children have I conducted interviews with since I began this work; how long does the process last and what does it mean to have an art therapist conduct the interview. She restated that I need to educate the court.

She summarized the process by saying that it is three parts; you and yourself; a general art therapy piece; and the specific case including the particulars as they relate to the child. She spoke about the need to be concise and informative despite the amount of information to address. With regard to an upcoming case, she allowed that it was going to involve not just one attorney – but a child advocate attorney as well who would support and collaborate with the city attorney. The advocate would conduct rehabilitation if necessary – in the event defense tried to box me into a hole and not let me provide information beyond yes or no responses. The solicitor described rehabilitation as a "benevolent shot to allow me to answer what I didn't get to answer". Also, the attorneys would ask me if there were any other observations to give me an open door so if something was missed, I would be able to clarify.

As one can imagine, the pressure to do well on my initial witnessing adventure was onerous to say the least. The challenge was obviously great. The best advice was to script (to be explained) and prepare with the calling attorney (the one who is responsible for requesting your presence in court) to alleviate some of the panic. As wonderful an idea as this is, in all practicality, it is not always feasible. Some attorneys, given their workload, are not amenable to meeting in advance or simply do not have the time to give. Sometimes a meeting is not prudent given shifts in assignments and court delays. On occasion, extensive prep may be minimized due to the extension of proceedings or delays due to conflictual or calendar commitments. Although prolonging a process erases one's nerves in the moment, in the long run a delay only serves to provoke the same measure of anxiety at a later date. In addition, the need to review and prepare again when a case finally reaches the docket requires investment in time and energy if preparation has to begin anew. Given the potentialities for delays and possible person-nel changes, preparatory meetings may be necessary with a new set of attorneys and others associated with the case, which subverts one's time and may impact memory and even presentation (despite having a report).

In spite of all of these obstacles, it is imperative that a potential witness make the time and request a meeting with the calling attorney, preferably in person. I cannot stress the importance of doing so for one's peace of mind as well as to promote a collaborative and supportive relationship with the attorney who is responsible for presenting your qualifications. Not doing this may result in a less-than-favorable performance by either or both the attorney who is presenting one's qualifications and the witness who is estab-lishing them.

I have had attorneys instruct me after the fact never to say something that I offered on the stand, and others have asked me questions that I purposely said I could not speak to while on the stand in the hopes that I would respond and meet a preconceived agenda. I do not think there is ever a perfect scenario as a witness, but I have learned some key insights through the years given various interactions and verbal exchanges when on the witness stand.

In order to avoid being seen as incompetent or unprepared, the best approach is to discuss in advance what you are willing and able to offer on the witness stand. In an effort not to be placed in a position that will compromise integrity, conviction or eth-ics, it is fundamental to be up-front and clear with regard to perception and expecta-tion. Although sometimes, no matter how vehemently one states what they are willing or not willing to commit to when on the witness stand, such a sagacious attempt to be clear may fall on deaf ears. When an attorney does not accept the limitations imposed for professional reasons or personal convictions (which may intermingle), one may appear to be at odds while in the midst of testifying with calling counsel. It happens. Although cross examination may be enjoying the exchange, there just may not be a solution except to say out loud, "Counselor, I believe we discussed this, and I have made my position very clear". The attorney may not be appreciative; however, if one has made their position known, there may be no other way to handle the situation. If this occurs in civil court, the witness may appeal directly to the judge. Sometimes a clear and concise conversation is sufficient to convince an attorney that you are not the best witness for a particular case. Although not always apparent, unearth the agenda and explore if there is a hidden one as to why you are being asked to testify. Know your limits and do not be afraid to express yourself in a preparatory meeting so that there is clarity instead of confusion in the event you are placed on the witness stand.

I was often asked if I thought a child was sexually abused even after explicitly expressing during prep that I could not speak to that question given my role as a child interview specialist (depending upon the nature of the case but mostly in civil court). I would offer that it was not my purview to make that assertion. I conducted the fact-finding process; however, it was up to each investigator to make a determination, as was previously detailed earlier in the text. Invariably, attorneys still asked me this question when on the stand despite having made my position clear in advance hoping I might take the bait. This always made for an awkward encounter when I would reiterate that it is not my purview to state such an opinion given my role in the case, which was to facilitate a fact-finding process and conduct an investigative interview on behalf of a team. Despite having a lengthy report that clearly indicated what occurred in the process coupled with recommendations that addressed investigative and interventive measures, this question always loomed when on the witness stand.

It was the responsibility of the investigative agents to determine if their respective burdens of proof were met in conjunction with the investigative process. My report included investigative as well as interventive information and recommendations leading to an inference; however, it was up to each investigator to make a determination via the information gathered and within the context of a team process. (It was not for me to tell someone which proverbial box to check, although I was asked to on and off the witness stand). The report also did not confer the status of the case.

My role is as a fact-finder, not an investigator. The distinction was that I facilitated and often conducted the interview on behalf of the team; however, I was not involved in investigative pursuits that extended beyond my role such as interviewing alleged perpetrators or external witnesses and other contacts. Evidentiary materials that were available to investigators beyond the investigative interview factored into decision making by the respective agents. It was incumbent upon the investigators to decide whether or not to indicate, substantiate, not substantiate, found or unfound a report (depending upon the mandate of the particular investigative entity) or the allegations subject to the burdens of proof of the respective agency.

I spent several hours on multiple occasions speaking with more than one attorney assigned to a case rooted in a specific community. We spent time scripting questions and answers. The attorneys were well versed on what to expect from me, and I knew the same with respect to them. Lines of communication were clearly established. As luck would have it, the primary attorney was on vacation when the case finally made it onto the docket (court roster). Unfortunately, the substitute attorney had no knowledge about the case and was inadequately prepared. We went in with a losing proposition given the dynamics and the attorneys that had appeared for the opposite side. Unbelievably, the attorney filling in for the prosecution did not spend five minutes speaking with me prior to the commencement of the proceeding; instead, he grabbed my CV and proceeded when I was seated on the witness stand to ask me about my first master's degree, which had no relevance and no bearing on the case or my status as an expert in child sexual abuse. My credibility blew up before I even had a chance to speak. Sad all the way around, especially given the amount of time and energy that had been invested previously in anticipation of the case moving forward to trial.

Important lessons derived from that unfortunate situation were the need to rework and adapt my CV so that it did not reflect my previous professional life that served no role regarding my status as an expert (in child sexual abuse, art therapy or related specialization). I also had to find my voice and not let someone filling in for another attorney negate all of the hours of planning, preparation, commitment and investment. To nullify my testimony was a travesty but a reality. The testimony that merited presentation on behalf of the client was not allowed, as my voice was muted and my expertise was silenced.

The outcome of that particular case and the manner in which the qualification process was handled were troublesome on so many levels and for so many reasons but life lessons were instilled. Never again, would I permit someone to be so cavalier and think that they were positioned to present my qualifications and my experience, as well as expertise, without a preparatory meeting whether in person or via phone. If my testimony was warranted and my status necessary, then respect was required not only for me but for the process and the client.

In preparing with the calling attorney, the information provided and included on a CV will be used to enhance credibility when presented on the stand. As detailed earlier, only the information that is relevant to the case merits attention. The purpose is to provide the jury with an understanding of the expert's credibility as it relates to the case. Even though credentials may be impressive, at times, certain ones may not be pertinent for the issues being addressed. As such, extraneous information need not be offered, presented or discussed on the witness stand, as this may convolute how a witness is to be viewed, presented or qualified.

A witness's credibility may be jeopardized by the inclusion of information that may appear irrelevant, as the jury may question why an expert in something unrelated (as noted) is on the witness stand. Sometimes too many credentials or professional qualifications may detract from the premise. After all, an expert need only be qualified on the matter before the court, not on every element of their CV no matter how extensive it may be.

Thus, one has to prepare as best as possible by learning the skills and techniques that are innate on the stand as well as respecting the limits of one's expertise. Familiarity with the semantics of the case one is testifying about cannot be underscored enough. Truly, the best way to understand and appreciate the process is to be an attentive witness when duly engaged on the stand. Preparing in advance and presenting oneself as level-headed will work to one's advantage, as will learning the process and the procedural trappings. Knowing how to handle and manage the strategies and intentions of cross examination is essential for effective presentation. The locus of control can shift in an instant on the stand but adequate preparation and anticipation of such will assist in effective witnessing or presentation.

Kate, as I will refer to her (not her name), asked me to send my CV to her in advance of meeting. Certain information should be contained and highlighted within a court CV. This, as explained, may require some revision so that relevant information for court is included and illuminated. This information will be a factor in qualifying as an expert and will be considered within the scripting exercise to be examined.

Kate very professionally informed me what the expectations were for me. The proceeding I was subpoenaed to participate in surrounded sexual abuse. The proceeding was to be held in juvenile court. Kate explained that I would be qualified as an expert. She discussed the process as well as the anticipated cross examination she projected as she read my CV.

She described the process of testifying as a three-part process: First the emphasis is on the witness, in this case, me. My qualifications were to be addressed, including my credentials, experience, training, education and background. Next, my professional work and experience in the realm of child sexual abuse and my use of art therapy with this population, as well as the interview guideline (CIG), would be the focus. Third, the specific case would be examined including my role. All of this would be used to help establish my credibility as an expert working with this population and with regard to the particularities associated with the case, and then my conclusions would be discussed. A semblance of the conversation for qualification that was scripted is illustrated here.

(*Continued*)

(Continued)

Exemplar of qualification prep and scripting

Name
Professional degrees
Educational background
Current position and length of employment there
Related professional experience
Continuing education
Professional development and contributions (publications, presentations, etc.)
Do you lecture, teach or instruct on related topics and where
How many children have you worked with in current capacity
Have you testified as an expert in court in the area of child sexual abuse
or art therapy
Kate instructed me to generally describe art therapy:
What it is
Provide background about the profession
How do I use art therapy
The significance of drawing in the interview process
The use of media
Describe a typical interview process
What is your standard operating procedure
Has this art therapy–based interview process been discussed in court before
How many times
Has it been stipulated to as accepted by the court
How do you know the child
When did you interview the child
How old was the child
Who brought the child to the interview
Why were you asked to interview the child
Were you provided with information in advance of meeting the child
What was the child's presentation like behaviorally, cognitively, socially
Describe child's verbal capacity
Describe her comprehension
Describe her affect/mood
What were the circumstances that precipitated the interview
Explain the interview process you conduct to assess allegations of sexual abuse
Is this the process you used with this child
What did the interview entail
What did it reveal
What type of media besides drawing was used
How were drawings introduced
Did child produce any drawings
Please describe them individually and show the court
What were child's associations to each drawing
Please describe anything unusual or significant in each drawing
What did child disclose about the allegations in relation to the drawings
What did the child disclose about the alleged perpetrator
Did the child disclose new information that was not previously reported
If so please explain
What findings did you make regarding what the child reported
Based upon your interview and interaction with the child what are your conclusions
What are the recommendations you made

Kate said to explain for the judicial officer what exactly art therapy is and how it works so the
    officer (judge) will understand what I do and why I do it. Kate re-emphasized that I needed
    to educate and enlighten in a manner that was comprehensible so that individuals with no
    background would have a working sense and an appreciation of the modality with the

population described and specifically with regard to the case. She explained that she wanted what I said about how art therapy is used and how it factors into the interview process to be on the record so it is clear and would provide testament to the benefits associated with using an interview process that juxtaposes forensics and art therapy and was investigative with therapeutic overtones. It would also serve as a record that could be referred to in later proceedings, especially if the judge accepted the profession as valid. The possibility of a special proceeding to determine the status regarding the use of drawing was explained to me by Kate (novel scientific evidence). Kate expressed her hope that the judge would accept my previous qualification as an expert as well as the acceptance of the interview process and the use of art therapy and drawings as previously stipulated to during previous court proceedings where I testified and was qualified as an expert.

Ethical Considerations

- testimony should be the same regardless of which side one is testifying for
- expert should be active practitioner in field to which ascribe expertise
- should not be full-time expert witness
- expert witness should only be a minimal part of professional activity
- avoid partisanship
- if relevant – advanced agreement is best about rates of compensation and travel expenses, including being on call (meaning if being held in reserve as a potential witness – external experts may charge for their time)
- not ethical to adopt an attorney's agenda if it conflicts with one's opinion and/or exceeds scope of expertise
- do not be manipulated into supporting an agenda
- do not let an agenda contradict professionalism, including ethics and integrity
- do not allow something you do not support to be deemed acceptable by you
- be aware of compromising objectivity and ethical standards
- know own biases

Qualification Preparation

Curriculum Vitae

An expert preparing to testify in court will need to present a curriculum vitae (CV) to the calling attorney. The information contained should be relevant and appropriate for testifying. As such, the CV may need to be revamped, as it is not intended for job seeking or an academic teaching position or any other professional position listing. The information contained in a court CV will reflect a potential witness's education; training; specialized skill (in area of and related to expertise); relevant internships; academic awards; professional affiliations; board memberships; board certification; licensure; professional memberships and committee assignments; consultant work; advisory boards; publications, including journal articles, book chapters and books; editorial positions; trainings and workshops conducted; keynote presentations; faculty positions; prior qualifications as an expert and in what type of proceeding; and any other pertinent information such as legislative testimony that may support and increase the expert's credibility.

Curriculum Vitae for Court and Expert Qualification

Include education, experience, training, knowledge and skill

Education

Degrees – relative to expert testimony
Dissertation/thesis titles if relevant to topic to be discussed
Teaching and research assistantships
Courses taught
Research projects
Internships (in what, where and with whom)
Postdoctoral work
Fellowships
Academic awards
Grants

Experience

Current position – role, duties, length of employment
Clinical Experience
Forensic Experience
Prior positions if related and relevant
Area of specialization(s) and experience (how acquired)
Academic positions
Board certifications
Licensures
Professional presentations
Trainings Conducted (education of peers/community/others)
Consultant work (in what area/field)
Supervisory role (for students/professionals/organizations)
Mentoring
Prior qualification in court as an expert witness (date, location and qualification designation)

Training

Specialized training related to presence in court (type of case such as child sexual abuse)
Professional conferences attended
Professional training related to topic of expertise
Continuing education (relevant to area of expertise/case) – attended or provided

Affiliations

Professional organizations (committees)
Board memberships – volunteer, appointed or elected

Advisory boards

Editorial positions

Volunteer positions (what organizations/mission – if relevant and contributory to proceeding)

Community involvement/engagement (if relevant)

Publications

Peer-reviewed journal articles

Book chapters

Books edited

Books authored

Presentations

Keynote addresses

Papers (where presented – audience, etc.)

Trainings and workshops conducted

Professional conferences – local, regional, national, international

Not all of this information will need to be discussed by the witness. However, the attorney might look to these areas and similar items, to determine what qualifications the particular witness possesses that will enhance the witness's credibility. In each case the attorney should emphasize only those credentials that are most germane to the issues relative to the trial or proceeding. Those that are addressed in court should be the ones that tend to give the jury greater reason to accept the teaching and opinions of the witness in the specific case. Information contained in the CV will be presented in an effort to bolster the witness's credibility and support the determination or conferring of expert witness status.

Scripting Exercise

Scripting eliminates the element of surprise, and appropriate prep can eradicate misperceptions and misunderstandings. Scripting is an exercise designed to understand the expectations as a witness primarily about direct testimony. It is also valuable in approaching possible areas that might be potential areas for cross examination. Identifying areas of weakness ahead of time may preempt and assuage attacks delivered on cross examination.

Scripting necessitates speaking with calling counsel and literally writing or scripting out questions and answers so that both the attorney and the witness are on the same page and understand the scope of testimony as well as the limits. Potential areas of conflict or weakness can be discussed and strategies for how to address in anticipation of cross examination occur.

This process is a dialogue that helps with planning and preparation. In the event the attorney is reassigned or the case moves slowly through the court system, preserving the script will maintain the information and minimize the need for another prep meeting, as the script can be shared with the calling attorney ahead of time.

Scripting means that the attorney and the witness understand the expectations with regard to testimonial capability as well as evidentiary presentation on the stand. This may originate with a list of foundational questions in anticipation of meeting with the calling attorney. Scripting enables advance preparation for proposed testimony. The best way to answer questions and present information is prepared by literally writing out questions and answers so that there are no surprises and no hidden agendas.

Scripting Tips

- give CV or resume in advance to calling attorney
- provide a list of foundational questions to the attorney pertinent to your background, education and training as well as your professional orientation
- may need to provide explanatory information if area of expertise (such as art therapy) is unknown or unfamiliar to the attorney/parties (professional literature)
- be prepared to provide information to help educate about your profession if not common
- document experience or expertise
- list prior cases testified in
- note how you want to be presented – if have multiple titles, names or degrees, what is best for the case (prudent to establish this ahead of time so there is no confusion as to how you are addressed on the stand)
- state what you do not want emphasized from your CV and explain why
- identify strengths and weaknesses to prepare how to present on the stand
- anticipate potential areas for cross examination to zoom in on (potential weaknesses)
- strategize and prepare for cross examination
- review report/findings in advance with the attorney so there is consensus and understanding regarding the dynamics as well as the findings and recommendations
- find out what areas will be targeted for discussion
- address agenda of calling attorney
- know biases and boundaries
- discuss ethical concerns about testifying
- do not exceed limits of expertise
- do not compromise integrity by agreeing to say something you cannot support
- ask about hidden agenda; if you suspect one, confront the attorney
- make clear what will happen if asked something that has been identified as something you are not willing to say on the stand – how will you respond
- be firm in what you will and will not be able to support

Voir Dire (Qualification) Scripting Exercise

During voir dire an individual presents their credentials in order to qualify as an expert. Questions are directed at the individual's knowledge, skill, training, experience and education. Scripting is only practiced and conducted with the calling attorney, not with the defense. The following is a generalized script that is reflective of questions that may be posed during voir dire to qualify an individual, oriented toward an art therapist, who conducts forensic interviews. The scope of questions and lines of inquiry are narrowed here but can be expanded in accord with the calling attorney's knowledge and understanding of the individual as a potential witness. In this capacity, the forensic art therapist is neither an advocate nor an adversary, but rather presents as neutral, impartial, objective and unbiased (Cohen-Liebman, 2003).

Sample Script

> State your name
> Please describe your education and background
> Postgraduate training
> What type of continuing education do you attend?
> What kind of certification or licensure do you have?
> What are your professional affiliations?
>
> Where do you work?
> How long have you been there?
> Describe what you do and the interview guideline/format you use
> What is the population you primarily see?
> How many children have you interviewed in this capacity?
>
> Define art therapy
> Describe the professional organizations that sanction art therapy
> Provide a brief history of the field and the development of the profession
> How is a forensic art therapy process conducted?
> What materials are used?
> How do you evaluate drawings?
>
> Do you know child X?
> When did you meet child X?
> Why did you see this child?
> Who referred the child and for what purpose?
> Prior to meeting child X, did you review other documents related to X?
> Explain what you did when you met with child X
> What was the process you conducted?
>
> How many drawings did child X make?
> Do you have the drawings – please explain the drawings (the attorney will most likely ask to have each drawing entered into evidence)
> What was child X asked to draw?
> What did child X draw?
> What did child X state about each drawing?
> What were your conclusions?
> What were your recommendations?

Remember that on cross examination attempts will be made to discredit you and your testimony. The more you educate the calling attorney and the more you prepare, the more you will be better equipped to interact, engage and respond to the cross examiner and manage cross techniques and strategies. In advance, it is best to identify which area of your testimony may be weak or less effective which may be targeted by cross. Identifying these areas ahead of time before defense does will help defend against cross attacks. Remember to maintain composure, master emotions and do not let the defense control or manipulate you. Remain calm, professional and convincing which will contribute to effective and persuasive witnessing.

Testimonial Preparation

- prepare for cross examination
- consider material from defense perspective
- strategize possible defense strategies with prosecutor
- cross examination prep and anticipation will help strategize for redirect examination
- on cross examination goal is to discredit the witness using any available strategy
- if question is presented with intention of a yes or no response but the answer merits explanation, find a way to say what you want (in civil proceeding speak to the judge directly and say something to the effect of, "Your Honor, if you will permit me, I would like to respond to counselor's question; however, it merits a narrative response or more than a yes/no answer"; always thank the judge for indulgence)
- cross examination is intended to confuse the trier of fact about direct testimony and raise doubt about credibility

---

Court Prep in Review

Prior to Court Date
after receive subpoena or request to appear in court
contact person or the entity that requested your presence or your records
find out why your testimony/presence is requested or why your records are being subpoenaed
ascertain expectations
determine hidden agenda
clearly define the limits of your role/expertise/ethics/purview
clarify and clearly express what you will and will not say or speak to

Speak With Attorney
educate about your involvement/role with the case
educate about your profession
provide relevant material so attorney can prepare accordingly
discuss your credentials
inform about your process – forensic or clinical
find out if expected to testify as expert or fact witness and understand the obligations

Curriculum Vitae – Court CV
review information with attorney
address gaps or inconsistencies/weaknesses/strengths
know what is included
be able to discuss/explain

Voir Dire – Qualification Process
conduct scripting with attorney
question and answer
practice and, if permissible, role play to prepare

Practice Tips

Preparation Tips

- request pretrial conference with requesting attorney – pretrial conference can learn strategy, anticipate questions and script
- if many witnesses are to be called – advisable for attorney to convene a conference of all potential witnesses to explore details of the case and to be sure that everyone has the same factual knowledge

- opinion about the case may vary – it is up to the attorney to assess the effects of differences between experts; as a group can plan direct examination and anticipate cross examination as well and discuss possible testimony by opposing experts
- the more insight garnered regarding trial strategy will be helpful

Presentation Tips

- avoid professional jargon
- dress professionally – presentation and demeanor are important
- do not hide on the stand – use personal space to advantage
- behavior, demeanor and affect are being observed both in and out of the courtroom – be aware of surroundings and interactions – eyes and ears are real

Behavior Tips

- be conscious of your surroundings while waiting to be called or when preparing
- do not talk in the hallway or near people who may overhear your conversation – due to possible affiliations with the defense, this may compromise your position and/or strategy
- do not speak with anyone – people may be potential jurors or witnesses
- you are being observed
- conduct yourself in a professional manner
- try to moderate anxiety and nerves
- do not portray lack of preparedness
- do not sit prominently reviewing your notes – shows lack of confidence
- everyone is judged consciously and subconsciously
- in the courtroom value judgements are being made – personality, sincerity
- remember not to personalize anything
- do not be seen flipping through notes and your report
- even if report is with you on the stand – unless you know clearly where to find something, do not page through it
- your behavior is front and center in the courtroom, and you want to be viewed as a consummate professional

General Preparation Tips

- be familiar with courtroom procedure
- present as a willing participant even if you are not
- prepare accordingly
- knowledge of notes, summaries, outlines so not looking for something while on the stand
- review materials so cognizant of essential details (especially given time delays)
- testifying is a verbal process – predicated upon verbal language
- be aware of nonverbal communications and potential impact
- possess thorough knowledge of the case facts
- be confident in conclusions drawn from the facts
- before testifying – meet with the attorney who solicited testimony
- review records and script

Testifying Tips

- be confident
- maintain control of testimony
- be prepared
- know the facts
- know what is in your report
- make eye contact with trier of fact
- use words to communicate the facts and convey impressions
- speak loudly and clearly
- avoid nonverbal responses
- do not nod – answer verbally – need to be aware of this because verbal testimony is being recorded
- speak directly to the jurors or trier of fact
- do not become argumentative
- never lose your temper
- avoid professional or discipline-specific language and technical terms
- if must use discipline-specific terminology – clarify and explain
- remain calm – do not outwardly show emotion
- pause before answering
- make sure you understand the question – if not, ask for clarification; this also buys time to formulate a response
- use specific analogies or everyday scenarios aimed at the jury's comprehension
- if you did not understand the question, most likely trier of fact or jury did not either
- statements should be declarative
- if you do not know the answer to a question – do not guess; say you do not know
- do not repeat the question back
- answer only what is asked – do not volunteer more information
- beware of questions specific to dates and locations
- control emotional and behavioral response
- be professional and courteous
- avoid use of notes or report on the stand – can have material available to refresh memory or for specificity but do not spend time flipping through papers on the witness stand
- never give an opinion or statement you cannot support
- be aware of current literature as well as viewpoints of professional organizations
- know counter arguments to major points so you are prepared if challenged

Tips for Cross Examination

- with cross examination – support position with facts or literature
- be concise – do not offer anything beyond what is requested
- anticipate the defense
- direct examination should not be repeated
- do not look to prosecutor or judge for help
- cross examination tries to cast doubt on expertise of witness
- you know more about your involvement in the case than the defense attorney – let that be known
- can disagree with defense in a proper manner (respectfully disagree)
- remember the defense attorney's role is to try and disprove the expert's credibility

- defense will use a variety of tactics to discredit
- cross examination will try to provoke by upsetting, embarrassing and unsettling
- once understand techniques and goals of cross examination – less anxiety and more effective witnessing
- cross examination will attack the weakest area of CV – so attempt to highlight or at least acknowledge weakness on direct examination to preempt
- vary responses to control cross examination
- listen with care to the structure of the question and use to your advantage
- disagree with cross examination when possible
- do not let cross examiner intimidate or control you
- if cross attorney has witness under control – the attorney will direct the flow of the testimony
- defense attorney has responsibility of defending her or his client – ethically bound to defend
- remember not to take anything personally (which can be difficult)
- everyone has a job to do within the scope of a court proceeding
- know you are participating in an adversarial process – proper mindset
- cross examination is intended to impeach the expert by whatever legal means are available (Myers, 1996)

John Myers (1996) uses the acronym HELP to organize the meta principles that underlie expert testimony to help jurors understand technical, clinical and scientific issues.

H – honesty – if an expert is not honest, this undermines the law. An attorney's job is to win the case for the client. The ultimate goal of the legal system is truth, but the theory of the adversary system is that the truth emerges through courtroom confrontation of adversaries; thus, attorneys are advocates for their clients and are not supposed to be objective.

E – evenhandedness – expert's role is not to win the case and not to be partisan; rather the role is to help the jury understand clinical, scientific or technical issues by educating. The degree of objectivity is compatible with honesty and professionalism. Expert must recognize bias and the role it has on shaping expert testimony.

L – limits of expertise – knowledge about child sexual abuse. Expert needs to know relevant and current literature. Appreciation and acknowledgement of the limits of one's knowledge, as well as that associated with the field, are necessary.

P – preparation – is the key to effective expert testimony.

References

American Bar Association. (n.d.). www.americanbar.org

American Mock Trial Association. (1985). Retrieved November 1999, from www.collegemocktrial. org/appendix1.htm

Barsky, A., & Gould, J. (2002). *Clinicians in court: A guide to subpoenas, depositions, testifying, and everything else you need to know.* The Guilford Press.

Brodsky, S. L. (1991). *Testifying in court: Guidelines and maxims for the expert witness.* American Psychological Association.

Brodsky, S. L. (2004). *Testifying in court: Guidelines and maxims for the expert witness.* American Psychological Association.

Brodsky, S. L. (2013). *Coping with cross-examination and other pathways to effective testimony.* American Psychological Association.

Brodsky, S. L., & Gutheil, T. G. (2016). *The expert expert witness: More maxims and guidelines for testifying in court.* American Psychological Association.

Cohen-Liebman, M. S. (2003). Drawings in forensic investigations of child sexual abuse. In C. Malchiodi (Ed.), *Handbook of art therapy* (pp. 167–179). Guilford Press.

Lilly, G. C. (1996). *An introduction to the law of evidence* (3rd ed.). West Publishing Co.

Myers, J. E. B. (1992). *Legal issues in child abuse and neglect.* Sage Publications Inc.

Myers, J. E. B. (1996). Expert testimony. In C. Jenny, J. Briere, J. Bulkley, L. Berliner, & T. Reid (Eds.), *The APSAC handbook on child maltreatment* (1st ed., pp. 319–326). Sage Publications, Inc.

Myers, J. E. B. (2002). Legal issues in the medical evaluation of child sexual abuse. In M. Finkel & A. Giardino (Eds.), *Medical evaluation of child sexual abuse: A practical guide* (2nd ed., pp. 233–250). Sage Publications Inc.

Myers, J. E. B. (2011a). Criminal prosecution of child maltreatment. In J. E. B. Myers (Ed.), *The APSAC handbook on child maltreatment* (3rd ed., pp. 87–124). Sage Publications, Inc.

Myers, J. E. B. (2011b). Juvenile court. In J. E. B. Myers (Ed.), *The APSAC handbook on child maltreatment* (3rd ed., pp. 53–66). Sage Publications, Inc.

Myers, J. E. B. (2011c). Legal issues in child abuse and neglect practice. In J. E. B. Myers (Ed.), *The APSAC handbook on child maltreatment* (3rd ed., pp. 361–376). Sage Publications, Inc.

Myers, J. E. B. (2011d). Proving child maltreatment in court. In J. E. B. Myers (Ed.), *The APSAC handbook on child maltreatment* (3rd ed., pp. 377–397). Sage Publications, Inc.

Myers, J. E. B. (Ed.). (2011e). *The APSAC handbook on child maltreatment* (3rd ed.). Sage Publications, Inc.

Vieth, V. (2000). Thirteen tips for cross examining child abuse defendants and defense witnesses. In *National center for prosecution of child abuse update* (Vol. 13, No. 6). American Prosecutors Research Institute. APRI.

Part V   The Art of Drawing to Disclose

A Forensic Art Therapy
Investigative Interview Process

Introduction

As a forensic art therapist, I utilize an investigative interview format predicated upon art therapy principles and practices that is juxtaposed with judicial canons. Investigating interpersonal violence and related issues, I interview victims and witnesses to uncover and explore information related to experienced events that may be traumatic in nature through the use of the Common Interview Guideline (CIG), an art therapy–based investigative interview process (Cohen-Liebman, 1999, 2017, 2020, 2021). Drawing functions as an open-ended prompt rather than as a secondary support or an ancillary tool used to confirm verbal statements in the CIG. The CIG consists of five fluid phases that incorporate nondirected or free drawing as a primary resource to enhance memory recall and facilitate fact-finding or evidentiary disclosure. The phases associated with the CIG are rapport building, developmental screening/skills assessment, anatomy identification, fact-finding and closure.

This chapter will present an overview of a recent study that explored the CIG and the effect of drawing within investigative interviewing from an art therapy perspective. The qualitative study addressed how drawing in the capacity of an open-ended prompt supports the facilitation of memory recall. The study was responsive to the call for research regarding "how, when, and whether drawing should be introduced in forensic contexts" (Pipe et al., 2004, p. 451) and will hopefully contribute to the determination of the relevance and appropriateness of the use of drawing in forensic interviews (Driessnack, 2005). The study explored drawing and its effectiveness in assisting children to communicate and recall information in an effort to contribute to the body of literature that exists surrounding what drawing does and, more importantly, how drawing works within investigative interviews (Faller, 2014; Olafson, 2012). As such, the study was a response to the evaluative call for research on the effect of drawing on the content of children's reports in forensic interviews (Patterson & Hayne, 2011, p. 119). A review of the associated literature that addresses the use of drawing in investigative interviewing, which has been described as contributory as well as conflictual, is provided.

The study approached the use of drawing from an art therapy perspective. Although interviews are considered verbal constructs, they may utilize or incorporate supportive measures such as props and tools as well as various techniques and strategies as adjuncts. How drawing functions in a primary capacity and the manner in which it supports the facilitation of fact-finding and thus contributes to disclosure of information was examined. This exploratory project offered a different perspective as to "why" drawing in these contexts. The onus attributed to art therapy substantiated a unique contextual basis for the investigation of the use of drawing as a means of facilitating and enhancing memory recall.

DOI: 10.4324/9781003225041-6

A platform for the application of drawing as an open-ended prompt will be discussed through exploration of the literature, including investigative interviewing, the underlying tenets associated with art therapy, the encoding of trauma in image form and forensic fundamentals. Finally, the use of content analysis and the resulting themes that emerged from the study will be examined in relation to the research question: *How does drawing facilitate disclosure of experienced events of school-aged children in an art therapy–based investigative interview process when compared to a verbal investigative interview process?* The rationale for studying the CIG, a forensic art therapy investigative interview process, was to assess the efficacy of an art therapy–based process and evaluate the use of drawing as an open-ended prompt to facilitate memory recall and facilitate fact-finding. Secondarily, the study considered the underlying mechanisms of the drawing effect from an art therapy perspective.

The rationale for using the CIG as the investigative tool for the study was to explore how drawing facilitates recall and disclosure (evidence) in investigative interviews (a dialogical process) of school-aged children when used as an open-ended prompt (imagery) in a forensic art therapy investigative interview (a relational process) as compared to a verbal process. Three ideas were considered: 1) if evidentiary disclosure is influenced when drawing is incorporated as a primary resource in an art therapy–based investigative interview process; 2) study of the CIG, a forensic art therapy investigative interview process; and 3) how the drawing effect and associated underlying mechanisms contribute to recall and disclosure within the context of an art therapy-based investigative interview process.

Drawing and Investigative Interviews

The literature on the use of drawing in investigative interviews represents inconclusive research about the value of drawing regarding facilitation of evidentiary disclosure (Faller, 2005, 2014; Gross & Hayne, 1998, 1999; Jolley, 2010; Katz & Hershkowitz, 2010, 2013; Lyon et al., 2009; Vieth, 2008; Williams, 2001; Williams et al., 2002). As such, empirically sound and forensically relevant research regarding the efficacy of free drawing within investigative interviews of children has been advocated in the literature (Driessnack, 2005; Everson & Boat, 2002; Olafson, 2012) and is endorsed by researchers exploring the context of forensic interviews of children (Driessnack, 2005; Everson & Boat, 2002; Jolley, 2010; Macleod et al., 2013; Olafson, 2012; Patterson & Hayne, 2011; Pipe et al., 2004).

The use of drawing and its effectiveness in assisting children to communicate and recall information in various contexts has been examined to decipher what drawing does and more importantly how drawing works. The use of drawing for various purposes from clinical assessment to investigative interviewing has been a source of study for many researchers in related and diverse fields. Yet according to the literature, the drawing effect and the underlying mechanisms attributed to it have been identified as "elusive" (Gross et al., 2009). Researchers that have investigated this topic for many years put forth in 2009 that their primary concern has shifted from "the practical issue of whether drawing works to the more theoretical issue of why it might work" (Gross et al., 2009, p. 967).

Although there are inherent limitations in traditional verbal methods of inquiry, the literature on the use of drawing in investigative interviews represents inconclusive research about the value of drawing with regard to evidentiary disclosure (Lyon et al., 2009). Advantages and disadvantages associated with the use of drawing in stimulating memory recall in a forensic context with children have been considered. In addition, the utility of drawing in investigative interviews has been studied in an effort to understand the function of drawing in facilitating children's recall and memory of events.

Researchers studying the use of drawing in forensic interviews report conflicting findings (Faller, 2005; Lamb et al., 2008; Vieth, 2008). Even within their own studies, researchers have identified differences in investigative interview protocols and the inclusion of drawing (Wesson & Salmon, 2001). Some studies support the use of drawing (Butler et al., 1995; Gross & Hayne, 1998, 1999; Salmon et al., 2003; Wesson & Salmon, 2001), while other studies are associated with a decrease in accuracy when drawing is incorporated (Salmon & Pipe, 2000).

Interventions that enhance children's self-report and thus their testimony are topics of importance (Katz et al., 2014). Empirically sound and forensically relevant research regarding the efficiency of free drawing within investigative interviews is advocated by researchers exploring the context of forensic interviews of children (Everson & Boat, 2002; Olafson, 2012). Increasingly, researchers have identified the need for empirical evaluation of the use of drawing within the process of forensic interviews (Faller, 1993, 2007; Katz et al., 2014; Lamb et al., 2007; Macleod et al., 2013). Through studying children's narratives before, during and after an investigative interview, the way in which drawing has "aided children's retrieval process" has been examined and continues to be a current area of inquiry (Katz & Hamama, 2013, p. 877).

Exploration of an Art Therapy Investigative Interview Process

The study presented here explored the use of drawing within an art therapy investigative interview process. The qualitative study addressed how drawing in the capacity of an open-ended prompt supports the facilitation of recall. The use of drawing within an art therapy investigative frame was considered. The study was responsive to the appeal for research on the effect of drawing on the content of children's reports in forensic interviews (Patterson & Hayne, 2011). Exploring the use of drawing and its effectiveness in assisting children to communicate and recall information in this and related processes is an attempt to respond to the need to decipher what drawing does and, more importantly, how drawing works within investigative interviews (Faller, 2014; Olafson, 2012).

The study approached the use of drawing from an art therapy perspective and considered imagery as a means of gaining access to preverbal memory. This corresponds to the encoding of traumatic memory (Lusebrink, 1990). The use of drawing within the investigative interview context as an open-ended prompt rather than a secondary support or an ancillary tool was the impetus for exploration. Within the scope of the interview process, drawing was incorporated in a primary capacity. Examination of drawing from an art therapy perspective and in the capacity of an open-ended prompt afforded a point of view not previously targeted or investigated in relation to forensic interviewing of children.

Study Overview

The debatable acceptance that currently surrounds the use of drawing within forensic investigative interviews of school-aged children contributed to the development of the study. Several topics associated with drawing as an interview strategy contributed to the rationale. Exploring how drawing facilitates communication, recall and elicitation of information pertaining to experienced events when utilized in the capacity of an open-ended prompt in an art therapy investigative interview process provided the impetus for the exploratory study.

The literature reviewed for the study encompassed topics related to forensic interviewing and the use of media within these processes. Topics included forensic interviewing practices and techniques, the use of props and cues, open-ended prompts, drawing as an interview strategy, forensic relevance and analogue research in the field of investigative interviewing. Examination of aspects related to art therapy, including basic tenets and inherent advantages of the modality, were also reviewed. Imagery as it pertains to the encoding of trauma was explored as well as the function of imagery and the practice of art therapy. Literature on memory and recall as it applies to the study were additional factors reviewed. Finally, the drawing effect and associated underlying mechanisms were considered, as was data gathered from the perspective of art therapy.

Study Parameters, Problem and Purpose

The purpose of this study was to explore how drawing as an open-ended prompt in an investigative interview facilitates evidentiary disclosure. More specifically, this study explored the use of drawing as an invitational prompt in an investigative interview process that is based on art therapy principles and practices. The study compared an investigative interview process with and without the use of a drawing strategy (drawing as an open-ended prompt) with school-aged children in an analogue setting. The purpose included the study of the CIG, a forensic art therapy investigative interview process. Secondarily, underlying mechanisms associated with the drawing effect were explored.

The problem addressed how to enhance children's abilities to communicate accurate information pertaining to experienced events in an investigative interview. How drawing enhanced memory recall and facilitated disclosure of experienced events when used in the capacity of an open-ended prompt in an art therapy–based investigative interview was considered in relation to the stated problem. Delineating the underlying mechanisms associated with the drawing effect from an art therapy perspective provided a means for understanding how drawing contributed to enhanced communication about an experience.

The CIG, a forensic art therapy investigative interview process, was both the investigative tool for the study as well as the object of study. It was used with and without drawing to gather comparative data. The CIG is predicated upon the juxtaposition of art therapy principles and practices with legal and forensic tenets (Cohen-Liebman, 1999; Gussak & Cohen-Liebman, 2001). The CIG incorporates nondirected or free drawing as a primary resource to facilitate fact-finding or evidentiary disclosure and memory recall. As such, drawing functions as an open-ended prompt within the interview process rather than as a secondary or confirmatory support.

This study compared the CIG, an art therapy–based investigative interview process that is predicated upon rapport building, attunement to a child's developmental capabilities, fact-finding and minimization of re-traumatization (Cohen-Liebman, 1999, 2003; Gussak & Cohen-Liebman, 2001), to a verbal process (Cohen-Liebman, 1999, 2003, 2017, 2021). Three central principles form the basis of the CIG. The underlying principles are 1) an open invitational drawing process; 2) a dialogic and relational process; and 3) the encoding, storage and recall of traumatic memory in image form. Although the CIG has been accepted in court as a valid investigative process (Cohen-Liebman, 1999), it had not been empirically or systematically studied until the described study was conducted (2017).

The study explored how an investigative interview using drawing differed from and compared to an investigative interview without drawing. The study sought to retrieve data that were rich and descriptive; thus, a qualitative comparative study was used. A significant aspect of this research was the use of an analogue design. Due to inherent difficulties, including legal, ethical and practical challenges to conducting a field study with sexually abused children, an analogue study was designed to address the research question. Analogue studies are frequently employed in investigative or forensic interview research, given that determination of feasibility and validity of an experienced event is limited in a field study (Ehring et al., 2011; Lamb & Thierry, 2005). Additionally, the use of an analogue design was intended to minimize risk to the participants.

In an effort to simulate a real and objective experience and provide the basis for an investigative interview situation, the analogue design meant that variables were known. This provided a means of comparison between the two interview conditions under investigation. The design included the presentation of two short animated videos about bullying featuring McGruff, the Crime Dog, which were presented to 12 school-aged children. After viewing the tapes, the children were assigned to one of two interview conditions: 1) interview with drawing or 2) interview without drawing. The analogue design allowed for a descriptive comparison between the two groups of school-aged children. Both verbal and imaginal data were collected to determine if evidentiary disclosure of an experienced or witnessed event was influenced when drawing was incorporated as a primary resource in an art therapy–based investigative interview process.

Statement of the Problem (Primary)
- how to enhance children's abilities to communicate accurate information pertaining to experienced events in an investigative interview

Secondary Problem
- what is the effect of drawing
- how does the "drawing effect" contribute to enhanced communication about an experience
- what are the underlying mechanisms associated with the "drawing effect" from an art therapy perspective

Study Purpose
- to study how drawing, when used in the capacity of an open-ended prompt within an art therapy investigative interview process, enhances memory recall and facilitates fact-finding or evidentiary disclosure when compared to an investigative interview without drawing

Study Explored
- if evidentiary disclosure is influenced when drawing is incorporated as a primary resource in an art therapy–based investigative interview process in comparison to a verbal interview process
- the CIG, a forensic art therapy investigative interview process
- the underlying mechanisms associated with the drawing effect from an art therapy perspective

---

Gap Analysis and Rationale

The rationale for this study stems from the debatable acceptance that currently surrounds the use of drawing within forensic investigative interviews of school-aged children. The literature on the use of drawing in investigative interviews represents inconclusive research about the value of drawing with regard to facilitation of evidentiary disclosure (Faller, 2005, 2014; Gross & Hayne, 1998, 1999; Jolley, 2010; Katz & Hershkowitz, 2010, 2013; Lyon et al., 2009; Vieth, 2008; Williams, 2001; Williams et al., 2002). Empirically sound and forensically relevant research regarding the efficacy of free drawing within investigative interviews is advocated by researchers exploring the context of forensic interviews of children (Driessnack, 2005; Everson & Boat, 2002; Jolley, 2010; Macleod et al., 2013; Olafson, 2012; Patterson & Hayne, 2011; Pipe et al., 2004).

The literature revealed that the use of drawing as a primary resource in the capacity of an open-ended prompt (rather than as a secondary resource) in investigative interviews of child victims and witnesses had not been addressed. An investigative interview process that is based on art therapy was not an area of former exploration. In addition, the drawing effect and the underlying mechanisms associated with the effectiveness of drawing have been referred to as elusive (Gross et al., 2009).

Literature Review Encompassed

- child sexual abuse
- investigative interviewing
- strategies to promote retrieval and recall
  - props and cues
  - open-ended prompts
- drawing
  - investigative interviewing
  - to facilitate communication
  - effect of drawing on children's reports
- analogue studies and investigative interviewing
- the drawing effect
  - underlying mechanisms that may account for the drawing effect
- field studies and recent research
- trauma
  - the brain
  - traumatic memory and sensorium
- art therapy
  - advantages
  - dynamic relationship
- forensic art therapy (FAT)
  - common interview guideline (CIG)
- bullying
  - parallels to sexual abuse
- content analysis
  - approach/models
  - art psychotherapy

Thus, the systematic study of the CIG and its associated theoretical and foundational art therapy principles were studied to address the identified gaps. The rationale for using the CIG as the investigative tool for this study was to explore how drawing facilitates recall and disclosure (evidence) in investigative interviews (a dialogical process) of school-aged children when used as an open-ended prompt (imagery) in a forensic art therapy investigative interview (a relational process) as compared to a verbal process.

Thus, five gaps in the literature contributed to the rationale for conducting the study: 1) the inconclusive information and debatable acceptance that currently surrounds the use of drawing in investigative interviews of school-aged children; 2) the identified need for research in forensic interviewing approaches for children; 3) the lack of systematic study of the CIG, an art therapy–based forensic interview protocol; 4) the need to explore the medium of drawing as an open-ended prompt within an investigative interview format and the use of imagery with regard to recall and disclosure; 5) the elusiveness of the drawing effect and the underlying mechanisms attributed to it from an art therapy perspective. Also, contributing to the rationale for the study was understanding the medium of drawing as a primary or central component within a traditional verbal process.

Overall, these gaps comprise the basis for studying the identified problem: how to enhance children's abilities to communicate accurate information pertaining to experienced events in an investigative interview. The study explored the problem through an analogue study to collect data from two interview conditions: 1) the use of drawing as an open-ended prompt in conjunction with a verbal process (associations) as compared to 2) a verbal process in which children relate their experience(s) without the use of drawing.

Gaps in the Literature That Contributed to the Rationale for the Study

---

1. the debatable acceptance that currently surrounds the use of drawing in investigative interviews of school-aged children
2. the identified need for research in forensic interviewing approaches for children
3. the lack of systematic study of the CIG, an art therapy–based forensic interview guideline
4. the need to explore the medium of drawing as a complement to a traditional verbal interview process
5. the elusiveness of the drawing effect and the underlying mechanisms attributed to it from an art therapy perspective

---

The study also was responsive to the call for research initiatives exploring the linkage between bullying and child maltreatment/victimization. This topic was considered through review of the literature on child sexual abuse. As such, commonalities and comparisons were identified that connected bullying and child maltreatment, and will be presented. Exploration and evaluation of this arena were derivative of the material that factored into the literature review and provided a linkage that expanded the scope of the study and contributed to recommendations.

In Brief

Based upon the stated purpose, problem and gap analysis, the study explored how evidence about experienced and/or witnessed events is disclosed in investigative interviews of school-aged children using the CIG with drawing as compared to the CIG without drawing. More specifically, the purpose was to study how drawing, as an open-ended prompt, within an investigative interview facilitates recall of experienced events and contributes to evidentiary disclosure by school-aged children.

The study sought to gather meaningful information through a comparative analogue process wherein the use of drawing was incorporated as an open-ended prompt within a relational context. Information pertaining to memory recall and evidentiary disclosure when drawing is used as a primary resource in investigative interviews of school-aged children was analyzed through content analysis.

The study provided data that will hopefully contribute to the debate regarding the use of drawing within investigative interviews through the systematic exploration of the CIG. As such, the study may impact understanding and create awareness of an art therapy–based investigative interview process for children. In addition, exploring and identifying the underlying mechanisms associated with the drawing effect may offer explanation and clarification regarding how drawing promotes verbalization and disclosure of information in investigative interviews that may or may not be premised on art therapy. This information may also promote cognizance and appreciation with regard to how drawing contributes to elicitation as well as facilitation of fact-finding within the investigative interview process.

As such, this study may impact the reception of an art therapy–based investigative interview process. Ultimately, it is hoped that the data collected in this research may generate understanding of an art therapy–based process and offer an alternative or perhaps a complement to traditional verbal fact-finding measures invoked in the investigation of allegations by positively impacting the process for victims and witnesses. The CIG juxtaposes art therapy principles and practices with judicial tenets and is designed to maintain forensic integrity while safeguarding the emotional well-being of children who are interviewed either because of victimization or the witnessing of an interpersonal experience that may be traumatic in nature.

Review of the Literature

The literature has addressed many issues, concerns and controversies associated with the practice of investigative interviewing of children for many years (Conte et al., 1991; Faller, 2014). A range of related topics have been pursued, including the use of aids, tools, props and media, as well as the use of drawing within these processes (Cohen-Liebman, 1999, 2002, 2003, 2017, 2020). The impact of various factors on children's abilities to communicate within an investigative interview, especially with regard to allegations of sexual abuse, are additional topics that have been considered (Sternberg et al., 1997).

Researchers have evaluated the use of drawing for various purposes, from clinical assessment to investigative interviewing, in an effort to decipher what drawing does and, more importantly, how drawing works. Historically, drawing has been studied with regard to facilitating children's reports of past events, typically within the context of clinical practice, including as a means to access traumatic memories. Several studies have focused on this type of research (Burgess & Hartman, 1993; Clements et al., 2001; Driessnack, 2005; Gross & Hayne, 1998, 1999; Salmon et al., 2003). Findings from studies within clinical and legal contexts have demonstrated that children can provide information about past personal experience that is accurate (Ceci & Bruck, 1993; Hershkowitz et al., 2012; Macleod et al., 2013).

Empirically sound and forensically relevant research regarding the efficacy of free drawing within investigative interviews of children has been advocated in the literature (Driessnack, 2005; Everson & Boat, 2002; Olafson, 2012). Research has also been directed toward empirically and judiciously studying the effect of drawing on the content of children's reports in forensic interviews (Patterson & Hayne, 2011). The need for research to determine the relevance and appropriateness of the use of drawing in forensic interviews has also been identified (Driessnack, 2005). "Given that drawing has shown such promise in research to date, it would be valuable to explore further how drawing could be helpful in both clinical and forensic settings" (Macleod et al., 2013, p. 571). This is especially true due to the significance attributed to accuracy of recall and comprehensive retrieval of information in investigative interviews of children (Jolley, 2010). Recent findings suggest a trend in both analogue and real-time studies directed at assessing whether drawing enhances forensically relevant information disclosed by children about experienced events (Macleod et al., 2013).

The literature review will address forensic interviewing practices and techniques, including the use of props and cues, open-ended prompts, drawing as an interview strategy, the effect of drawing and analogue research in the field of investigative interviewing. The variable acceptance of the use of drawing within investigative interviews, typically verbal processes, is also considered. A brief explanation of art therapy, including basic tenets and inherent advantages, is also presented. The underlying principles associated with art therapy, including the nature of imagery and meaning making, are also addressed. Examination of the literature relevant to trauma and memory as it pertains to the study, including retrieval and recall of sensory-based memory, follows. Finally, a brief overview of forensic art therapy is provided. The examination of these topics is consistent with the gaps previously identified, which underlie the basis for the study.

Investigative Interviewing of Children

Allegations of sexual abuse are difficult to investigate, given that corroborative evidence is often unavailable (Faller, 2014; Lamb & Brown, 2006; Lamb et al., 2008; Macleod et al., 2013; Myers, 1998; Orbach et al., 2000; Poole & Lamb, 2009). Thus, investigators and forensic interviewers are reliant upon the information imparted in forensic interviews by children (Lamb et al., 2008).

Methods for extracting viable information from children became a pivotal aspect of investigation in the late 20th century, given the resurgence of awareness and renewed recognition of child maltreatment (Faller, 2014; Miller-Perrin & Perrin, 2013). Forensic interview practices are based on extensive research and study of technique, practice and method (Everson & Boat, 2002; Cheit, 2014; Olafson, 2012). Reportedly some practices evolved in response to the backlash regarding standards of acceptable interviewer practice, related to questionable techniques such as leading and repetitive questioning stemming from sensationalized cases (Cheit, 2014).

The central component of a child sexual abuse investigation is an interview of the alleged victim by a highly skilled child interview specialist or law enforcement agent. Specialized interview training and skill contribute to best efforts to obtain credible and reliable accounts from children given that self-reporting by child victims is often the primary source of information when sexual abuse is suspected (Faller, 2014; Lamb & Brown, 2006; Lamb et al., 2008; Macleod et al., 2013; Myers, 1998; Orbach et al., 2000; Poole & Lamb, 2009). Investigators are tasked with the responsibility of eliciting factual and detailed information from child victims and witnesses in investigative interviews (Faller, 2014; Katz et al., 2014; Malloy et al., 2011; Patterson & Hayne, 2011). To accommodate such undertakings and address the myriad of responsibilities associated with the multiple investigative agencies involved, best practice centers on the use of interview protocols or guidelines to direct the process (Kemp, 2017). This contributes to the alleviation of interviewing issues that have vexed or plagued the field since its inception.

Through the years, as investigators attempted to improve and streamline investigation, emphasis shifted. Initially, focus was directed at prosecution and finding alleged offenders guilty. The most creative solution early on (in the late 1980s) was to bring the systems together and conjointly conduct an investigative interview. To accomplish this goal and to obtain as much information in a single interview that was broad enough to meet the respective burdens of each system, reliance was placed on eliciting facts from the single most important aspect of the process: the child and the child's narrative. Subsequently, multidisciplinary interviewing centers that promoted interagency collaboration and team cooperation in an effort to minimize repetitive interviews while maximizing the information provided by children emerged and became the dominant approach to investigation (Cohen Liebman, 1999; Davies et al., 1996; Sheppard & Zangrillo, 1996; Sorenson et al., 1997). These efforts and the outcomes were detailed in Part I.

Forensic interviews adhere to rules of evidence in accordance with judicial standards (Gould & Stahl, 2009). Competency, credibility and the exploration of alternative hypotheses are factors that distinguish a forensic interview from a clinical interview. These elements are critical features of forensic interviews of children given that disclosure by a child is considered the single most significant method by which some crimes such as sexual abuse are discovered (Goodman-Brown et al., 2003; Lippert et al., 2009). Accurate memory recall and disclosure of experienced and witnessed events are challenging due to the effects of trauma inherent in these experiences.

Many factors contribute to the acquisition of a reliable verbal account from a child in an investigative interview, and factors may also impede or contribute to a lack of disclosure within a verbal format, including communication skills, interactive patterns, witness memory and management of information (Melinder et al., 2010). Understanding what factors might facilitate children's verbal disclosures have been considered in addition to impediments within the forensic interview context. Children may lack the cognitive capability or the verbal capacity to articulate their abusive experiences (Cohen-Liebman, 1999). They may be too ashamed or embarrassed to disclose verbally. They may be intimidated by the process and by the interviewer. Research has been directed at identifying considerations that may contribute to a child's lack of disclosure, including cognitive, social and emotional factors (Lippert et al., 2009; Melinder et al., 2010).

Open-Ended Prompts in Investigative Interviews

A definitive way to interview children has not been devised. There is not a singular protocol that has been determined as the standard for interviewers. The literature suggests that the use of open-ended prompts and questions within a forensic investigative interview format is the preferred method to acquire accurate information and evidentiary disclosure from school-aged children (Jolley, 2010; Lamb et al., 2008; Lyon et al., 2012; Orbach et al., 2000; Sternberg et al., 1997; Sternberg et al., 2001). As such, the use of open-ended prompts is gaining acceptance as best practice for eliciting information in forensic investigative interviews (Lamb et al., 2008). An open-ended prompt is an invitational prompt which invites a narrative response. In contrast, a focused or closed prompt implies a specific response. Open-ended questions are defined as "ideally ones that elicit true disclosures from actually abused children" (Saywitz et al., 2018, p. 317).

Free recall via open-ended questions tends to be more accurate than responses to direct questions according to various researchers (Bruck et al., 2000; Gentle et al., 2014; Lamb et al., 2008; Lindberg et al., 2003). Research studies directed at assessing children's responses to prompts freely given, as well as focused, revealed that free prompts elicited enhanced information and accuracy while decreasing suggestibility (Lamb et al., 2008; Lyon et al., 2012) by facilitating free recall; thus, disclosure of information in forensic interviews is augmented (Lyon et al., 2012).

Open-ended prompts tend to elicit free recall, which may not be as detailed; however, the information provided in response to open-ended prompts tends to be more accurate than responses to focused prompts (Orbach et al., 2000; Pipe et al., 2004; Sternberg et al., 1997; Sternberg et al., 2001). An open-ended prompt in the form of drawing corresponds to a free or unstructured drawing process, meaning the child chooses what to depict without the interviewer leading or focusing the content of the drawing (Cohen-Liebman, 1999).

Focused prompts or questions prompt "recognition memory and may induce errors" (Pipe et al., 2004, p. 448). They may prompt recognition memory rather than recall memory, which can impact what is disclosed (Lamb & Brown, 2006). Open-ended prompts followed by nonspecific utterances by interviewers promote disclosure of information. Thus, the manner in which children are questioned can impact accuracy of recall (Pipe et al., 2004). Accuracy is difficult to establish in field studies as compared to analogue studies. Brown explains (with regard to the National Institute of Child Health and Human Development [NICHD] protocol), "the accuracy of information obtained in field studies can usually be inferred only by extrapolating from laboratory studies on the relative efficacy of different types of prompts in eliciting accurate information" (p. 368). "Field studies have obvious advantages in that the interviewing techniques are studied in the actual forensic contexts to which generalization is sought, but analogue studies in which known experiences are described are also necessary" (Brown et al., 2013, p. 369).

It has been determined that even very young children can provide reliable information in response to free recall prompts (Pipe et al., 2004). Younger children provide typically fewer details than older children in free accounts of experienced events (Lamb et al., 2008). This may be attributed to an inability for children to produce their own internal retrieval cues, which support the recall of information (Gentle et al., 2014; Katz & Hershkowitz, 2012; Lamb & Brown, 2006). In a study conducted by Butler et al. (1995) whether the problem with children's recall had to do with the encoding of information rather than the retrieval of information was considered. It has been determined that the retrieval of information is influenced by the manner in which a child encodes information (Salmon, 2001). Accordingly, what children say is related to how they retrieve information as opposed to how they interpret what is being asked of them, which may inhibit verbalization (Driessnack, 2005).

Forensic or Investigative Interviews

Forensic interviews conducted with children are typically verbal processes which focus on the acquisition of accurate and reliable information about experienced or witnessed events for legal and protective purposes (Carnes, 2000; Hoffman, 2005; Lamb & Brown, 2006; Macleod et al., 2013). Accuracy is important with regard to the information or memories elicited (Barlow et al., 2011; Macleod et al., 2013). These processes are fact-finding endeavors directed at facilitating a child's recall of experienced events (Lamb & Brown, 2006). "Forensic interviews with children probe their episodic memory, often for personal episodes with highly emotional content" given that "the ensuing investigative and legal process may be critically dependent on the quality and quantity of the children's memory reports" (Thoresen et al., 2009, p. 999).

Forensic interviews strive to achieve a balance between "sensitivity", meaning strategies that correctly identify sexually abused children, and "specificity", which refers to exclusion of children who have not been abused (Faller, 2014, p. 57). Forensic interviews adhere to rules of evidence in accordance with judicial standards (Gould & Stahl, 2009). The emphasis differs from a clinical process in that the focus is on obtaining information or fact-finding rather than a subjective focus, which is more attuned with addressing how one feels. Forensic interviews require the acquisition of accurate information, while mental health processes promote expression of thoughts and feelings (Carnes, 2000).

Distinctions Between Forensic and Clinical Interviews

The task of the forensic interviewer is to identify "the most effective means of getting an accurate, complete report" (Everson & Boat, 2002, p. 383). The task of the clinical interviewer is to "match the interview with the individual client in order to maximize the child's ability to convey significant information" (Salmon et al., 2003, p. 65). The clinical process addresses the safety and well-being of the child, including protective, medical and emotional needs (American Academy of Child and Adolescent Psychiatry, AACAP, 1990).

The goal of a forensic investigative interview is to gather information in a nonthreatening manner while minimizing secondary trauma (Cohen-Liebman, 1999, 2016; Gussak & Liebman, 2001). Accordingly, forensic and clinical processes differ with regard to the role of the interviewer, intent, context, the collection of data and management of information as well as style (Cohen-Liebman, 1999; Steinmetz, 1997). Additionally, elements that differentiate a forensic investigative interview from a clinical process include the assessment of competency and credibility as well as the exploration of alternative hypotheses or explanations. These elements are critical features of forensic interviews given that disclosure by a child is considered the single most significant method by which certain crimes, (specifically sexual abuse) are uncovered (Goodman-Brown et al., 2003; Lippert et al., 2009, 2010).

Forensic interviews are predicated upon obtaining a verbal statement from a child; however, a host of barriers may contribute to the acquisition of a reliable verbal account from a child. Issues or difficulties that may contribute to a child's lack of disclosure, as previously noted, include cognitive, social and emotional factors (Lippert et al., 2009; Melinder et al., 2010). Additional impediments that have been investigated include interactive patterns between the interviewer (adult) and the interviewee (child), including delivery of cues and prompts. Additionally, witness memory and management of information are issues that arise in investigative interviewing. Whether these issues contribute to a lack of verbal disclosure is under investigation (Melinder et al., 2010).

Forensically valuable information is sought from a child in a forensic setting, which is in contrast to a clinical process. In the latter, evaluative information is sought to garner understanding regarding a child's thoughts and feelings in relation to an experience. In a forensic process, information or details regarding an event are needed in an effort to determine episodic details including who, what, how and when (Macleod et al., 2013). Research has demonstrated that "what type" of information is reported by children is unclear with regard to the use of drawing in these settings (Macleod et al., 2013). As such, research has been devoted to assisting children with accurate recall of memories and the development of methods to optimize retrieval of information (Barlow et al., 2011).

Origins of Forensic Investigative Interviewing

Forensic interviewing originated in the 1980s as a strategy to help investigators address the problem of child sexual abuse (Cheit, 2014; Faller, 2014). Investigative interviewing emerged as a method to help alleged child victims of sexual abuse "relate their experiences accurately and completely" (Poole & Lamb, 2009, p. 3). The need for research and data regarding forensic interview practices increased in response to high-profile multi-victim cases that garnered media coverage and public awareness (Cheit, 2014; Faller,

2014; O'Donohue, & Fanetti, 2016). Recognition of this societal issue (Kempe, 2007) resulted in the creation of research initiatives directed at exploring various aspects of investigative interviewing and influenced the development of investigative interviewing protocols (Faller, 2014; Lamb et al., 2008; Poole & Lamb, 2009).

Knowledge about child development, including memory and cognition, as well as suggestibility, have contributed to improvements in the way child victims of sexual abuse are interviewed. As a result, the development of strategies and techniques to support the process and promote the elicitation of accurate information has burgeoned (Harris, 2010). Specialized interview training and skill building, as well as interview protocols and guidelines, contribute to best efforts to obtain credible and reliable accounts from children.

Investigative Interviewing and Child Sexual Abuse

Sexual abuse is considered a complex event that children are ill prepared to describe (Everson & Boat, 2002). An objective scientific standard for the determination of child sexual abuse does not exist (Allen & Tussey, 2012; Brooks & Milchman, 1991). Investigators and forensic interviewers are reliant upon information imparted by children given that little, if any, corroborative evidence is available in child sexual abuse cases (Faller, 2014; Lamb & Brown, 2006; Lamb et al., 2008; Myers, 1998; Poole & Lamb, 2009) and a child may be the only witness or victim of such a crime (Macleod et al., 2013). "Children's conversational skills therefore take on particular significance in such investigations" (Lamb & Brown, 2006, p. 216), especially since the amount of detailed information necessitated by a forensic investigation is not always provided by a child (Hershkowitz et al., 2012; Orbach et al., 2000).

Thus, an investigative interview is the primary method used to acquire factual and detailed information from child victims and witnesses. Investigation often hinges upon information elicited in an investigative interview, and sexual abuse is often determined from a child's statements (Faller, 2003, 2014). Investigative interviewing evolved out of a need "to help avoid false accusations and ensure justice in these cases to strengthen law enforcement's ability to elicit accurate information from children" (Harris, 2010, p. 12).

Strategies and interventions that enhance children's self-report in investigative interviews, and correspondingly, children's testimony drive research and influence practice (Faller, 2014; Katz et al., 2014; Patterson & Hayne, 2011). Continued exploration and redress are advocated in the literature with regard to interview strategies in an effort to improve outcomes both with regard to investigation and prosecution (Everson & Boat, 2002; Hiltz & Bauer, 2003). Methods for extracting viable information from child victims of sexual abuse remain a focal point of research and study (Everson & Boat, 2002; Olafson, 2012; Wakefield & Underwager, 1998). Some researchers advocate that "arguably, the disclosure of sexual abuse of a child is the most important or at least one of the most important aspects of the field" (Conte & Vaughan-Eden, 2018, p. 101). As such, the need to improve outcomes with regard to investigation and prosecution have been construed as pivotal for study and research.

Forensic interviewing is considered a dynamic and evolving profession by many researchers (Everson & Boat, 2002; Faller, 2014; Olafson, 2012; Poole & Lamb, 2009). Others contend that investigative interviewing is still in its infancy or formative stage despite the proliferation in the 1990s of the development of guidelines and protocols (Poole & Lamb, 2009). Forensic interviewing practices are based in part on extensive research and study of technique, practice and method (Cheit, 2014; Faller, 2014; Poole & Lamb, 2009).

Children are considered capable of providing information that is accurate about experiences; however, the information communicated is impacted by "types of retrieval mechanisms employed and the quality of the communication between them and their interlocutors" (Pipe et al., 2004, p. 441). Children's meta-linguistic abilities are particularly important in forensic interviews because children need to recognize what interviewers want to know and report information coherently. Additionally, interviewers must monitor the success of the conversations and modify interview strategies (Lamb & Brown, 2006). The "utilization of innumerable cognitive functions by a child" (Anderson et al., 2010, p. 204) is required in an investigative interview.

When interviewers are mindful to the meta-linguistic tendencies of children and accordingly adapt their "capacities, tendencies, and limitations", they can "shape children's performance in forensic interviews" (Lamb & Brown, 2006, pp. 223–224). "The risks and potential benefits of specific interview techniques are a function of children's life experiences, their levels of cognitive maturity and the potential impact of the information on other individuals" (Poole & Lamb, 2009, p. 5). This makes it essential that interviewers possess knowledge, training and experience to meet the needs of a child (Poole & Lamb, 2009). "It takes a sophisticated understanding of cognitive and social development to formulate appropriate alternative hypotheses about children's behavior and language during an interview" (Poole & Lamb, 2009, p. 5).

Relational Conversational Context

Within a forensic investigative interview, significance is placed on the child's ability to communicate experience or self-report. Children are reliant upon the interviewer to convey the premise as well as explain the process in order to effectively communicate (Lamb & Brown, 2006). The strategies employed by interviewers are fundamental in shaping how children retrieve and report information (Lamb & Brown, 2006; Wakefield & Underwager, 1998). The effectiveness of the information elicited is dependent upon the interaction and interactive patterns behaviorally and communicatively between interviewer and child. Accordingly, children are dependent upon interviewers "to provide retrieval cues, signal what information is important to recall and report, and structure their reports using prompts and questions" (Lamb & Brown, 2006, p. 219). Interviewers have the responsibility to "help children function as informative conversational partners without compromising the accuracy of the information elicited" (Lamb & Brown, 2006, p. 217).

Research has been directed at examining forensic investigative interviews within the framework of a "unique conversational context" (Lamb & Brown, 2006, p. 223), which has resulted in a paradigm shift given the fact-finding nature of the process. Unlike a clinical process in which children are engaged in a conversation or questions are asked and responses assessed (Faller, 2014), forensic processes demand minimization of suggestibility. The interviewer encourages true accounts of experienced events at the onset of the process (Pipe et al., 2004).

Fact-finding, which is the primary objective of an investigative interview, improves when approached within a format that is commensurate with a child's developmental skill level and interactive patterns leading to enhanced recall and disclosure (Cohen-Liebman, 1999; Melinder et al., 2010). The manner in which a child is interviewed may enhance disclosure of information that is forensically useful (Wakefield & Underwager,

1998). Guidance for both interviewers and interviewees extends beyond question format and includes the use and introduction of props, tools and media, which are deemed essential for fact-finding purposes (Faller, 2014; Lamb & Brown, 2006). A key concern is how to best introduce or ask questions. "If children do not spontaneously mention abuse, introducing the topic is a sensitive and pivotal moment" (Saywitz et al., 2018, p. 317). Moreover, "further research is needed to find tools that are nonleading and productive" (Saywitz et al., 2018, p. 317).

Strategies to Promote Retrieval and Recall

To enhance children's abilities to provide information in investigative interviews, research studies have explored various aspects and ancillary strategies associated with the process (Faller, 2014; Poole & Bruck, 2012; Poole & Lamb, 2009). The use of media, including aids, tools and props, have long been identified as contributory as well as controversial within the practice of forensic interviewing (Barlow et al., 2011; Kendall-Tackett, 1992). Interviewing aids have been associated with dolls both with and without genitalia, stuffed animals, toys, doll houses, sand trays, puppets and anatomical drawings or body schematics.

Interview techniques and strategies have been studied in an effort to determine if they contribute to enhanced reporting by children with regard to personal experience (Gee & Pipe, 1995; Salmon, 2006; Wesson & Salmon, 2001). Wakefield and Underwager (1998) characterized the various media that are utilized to interview children about allegations of sexual abuse as "image-based". This includes the use of dolls, puppets and other aids that provide a means of communication in which an image or a symbol convey something else. Many of these aids are considered controversial due to the manner in which they are used within interviews, while others "appear valuable for assisting young children to provide forensically useful information" (Wakefield & Underwager, 1998, p. 177).

In simulated contexts such techniques have been evaluated to assess whether children report information without compromising accuracy when media is incorporated into the design. In developing a new interview technique, "it is important that an increase in the amount of information that children report does not occur at the expense of accuracy" (Patterson & Hayne, 2011, p. 119). How "image-based" techniques are incorporated will have a corresponding impact on the interview process (Wakefield & Underwager, 1998). According to Lamb et al. (2008),

> Despite widespread beliefs that young children will benefit from opportunities to express themselves using dolls or drawings to augment their verbal limitations, the evidence suggests that that these aids do not necessarily help children and that their effects depend on the way they were used.
>
> (p. 164)

Although endorsement of media within the interview process exists, it has been suggested that interviewing aids, props and tools to enhance communication came into being without empirical study, including the use of drawing (Macleod et al., 2013; Poole & Lamb, 2009). It has been proposed that interview aids came into practice when practitioners were responding to rapid changes in the number and complexity of abuse cases generated in the latter part of the last century (Poole & Lamb, 2009). As a result, minimization of media within the structure of investigative interviews has been advocated by some researchers (Lamb et al., 2007) and discouraged by others. "Techniques using images vary greatly as to whether they introduce potential error into the investigation or whether they are useful aids to accurate recall" (Wakefield & Underwager, 1998, p. 179).

Some researchers allow that despite a lack of systematic evaluation, various interview techniques and strategies have been incorporated by interviewers (Poole & Lamb, 2009). The technique that has been recognized as facilitating increased reporting within experimental designs is drawing (Macleod et al., 2013). Drawing has been identified as an ancillary support for interviewers (Poole & Lamb, 1998). The use of drawing has been studied to assess effectiveness as a retrieval tool. Studies have considered drawing in relation to the age of the child, type of event to be recalled and length of delay between the event and the retrieval, as well as the use of free recall prompts (Butler et al., 1995; Gross & Hayne, 1998, 1999; Jolley, 2010; Katz & Hershkowitz, 2010, 2013; Salmon et al., 2003; Wesson & Salmon, 2001).

Ancillary Props, Cues and Retrieval Aids

A "diverse array" of ancillary techniques have been developed for eliciting and interpreting children's responses in forensic interviews. Cues or retrieval aids are used to assist children with recall and are studied in an attempt to understand their effect and value (Poole & Lamb, 2009). These ancillary supports are supportive measures that are utilized due to the drawbacks associated with verbal cues (Jolley, 2010).

Cued invitations "constitute effective ways of triggering recall of information" (Pipe et al., 2004, p. 454). Cued invitations are used within forensic interviews to remind a child of something previously expressed. They are incorporated as a method of facilitating recall of material by providing children with an opportunity to provide additional narrative information and to enhance what a child remembers. The NICHD protocol encourages interviewers to "use invitations and cued invitations preferentially throughout the interview, perhaps complemented, when necessary, by more focused questions paired with follow-up invitations" (Lamb et al., 2018, p. 189).

Several studies have focused on cues and props (Gee & Pipe, 1995; Pipe & Wilson, 1994; Salmon et al., 1995; Salmon & Pipe, 1997), with findings mixed. The use of retrieval aids, according to Poole and Lamb (2009), have to be considered in relation to whether or not they promote recall or prompt children to offer information that is not accurate. In addition, concern is noted that children may respond to the use of such aids by not referencing experienced events but from inherent knowledge, thus mitigating the effectiveness of the usage of cues and props. Poole and Lamb (2009) addressed these concerns by stipulating that props and cues should be used with great caution given the nature of the techniques to facilitate memory, retrieval and recall (p. 198). It has also been proposed that cues should only be used to help a child provide additional information about material already disclosed in order to prevent suggestibility (Poole & Lamb, 2009), essentially functioning as secondary resources to confirm previous statements or to provide clarification with regard to a verbal statement.

Supportive Interviewer Behavior Within Draw and Tell Strategies

Bourg et al. (1999) state that communication with tools (such as drawing) cannot effectively substitute for statements, but they can provide value for clarity when verbalization is limited. Macleod and colleagues (2013) identified "the major factor associated with an increase in the amount of information reported during drawing interviews is the interviewer's supportive verbal behavior" (p. 565). As such, interviewers were found to use more minimal responses, which were identified as "non-directive encouragers to maintain rapport and the flow of conversation" (Macleod et al., 2013, p. 565) in draw interviews as opposed to tell interviews.

These findings were identified from the literature on draw and tell interviews of which there are several studies (Gross et al., 2009; Patterson & Hayne, 2011; Salmon et al., 2003; Wesson & Salmon, 2001). Although the correlational nature of the relationship between minimal responses and drawing is difficult to discern, the literature indicates that through the addition of a drawing strategy, "the interviewer makes more minimal responses, and these responses are associated with augmenting children's reports" (Macleod et al., 2013, p. 565). Barlow et al. (2011) provided that drawing may account for the correspondence between duration (length of the interview) and information (disclosed) due to the impact of drawing on the interviewer's behavior, which may promote more dialogical interaction. Interviewer verbal behavior has been categorized into two groups: interviewer minimal responses or interviewer prompts. Prompts included "a directive question, probe or instruction". Minimal response was identified as "a non-directive encourager or response to maintain the flow of the conversation" (Macleod et al., 2013, p. 567).

In a study that "replicated and extended prior research on drawing with 5–12-year-old children", findings revealed that developmentally, younger children had more difficulty when asked to discuss negative emotional experiences (Macleod et al., 2013, p. 569). The researchers pointed out that in a forensic interview context, children are typically interviewed about experiences that are generally negative. The results were identified as promising because "[d]rawing was as effective in increasing the amount of information that children reported as it was when compared to discussing positive experience" (Macleod et al., 2013, p. 569). Consistent with prior research, the study conducted by (Macleod et al., 2013) revealed that interviewers used more minimal responses when children drew, and the number of minimal responses was correlated with the amount of information that children reported.

On the surface, the data support the conclusion that drawing increases interviewers' minimal responses, and the minimal responses increase the amount of information that children report. Hence "drawing works via its effects on minimal responses" (Macleod et al., 2013, p. 570). Macleod et al. (2013) also reported that these processes were longer in duration than tell-only conditions. In essence, the impact of minimal responses on the information reported was difficult to determine, given that the additional time in the process may have accounted for the additional information disclosed. They summarized, "By definition minimal responses must occur in response to something else". They continue, "In our view, drawing works because it provides a natural context within which interviewers can provide minimal responses as the child draws or talks about what he or she is drawing" (Macleod et al., 2013, p. 570). In a draw and tell interview, minimal responses are made by the interviewer in an effort to promote verbalization from a child without prejudice from the interviewer's use of leading or suggestive questions. These utterances have been referred to as "non-specific encouragement" to promote additional or enhanced communication or verbalizations by the child (Macleod et al., 2013).

Whether or not drawing has an impact upon the interviewer's behavior has been a subject of study, with emphasis being placed on interviewer utterances and cues. The manner in which the interviewer asks questions is measured, including "facilitative, non-directive prompts" or minimal utterances (Lamb & Brown, 2006). An example of such would be if an interviewer repeats a child's words verbatim or rephrased what the child said. Also, "uh huh" or "what else" are facilitative utterances. They are used to promote free recall by a child, which is a verbal technique that promotes an elaborate response, rather than a brief response, which relies upon recognition memory (Lamb & Brown, 2006). These correspond with more frequent usage in drawing conditions (Salmon et al., 2003; Wesson & Salmon, 2001) and include any response provided as a result of an open-ended prompt as opposed to a direct question. Wesson and Salmon (2001) found that interviewers used more of these in draw conditions, and children reportedly gave more information in response when these utterances were used in tell-only conditions. Facilitative utterances were found to correlate to the amount of information provided by children (Gross et al., 2009; Patterson & Hayne, 2011).

Drawing Retrieval and Recall

Drawing is a contested topic that has generated much debate within investigative interviews of children (Poole & Lamb, 2009). Consensus about the implementation of drawing in investigative interviews of children is still undecided (Lyon et al., 2009; Wesson & Salmon, 2001). Inconclusive information and dubious acceptance surround the use of drawing within investigative interviews given conflicting findings in the literature (Faller, 2005; Jolley, 2010; Vieth, 2008). Some researchers have hypothesized that drawing in a forensic interview facilitates specific retrieval cues leading to enhanced verbalization (Gross & Hayne, 1998; Jolley, 2010; Williams, 2001; Williams et al., 2002). Some contend that drawing in the context of an investigative interview process may promote enhanced disclosure due to stimulation of memory, retrieval of information and recall of salient details (Cohen-Liebman, 2017; Katz & Hershkowitz, 2010, 2013; Faller, 2014).

The liaison between retrieval and recall of memories in relation to drawing has been a topic of recent study. Whether or not drawing has a facilitative effect on children's recall during an interview has been considered (Williams, 2001). In addition, the effectiveness of drawing as a recall aid (Williams et al., 2002) has been explored. Bruck et al. reported (2000) that until recently there has been a paucity of data "on the effectiveness" of drawing despite being used as an interview strategy by investigators and therapists and continues to be an area of interest for researchers (Salmon & Pipe, 2000).

Drawing as a Communicative Facilitator

The effectiveness of drawing as a method for communication and recall of information has been studied (Patterson & Hayne, 2011). Drawing has been identified as a means to facilitate communication and enhance disclosure of experience (Brown & Lamb, 2009; Burgess & Hartman, 1993; Gross & Hayne, 1998; Patterson & Hayne, 2011; Wesson & Salmon, 2001). Within investigative interviews, drawing and drawings have been determined to enhance children's reports in one of two ways. The first is as direct communicative aids, where children draw and talk about experienced events (Butler et al., 1995; Gross & Hayne, 1998, 1999; Salmon et al., 2003; Wesson & Salmon, 2001). The other method for using drawing is as a representational aid wherein children are given drawings that depict something such as a person or an object. Children are then asked to discuss the drawings and relate information about them (Aldridge et al., 2004; Brown et al., 2007; Willcock et al., 2006).

Drawing may facilitate rapport, reduce anxiety and create a comfort level in which children remain more receptive to talking, thus possibly contributing to additional retrieval of information and ultimately additional disclosure (Gross & Hayne, 1998; Poole & Lamb, 2009; Salmon et al., 2003). The safety of comfort drawing during investigative interviews has also been evaluated (Poole & Dickinson, 2014). Some researchers contend that the more concrete and realistic a child's drawing is, the more amplification of retrieval cues occurs (Butler et al., 1995). Others allow that "a drawing can be entirely child generated and independent of (potentially biasing) input from the interviewer" (Thomas & Jolley, 1998, p. 137).

According to some researchers, children provide more information about actual experiences when given the opportunity to draw and verbalize simultaneously (Brown & Lamb, 2009; Gross & Hayne, 1998, 1999; Katz & Hershkowitz, 2010). These findings were found to be consistent regardless of age and did not compromise accuracy (Brown & Lamb, 2009; Gross & Hayne, 1998, 1999; Katz & Hershkowitz, 2010). Other researchers have explored the use of drawing as a secondary retrieval strategy within forensic interviews. As such, drawing is introduced after children describe abusive events in response to open-ended questions as a means of confirmation or explanation of verbalizations (Katz & Hershkowitz, 2010, 2013; Poole & Lamb, 2009). In this capacity, drawing is not presented in a primary context.

Drawing has been characterized as a robust interview strategy by various researches in both clinical and forensic applications (Clements et al., 2001; Driessnack, 2005; Salmon et al., 2003). Drawing is commonly used in clinical interviews to help children talk about their experiences despite a lack of "solid scientific evidence" to explain why or how drawing works (Williams, 2001). The goal of a draw and tell clinical interview is to "extract clinically relevant information" (Macleod et al., 2013, p. 570) and to enhance "evaluative information" in forensic processes (p. 571). Salmon et al. (2003) found that more verbal information was elicited through drawing in experimental designs than through telling or re-enactment conditions. Also, verbalizations were found to be enhanced when a drawing strategy was provided (Salmon et al., 2003).

Clements et al. (2001), in a study of 13 children, reported that in conjunction with an interview, a series of drawings provided "robust data" (p. 14) with regard to the impact of sudden death and barriers to recovery. Drawings provided a means for communication of information within the context, which was conceived for clinical purposes. The drawings enhanced and enriched children's communication. In addition, drawing provided a means for understanding sensory factors or "sensory memory", which was identified as anything that the child may have heard, saw or felt with regard to the event (Clements et al., 2001, p. 14). The narratives provided by the children in tandem with the drawings revealed memories affiliated with the sensorium, resulting in "multidimensional and multilevel data that promoted deeper exploration and explanation of the reality" of the event under exploration (Clements et al., 2001, p. 14). According to the authors, the children's drawings "helped identify and assess the acute issues" that the children were confronting at the time of retrieval (Clements et al., 2001, p. 14).

Driessnack (2005) conducted a meta-analysis and identified six studies which "found that drawing facilitates children's abilities to talk" about "events or concepts they might otherwise find difficult to describe" (p. 416). The facilitative effects of "offering children the opportunity to draw as an interview strategy" as compared to a verbal process was considered in the meta-analysis (p. 415). The goal of the meta-analysis was to determine if drawing can facilitate communication with children and if evidence could support the inclusion of drawing in research and clinical protocols as well as practice (Driessnack, 2005, p. 415).

According to Driessnack's meta-analysis, drawing "provides strong and definitive results that support the use of drawing to facilitate communication with children" (p. 421). Despite this conclusion, however, the meta-analysis identified limitations in the various studies (such as small sample size) as well as with the analysis itself. The studies were predominantly conducted by a small group of researchers from the field of psychology. The studies were "quantitatively based and limited, by the inclusion criteria, to those using an experimental design" (Driessnack, 2005, p. 421). The meta-analysis included studies by Gross and Hayne (1998, 1999); Gross et al. (2006); Salmon et al. (2003); and Wesson and Salmon (2001). Driessnack's meta-analysis determined that "introducing the opportunity to draw is a relatively robust interview strategy relative to a verbal interview" (Driessnack, 2005, p. 420). Overall, Driessnack found that children who draw and tell about emotional experiences provided accurate information similarly to children that related their emotional experience verbally (Driessnack, 2005; Gross et al., 2006). This finding was found to be consistent throughout the various studies included in the meta-analysis (Salmon et al., 2003; Wesson & Salmon, 2001). When children were asked to draw during an interview, self-reports were more detailed and accurate (Gross et al., 2006).

Driessnack (2006) conducted a secondary study, which confirmed the findings from her meta-analysis (2005) that drawings functionally facilitate communication by children. Other researchers have determined that children's abilities to recall information are enhanced with a draw and tell scenario in comparison to a tell-only condition (Butler et al., 1995). When children were allowed to draw during an interview, they provided more information than children who were only asked to talk or tell about their experiences, and accuracy was not affected (Butler et al., 1995).

Significant to these studies, only verbal behavior was coded. Pictorial content was not coded (Driessnack, 2005). Contemporary research and analogue studies pertaining to the use of drawing in interviews tend to focus exclusively on what children said rather than address the content of the material drawn (Patterson & Hayne, 2011). As Williams (2001) in her doctoral dissertation stated, "[I]t is not the content of children's drawings primarily, but the production of a drawing as an aid to recall that is the main focus of experimental work" (p. 17).

Driessnack (2005, 2006), in her systematic meta-analysis of the literature, identified that the studies in her analysis were concerned with the variable amount of information disclosed by children rather than the content of the material communicated. As she pointed out, "Although it appears that children speak more freely when given the opportunity to draw first, it also appears that we know very little about what it is that they then say" (Driessnack, 2006, p. 1416). In her follow-up study to her meta-analysis, her research was directed at what children say about their drawings. "The draw and tell conversation is introduced as a child-centered and child directed approach to self-report that incorporates children's drawings for their facilitative effect rather than as a direct method for interpretation" (Driessnack, 2006, p. 1416). Driessnack concluded that "too often, clinicians and researchers disregard children's words used to explain or accompany their drawings and instead substitute their own explanations" (Driessnack, 2006, p. 1416).

In their own study, Patterson and Hayne (2011) stated, "We did not try to interpret what children had drawn. To date, there is no empirical evidence to support the use of drawing as an interpretive or a projective tool" (p. 125). Clements et al. (2001) reported that there is not a consistent statistical scoring mechanism to determine the validity and reliability of children's drawings in the literature for research purposes. Studies, however, do provide findings that describe how drawings have been successful in helping children relate traumatic events (Gross & Hayne, 1998, 1999; Jolley, 2010).

Emotional Response and Pictorial Content

In certain conditions interviewers may ask children to describe events that evoke more of an emotional response. This approach is consistent with a legal context or a forensic interview objective in which interviewers may need to question a child around an issue that may be more emotional in nature (Gross et al., 2006). As such, Gross and Hayne (1998) directed their research to focus on events that may promote an emotional impact on the subjects. They found that drawing appeared to enhance the amount of information that was retrieved. They identified that the effect of children's drawings on emotional experiences had not been considered, given that experimental designs (analogue or laboratory studies) tend to include educational or entertainment (such as a magic show) rather than focus on experiences that may provoke an emotional response (Gross & Hayne, 1998).

Gross and Hayne (1998) determined that drawing does increase children's verbalizations about their own experiences regardless of age or the content of the event and the corresponding emotional impact on the child. Given that accuracy was not compromised (in their research), they proposed that "drawing may be particularly valuable in evidential interviews with children, where the accuracy of their accounts is paramount" (Gross & Hayne, 1998, p. 174).

Several research studies have indicated that children tend to provide enhanced information while drawing that includes generalized information rather than situational or contextual information (Barlow et al., 2011; Gross & Hayne, 1998; Katz & Hershkowitz, 2010; Wesson & Salmon, 2001). Macleod and colleagues (2013) sought to understand what kind of information children report when drawing in an interview. They were interested in finding out if drawing would help "children to report forensically relevant episodic details and to report clinically relevant evaluative information about their emotional experiences" (Macleod et al., 2013, p. 565). Their study included a total of 60 children with half in the 5- to 6-year-old range and half in the 11- to 12-year-old age range. They examined "event" information, which was characterized as "concrete, factual aspects of a child's emotional experience that added to the interviewer's understanding of what, when, how, or why an event occurred" (Macleod et al., 2013, p. 567). They further broke down the information into two categories: object or episodic information. The former was identified as "object, thing, place or physical component", whereas episodic was identified with regard to whether or not the child provided details about the experience as well as the identification of a person (Macleod et al., 2013, p. 567).

Drawing Dichotomy Within Investigative Interviews

Drawing in investigative interviews has been revered by some researchers and rejected by others, demonstrating the variability of acceptance that has and still exists as addressed in research, study and the literature. The utility of drawing as an interview strategy that maximizes disclosure of abuse-specific information by children has been acknowledged by some exploring the topic (Everson & Boat, 2002; Faller, 1993, 2007; Katz et al., 2014; Katz & Hershkowitz, 2010; Lamb et al., 2007; Lyon et al., 2009; Olafson, 2012). Drawing and drawings in investigative interviews have been referred to as "potentially risky tools" by some researchers (Lamb et al., 2007, p. 1212; Lamb et al., 2018), while others (Faller, 2005; Vieth, 2008) have strongly advocated for the use of drawing or drawings within the investigative interview format as well as for courtroom acceptance (Cohen-Liebman, 1995) and as a means of enhancing eyewitness testimony (Williams et al., 2002). A child's experience can often be expressed pictorially through a drawing, which can later serve as evidentiary material (Burgess et al., 1987; Cohen-Liebman, 1995; Faller, 1993), since drawing concretizes a child's experience in a context that is viable for court (Cohen-Liebman, 1999; Gussak, 2013; Gussak & Cohen-Liebman, 2001). The American Bar Association supports the use of drawings to facilitate children's testimony (Cohen-Liebman, 1995).

Drawing in investigative interviews has been observed to empower child victims (Cohen-Liebman, 1999, 2016; Jolley, 2010; Katz et al., 2014). Children may not only be empowered but also maintain control of what they are marking on paper (Cohen-Liebman, 1999; Cox, 2005). Free drawing has also been found to provide uncontaminated accounts that were self-cued by children in direct response to open-ended prompts. Katz and Hamama (2013) determined that as a self-report tool, drawing is a "natural, accessible language that children can use for emotional expression" (Katz & Hamama, 2013, p. 877). Drawing as a means to induce verbal elaboration has been acknowledged (American Prosecutors Research Institute and National Center for Prosecution of Child Abuse, 2004; Poole & Lamb, 2009). Poole and Lamb (2009) discuss as well that within the context of investigative interviews drawing may "facilitate reporting by easing stress, by extending the length of the interview and providing more opportunity for details to surface, or by introducing topics that can be explored verbally" (p. 183).

Drawing during investigative interviewing has also been deemed controversial for a host of reasons. Poole and Lamb (2009) indicated that such practice might provide a means of distillation for anxiety and encourage rapport, allowing more information to be disclosed yet they have also referred to drawing as "innocuous". They furthermore emphasized that some interviewers "allow children to continue to draw during the substantive portions of the interview, without explicit instructions to draw the events in question" (Poole & Lamb, 2009, p. 183), which may promote the use of leading questions by interviewers in an effort to refocus a child's attention. Moreover, they asserted that children may provide an inconsequential response in an effort to focus on the drawing rather than on the exchange with the interviewer. They expressed that "[u]ntil firm data are available, it would be prudent to remove drawing materials and encourage children to devote their full attention to the interviewer" (Poole & Lamb, 2009, p. 183). Another negative they have expressed is that drawing may distract children from providing coherent narratives because "drawing could reduce the quality of the narrative by distracting children or by encouraging creativity and fantasy" (Poole & Lamb, 2009, p. 183).

Drawing has been considered useful as "an associative tool for assessing and accessing traumatic memories" (Burgess & Hartman, 1993). Proponents of including drawing within clinical and forensic interview processes have reported that children can pictorially express abuse-specific information through drawing (Burgess & Hartman, 1993; Burgess et al., 1987; Cohen-Liebman, 1999, 2003; Gussak & Cohen-Liebman, 2001). Free drawings have also been analyzed through content analysis to discern the possibility of abuse (Miller et al., 1987; Yates et al., 1985). In addition, several national organizations have addressed the use of drawing within the assessment or evaluation of sexually abused children through published guidelines (American Academy of Child and Adolescent Psychiatry, 1990; American Professional Society on the Abuse of children, 1990).

Analogue Studies and the Effect of Drawing on Children's Reports

To date, the majority of the empirical research on the effect of drawing on children's reports has involved analogue studies of nonclinical populations (Patterson & Hayne, 2011, p. 125). The use of analogue studies as a means of researching aspects of interviewer practices and techniques, including the use of drawing, has been used extensively given difficulties with conducting real-time experimental studies on these topics as has been noted in the respective literature and research (including Ehring et al., 2011; Lamb & Thierry, 2005; Poole & Lamb, 2009). Through analogue designs, participants are asked to report in an interview context about an event (staged or naturally occurring within a controlled setting). These studies are intended to replicate forensic interview conditions in which children are asked to discuss an experienced or witnessed event (Faller, 2014). Analogue studies provide an analogous scenario in which to conduct an experiment by providing a real and objective experience as the basis for the experiment; however, analogue studies tend to differ from real-world experience, especially with regard to a traumatic event (Lamb & Thierry, 2005). Exposing children to a traumatic event within the exploratory context is not in the best interest of children and as such, an analogue design may incorporate an event or a simulated experience that is not intended to be stress inducing and does not replicate a real-world scenario that may possibly trigger an emotional response.

Analogue studies have addressed the use of drawing as a means of helping children recall and remember experienced events. Studies directed at assessing if drawing facilitates recall and disclosure are limited to nonclinical or non-forensic populations in which circumstances are controlled (Patterson & Hayne, 2011). Studies have explored whether children's accounts can be manipulated as well as how material may be retrieved (Poole & Lamb, 2009; Lamb & Thierry, 2005). The facilitative effect of drawing on memory when children are asked irrelevant as well as relevant questions has been considered (Williams et al., 2002). Additionally, interviewer behavior and strategies interviewers employ have been studied to assess accuracy and reliability of the information recalled by children (Macleod et al., 2013; Pipe et al., 2004).

Analogue studies aimed at exploring issues related to forensic interviewing of sexually abused children have been viewed both positively and negatively. Analogue studies offer a means of application within forensic interview contexts given the study of strategies to enhance recall (Pipe et al., 2004). Although laboratory or analogue studies play a role in understanding how children report their experiences, these studies cannot replicate in their research designs the trauma, secrecy and stigma associated with sexual abuse (Lamb & Thierry, 2005). Ecological validity in which findings can be generalized to real life is an issue in analogue studies, given that the scenarios that children experience in laboratory studies are not typically congruent with traumatic events such as sexual abuse.

In addition, determination of feasibility and validity of an experienced event, especially with respect to measuring trauma memory characteristics, is limited in field or real-time study (Ehring et al., 2011). Moreover, studies often do not reflect the challenges experienced in the field by actual forensic interviewers (Faller, 2014). As such, analogue studies have been criticized because interview techniques are considered to be less congruent with forensic interviewing techniques.

Analogue studies have been conducted to evaluate the usefulness of drawing on children's memory and recall in investigative interviews. Experiments have been conducted to assess if drawing facilitates recall of information by children through four different approaches according to Barlow et al. (2011). The four methodological experimental approaches that have been implemented to explore if drawing facilitates verbal recall of an event and to determine the "usefulness of drawings as memory cues within each methodological approach" (Jolley, 2010, p. 222) include recall of staged/naturally occurring events, emotional memories, item recall and video information (Barlow et al., 2011; Jolley, 2010).

Drawing Within Analogue Studies: Mixed Findings

The function of drawing in facilitating children's accurate recall and memory of events has been explored in analogue studies. Accurate recall has been recognized when drawings were used (Butler et al., 1995; Gross & Hayne, 1998, 1999; Salmon et al., 2003; Wesson & Salmon, 2001). Other studies revealed that drawings have been associated with a decrease in accuracy, most notably after a delay in questioning (Salmon & Pipe, 2000). Under "ideal conditions" meaning "when asking children about true events using non-suggestive questioning" (Lamb et al., 2008, p. 46), children recalled more information and accuracy was not tainted (Butler et al., 1995; Gross & Hayne, 1998, 1999; Salmon et al., 2003; Wesson & Salmon, 2001). Analogue research has also suggested that children report erroneous information or report things that never happened (Bruck et al., 2000; Gross et al., 2006; Strange et al., 2003).

In reference to the literature, Lamb et al. (2008) concluded, "Taken together, these studies suggest that drawing and talking may generally increase children's responsiveness about both true and false events" (p. 46). Children actively engaged versus passively engaged in analogue research have been found to provide more accurate recall. Lamb and colleagues (2008) contend that within analogue studies, free drawing may help children "reconstruct experienced events and thus report them more fully" (p. 162). They provided that "researchers have consistently shown that free drawing while being questioned leads children to report more information" (Lamb et al., 2008, p. 162). They state that in some studies, researchers found "two and three-fold increases in the amount of information reported" (Lamb et al., 2008, p. 162). "Whether or not this information was accurate depended upon the types of questioning with which the drawing was associated" (Lamb et al., 2008, p. 162).

Similarly, Tobey and Goodman (1992) found that when children were participants in an event, resistance to suggestion was apparent compared to children who watched a video about an event. While freely drawing, children tended to report more information; however, accuracy of the information reported was dependent upon the type of questions asked in concert with the child drawing. If the drawing was accompanied by free recall prompts in the studies, the respondent information tended to be accurate, and the amount of accuracy did not diminish even with increased disclosure or reporting (Lamb et al., 2008). Summarily, Lamb et al. (2008) determined that when drawing was used with suggestive or leading questions, accuracy declined.

The impact of the interviewer's style and response to a child's interactions with regard to cultivating suggestibility are additional areas under study (Pipe et al., 2004). Pipe et al. (2004) conducted an extensive review of the literature pertaining to suggestibility and tainting of children's recall within the experimental literature. They provided that "suggestibility involves complex social, communicative and memory processes" (Pipe et al., 2004, p. 449). In their consideration of the literature, they reported that "social, cognitive and individual difference variables may account for suggestibility" (Pipe et al.,

2004, p. 449) and for understanding why children may report the things they do. Poole and Lindsay (1996), as noted by Pipe et al. (2004), reported that "suggestibility declines when children are counseled only to report experienced events" (p. 450). Children provided increased amounts of information when interviewed under ideal conditions, and the information children reported while drawing appeared to be highly accurate (Pipe & Salmon, 2009).

In a study conducted by Gross et al. (2006) conditions under which a child might describe events or experiences that they had not encountered were studied. Whether or not children would integrate false information included in drawings was considered (Gross et al., 2006). Although an increase in inaccurate information was recorded, the design was not meant to be a forensically similar process, but rather assessed whether or not a visual representation of a false event would increase suggestibility or, rather, susceptibility to suggestion (Gross et al., 2006, p. 124). It was determined that under ideal interview conditions "the opportunity to draw during an interview facilitates children's verbal reports of their past, personal experiences without decreasing accuracy" (Gross et al., 2006, p. 119). This has been determined in other research studies as well (Gross & Hayne, 1998, 1999; Pipe & Salmon, 2009; Wesson & Salmon, 2001).

Studies have been undertaken to determine if drawing would "enhance or impede" children's verbal accounts in less-than-ideal interview conditions, meaning coercive or suggestive techniques were incorporated by the interviewer (Ceci & Bruck, 1995; Gross et al., 2006). Bruck et al. (2000) undertook the task of assessing whether children were more willing to integrate false information of an event based upon the use of a drawing. Children (N = 87) between the ages of three and six participated in a magic show. The children were interviewed in suggestive or leading interviews at two- and four-week intervals. Both real and false information was given to the children in what is termed a suggestive interview with regard to the event. Children were more likely to incorporate false information when accompanied by a drawing based upon the known variables of the interview context as designed in the analogue setting (Bruck et al., 2000). The children were intentionally misled about elements of the event they had experienced in an effort to determine if they could be suggestible, especially when a drawing condition was used to help them relay information about their experience. Tantamount to these findings was the belief that such suggestibility may impede a child's credibility on the witness stand or when being interviewed.

A pilot study conducted as part of a dissertation (Williams, 2001) explored if errors would increase when children (N = 14, ages seven and eight) drew during an interview if asked specifically about an event that never occurred. Analysis of the data revealed "little evidence to support the claim that drawing during an interview increased errors when the questioning is about something that did not happen, as is often the case in legal settings" (Williams, 2001, p. 78). With regard to this experiment the author wrote,

> The effectiveness of including drawing during an interview with children is wholly dependent on further researching this question. In theoretical terms it may influence the literature on children's representational minds and their cognitive ability. In application terms it may be possible to recommend or deter the use of drawing in real clinical or forensic interviews. Further research with improved methodology will also help make real the possibility of making interviews with children more focused to their needs.
>
> (Williams, 2001)

Reflecting upon the results in another experiment associated with her research, Williams determined that her data indicated no differences between drawing and telling for direct questions, and accuracy remained constant. She wrote that her findings were contrary to the research conducted by Butler et al. (1995), where "a facilitative effect of drawing" was identified in association with direct questioning. She offered what has been stated by other researchers that the effect may be attributed to mechanisms associated with drawing, including comfort (Poole, & Dickinson, 2014) and control. Moreover, she indicated that retrieval may have been prompted by drawing, which may have increased recall due to self-generated cues by the participants (Williams, 2001). Researchers have suggested drawing may cue and as such reduce reliance on external retrieval cues (Butler et al., 1995; Jolley, 2010; Wesson & Salmon, 2001; Williams, 2001).

According to Gross et al. (2006), whether or not drawing will promote verbalization of a false event is still unknown given the limited studies surrounding this issue. In relation to an investigative interview process, a child who is asked to depict an erroneous event or provide pictorial details of such must then describe fictitious events in the interview verbally and that in order to do so, they must "generate the false information themselves" (Gross et al., 2006, p. 123). As a result, children may construct a less detailed narrative. Gross et al. (2006) contend that these children may be less likely to offer material about "a false event in a subsequent interview" (p. 123). They concluded, "In this way, drawing could actually buffer children from the effects of inappropriate questioning" (Gross et al., 2006, p. 123). Pipe et al. (2004) stated,

> In sum, many researchers have conducted laboratory-based and analogue studies designed to document the vulnerability of children's eyewitnesses' accounts to misleading questioning and suggestions and increasing numbers have explored alternative means of enhancing children's reports without decreasing accuracy. In general, definitive conclusions about such techniques as having children draw during the interview or refer to human figure drawings must await further research, especially research in field contexts.
>
> (p. 453)

Suggestive Techniques and Drawing

Experiments that assessed whether self-created drawings "increased or decreased the effects of misinformation" (Gross et al., 2006, p. 124) were consistent with the findings from other studies (Bruck & Ceci, 1999; Ceci & Bruck, 1993, 1995; Poole & Lindsay, 2001, 2002) that "children are often susceptible to the effects of misinformation" (Gross et al., 2006, p. 141). The researchers reported that "drawing does not buffer children against the negative effects of inappropriate and misleading questioning" (Gross et al., 2006, p. 140). According to Gross et al. (2009) research conveyed that when suggestive techniques and drawing were combined, accuracy of reports declined. They cited the following studies as demonstrating such findings: Bruck et al., 2000; Gross et al., 2006; Strange et al., 2003.

Gross et al. (2009) emphasized that enhancing children's reports of experienced events has implications for legal purposes such as testifying and for understanding children's memory. They indicated that unless interviews in both clinical and forensic settings do not include misinformation on the part of the interviewer, there is a risk that the children will "incorporate the incorrect information in a subsequent account of an event" (Gross et al., 2006, p. 142).

As others have determined, Gross et al. (2006) provided that drawing can facilitate memory performance when children are interviewed under conditions that are directed at maximizing accuracy (Butler et al., 1995; Gross & Hayne, 1998, 1999), such as through the use of nonleading and open-ended questions (Macleod et al., 2013). When interviewed under less ideal conditions, i.e., when accuracy is unlikely to be maximized, the "opportunity to draw does not inoculate children against the effects of misleading information" (Gross et al., 2006, p. 142).

Similarly, Strange et al. (2003) examined if drawing something that did not happen or that children had not experienced within a given scenario would motivate children to say that the event had occurred. They explored whether children would draw the event as if it had taken place. Their results indicated that five- and six-year-old children that drew false events were more likely to say that these events had actually happened to them.

Gross et al. (2009) reported that when suggestive techniques and drawing are combined, accuracy of reports declines. Research has shown that drawing does not protect children from "the negative effects of interviews that are highly suggestive, leading or misleading, and drawing does not prevent children from reporting false information that they have obtained from another source (Bruck et al., 2000; Gross et al., 2006; Patterson & Hayne, 2011; Pipe & Salmon, 2009; Strange et al., 2003). Thus, some researchers have found and assert that under less-than-ideal conditions, drawing may enhance errors (Macleod et al., 2013; Patterson & Hayne, 2011).

Although studies have demonstrated "that in addition to encouraging more complete recall of true events, drawing may also encourage children to report information about events that never occurred" (Bruck et al., 2000; Gross et al., 2006; Strange et al., 2003), Brown asserts,

> Taken together, these studies suggest that drawing and talking may generally increase children's responsiveness – about both true and false events. Thus, as with other supplementary techniques, the context in which children are asked to draw is a paramount consideration when used with school-age children and in conjunction with appropriate verbal questioning (i.e., open-ended prompting) drawing appears to aid children in recalling and reporting their experiences. When accompanied by misleading information or suggestive questioning, however, the additional information elicited is likely to be highly unreliable.
>
> (Brown, 2011, p. 236)

Some researchers have determined that drawing has the potential to be useful in clinical and forensic contexts (Brown & Lamb, 2009; Clements et al., 2001; Driessnack, 2005; Gross & Hayne, 1998, 1999; Katz & Hershkowitz, 2010; Patterson & Hayne, 2011). It is a developmentally appropriate tool; is an activity that children of all ages enjoy; and under optimal interview conditions, it elicits accurate accounts and increases the amount of information that children report (Driessnack, 2005). Furthermore, some studies indicated that when children are given the opportunity to draw, interviewers asked more open-ended questions, which was associated with higher accuracy according to some researchers. "Questions structured in a supportive and opened manner most likely will elicit responses without leading children to give explanations thought to be desired by the interviewer" (Clements et al., 2001, p. 16).

Given that drawing cannot protect children from questioning techniques that are suggestive or misleading, and that drawing may in some instances enhance children's tendency to report false information, recommendations that drawing be used in clinical or forensic contexts require careful consideration.

(Patterson & Hayne, 2011, p. 125)

Gross et al. (2006), explained:

> In the final analysis, a given interview technique is only as good as the professional who uses it. In the right hands, drawing may facilitate children's accounts without increasing errors. In the wrong hands, however, drawing may also induce children to make serious mistakes.
>
> (Gross et al., 2006, p. 142)

Use of Drawing to Express Personal Experience

The use of drawing to express personally meaningful experiences has been addressed and explored experimentally (Butler et al., 1995). In addition, whether drawing helps children to report material pertaining to emotionally laden experiences has also been considered (Gross & Hayne, 1998, 1999; Wesson & Salmon & 2001). Although these topics are considered relevant for both forensic and clinical situations (Salmon et al., 2003; Wesson & Salmon, 2001), the lack of a nondrawing control group in many studies has been identified as a methodological flaw by some studying the use of drawing within interview contexts (Jolley, 2010).

A study conducted in 1995 by Butler, Gross and Hayne was a seminal piece of research with regard to the effect of drawing (Gross & Hayne, 1998; Thomas & Jolley, 1998). This study was identified as the first "to provide empirical evidence that drawing can facilitate young children's verbal accounts of a past personal experience" (Gross & Hayne, 1998, p. 165). The research involved asking children to draw a picture about a personally meaningful experience. Reportedly, participants disclosed enhanced amounts of information when questioned about the features of drawings. A correspondence between increased information and pictorial realism was identified. The researchers found that the representational quality of the drawings was related to the children's verbal performance (Gross & Hayne, 1998; Thomas & Jolley, 1998).

Other research has contributed to an emergent growing corpus of study that "indicates that drawing facilitates children's abilities to talk about the past" (Gross & Hayne, 1998, p. 176). Gross and Hayne (1998, 1999) have studied the phenomenon of drawing as a means of communication for many years. In their original study, children between the ages of three and five were assigned to one of two groups: draw and tell or just tell. The data revealed that regardless of the delay between the actual experience of the staged event, the draw and tell group reported almost twice as much information as children in the tell group. Moreover, accuracy was consistent across the groups. Data confirmed that drawing facilitated children's verbal reports over short delays (Gross & Hayne, 1999). Continued study of this phenomenon by these researchers revealed that accuracy was not affected when a longer delay ensued between the experienced event and the interview (Gross & Hayne, 1999; Patterson & Hayne, 2011).

In a separate study that considered if drawing impacted the accuracy of children's verbal statements, Gross and Hayne (1998) explored the use of drawing and potential influence on fantasy or embellishment of detail. The study also investigated the effect of drawing on the accuracy as well as the amount of verbal accounts of an emotional experience (Gross & Hayne, 1998, p. 171). This study included 20 children between ages five and six. The study was directed at researching if drawing was able to facilitate recall of past personal experience rather than emotional experience. Gross and Hayne (1998) stated that no prior studies had used a control group in which children only told and did not draw for comparative purposes. Accordingly, no empirical data existed prior to the study that indicated the facilitative effect of drawing on verbal accounts (Gross & Hayne, 1998).

Use of Drawing to Express Emotionally Laden Experience

Researchers contend that when children self-select emotionally laden events, the use of a drawing strategy may maximize recall of information because the events the children choose to report on have salience for the particular child. Researchers have found that drawing such subject matter allows children to be removed from the intense emotional nature of the interview context (Thomas & Jolley, 1998), allowing for a narrative account of an event (Salmon et al., 2003). "Drawing may help children generate their own retrieval cues in the context of highly distinctive episodes" (Wesson & Salmon, 2001, p. 303).

Gross and Hayne (1998) studied whether or not drawing facilitated "verbal reports of emotionally laden events". In a study of 40 children, half of whom were three to four years old and the other half five to six years old, the children were randomly assigned to either a draw or tell condition. The children assigned to the draw condition were asked to draw about a time when they were happy, sad or scared, while the children in the other condition were asked to tell about such a time. The study results revealed that the children in the drawing or experimental condition provided more information than children assigned to the control group. The results were significant in that the experimental group, or draw condition, provided twice as much material as the tell condition according to the data. Additionally, accuracy was not compromised (Gross & Hayne, 1998). The following year, these same authors assessed whether drawing facilitated children's verbal reports of emotionally laden experience after a delay (Gross & Hayne, 1999). The study consisted of two separate experiments. The initial study assessed children's memory after an experience (a trip to a chocolate factory). Fifty-five children ages five to six were assigned first to one of the two timed delays (either one day or six months). The results found that the experimental group reported more information than the control group.

In 2001, Wesson and Salmon also assessed whether drawing facilitated children's verbal reports of emotionally laden events. In effect, their study was based upon the earlier work by Gross and Hayne (1998, 1999); however, they added a third interview condition. A total of 30 children participated with half between the ages of five and six and half between the ages of eight and nine. The children were randomly assigned to one of the three conditions: draw, tell or show (meaning re-enact everything they could remember) about a time when they were happy, sad or scared. The results revealed that the older children provided significantly more information than the younger children. Children within the experimental group used drawing and provided more than twice what the control group offered. Wesson and Salmon (2001) found that drawing augmented verbal descriptions, and information disclosed was accurate even after a delay. The data and results revealed that the drawing and re-enactment conditions elicited more descriptive information; however, more verbal information was elicited through drawing than through telling or re-enactment. As such, Wesson and Salmon (2001) determined recall may be enhanced in response to drawing and re-enactment due to the effectiveness of these retrieval cues. The study was directed at obtaining information for interviewing children in clinical contexts (Wesson & Salmon, 2001).

Another study conducted in 2003 considered drawing as a means for facilitating communication with children (Salmon et al., 2003). The study included 58 children between the ages of five and seven. The children were randomly assigned to one of three interview conditions: tell, draw or re-enact. The findings in this study were similar to the previous studies reviewed, which suggested that drawing promoted enhanced verbalization without compromising accuracy under ideal conditions (Gross & Hayne, 1998, 1999; Wesson & Salmon, 2001).

Video and the Facilitative Effect of Drawing

In a study that utilized a video segment as a source for the event to be recalled, Barlow et al. (2011) utilized an interactive interview process to evaluate the facilitative effect of drawing. In their study, which included 80 children between five and six years old, they assigned the children to one of four conditions: tell-only, draw and tell, interactive draw and tell and interactive tell. The interactive conditions included five questions to provide an opportunity for children to elaborate upon previously mentioned material in the interview. Accordingly, the questions were incorporated to provide children with an opportunity to elaborate on each piece of information that was said or drawn. The study utilized video as a methodological experimental approach to explore the facilitative effect of drawing.

The study emanated in response to Jolley's work (2010) in which he asserted that the "optimum drawing conditions for recall have yet to be established" despite "the effectiveness of drawing as a retrieval cue" (Barlow et al., 2011, p. 481). The premise sought to explore the supposition that if given more verbal support, perhaps children would offer more information in investigative interviews. Although facilitative utterances by the interviewer appeared to promote more interaction in situations where direct questions or focused questions were asked, previous research had not encouraged children to expand or elaborate upon their responses. As Barlow et al. (2011) stated, these questions were not "reactive" to what the child said or drew (p. 481).

Thus, the study considered the "optimum verbal support" from an interviewer to assist in the retrieval of information while drawing in an interview (Barlow et al., 2011, p. 485). Children were asked to verbally expand on information they had "spontaneously drawn or articulated" (Barlow et al., 2011, p. 485). Findings revealed that more accurate information was recalled in the interactive draw and tell condition. This effect was attributed to drawing in concert with the interactive/elaborate questions. The findings, in conjunction with other studies (Butler et al., 1995; Gross & Hayne, 1999), supported that drawing alone "is not as strong or reliable a recall cue than when accompanied by direct questions from the interviewer" (Barlow et al., 2011, p. 485). The nature of the questions included were in reference to the context of what was drawn or said. The questions were child cued in contrast to predetermined questions, whether general or specific, that were directed at what a child drew or said (Barlow et al., 2011). Given the interactive questions included in the design, interviewers had flexibility to expand upon the information that children provided due to the synergistic nature of the interview. The combination of interactive questions with drawing appeared to provide a positive retrieval cue (Barlow et al., 2011).

> The child's developing drawing provides a publicly shared resource that affords the interviewer useful opportunities to ask the child questions about the event. The

child's verbal responses then give the interviewer further opportunity to ask the child to expand upon a point or give further details about what happened next, or even to draw further, setting up a circular memory cue of draw-talk-draw (and so on). Furthermore, because the drawing is a permanent and public record, unlike speech, the interviewer can refer the child's attention back to a previously drawn item that is presently available, thereby probing further the child's memory.

(Barlow et al., 2011, p. 485)

The study also confirmed that interview duration correlated with accurate recall. These findings were noted in other studies (Butler et al., 1995; Wesson & Salmon, 2001). Barlow et al. concluded that incorporating interactive questions enhanced recall; however, they were unable to identify if other "retrieval facilitators", such as focus and duration, accounted for their findings (Barlow et al., 2011). Barlow et al. (2011) suggested empirical study of these other factors independently to determine if enhanced recall may be attributed to these other factors when an interactive questioning condition is a part of the design. They reported:

Our findings are of particular interest to those who interview children in a number of applied settings. Studies on using drawing as a memory aid for children have sometimes been presented in a context of improving children's eye-witness testimony, although researchers have rarely discussed how their findings may apply in legal interviews with children.

(Barlow et al., 2011)

Furthermore, Barlow et al. (2011) offer that the interactive draw-and-tell interview technique presented in their study paper may "represent therefore a useful initiative to derive an interview framework for how drawings and questions are combined to optimize children's verbal recall" (Barlow et al., 2011, p. 486). Barlow et al. (2011) continued by acknowledging art therapy. They provided that

[d]rawing may enable children to recreate an event from a position of power and control (a fundamental basis of art therapy), helping vulnerable children give evidence on issues they may not have felt comfortable doing in a conversation-only interview.

(Barlow et al., 2011, p. 486)

Barlow et al. (2011) identified that in some studies (Butler et al., 1995; Jolley, 2010; Salmon, 2001) drawing was deemed "a non-threatening and enjoyable activity", which may in and of itself be recognized as contributory to the facilitative factor associated with drawing in the interview context. Barlow et al. (2011) expressed that what they have referred to as the interactive draw and tell interview "[h]as all the recall benefits of the draw-and-tell method, but provides further verbal structure enabling the child to retrieve additional information" (Barlow et al., 2011, p. 486).

Drawing and Developmental Considerations

Developmental effects and the impact of drawing with younger children as well as older children have been considered in the investigative interview literature (Gross & Hayne, 1998, 1999; Patterson & Hayne, 2011). Drawing has been identified as a means for overcoming cognitive and language developmental limitations, which may impact expressive communication and memory recall (Patterson & Hayne, 2011). Research has demonstrated that even young children with limited vocabulary and cognitive skills can reveal information pertaining to lived experiences that is accurate and detailed (Aldridge et al., 2004; Lamb & Brown, 2006; Patterson & Hayne, 2011). Researchers have also studied whether drawing impacts children's abilities to recall information after short delays (Butler et al., 1995) and after longer delays (Gross & Hayne, 1999), as well as between time of experience and interview. Findings have indicated that when using a drawing strategy, children reported more information regardless of the interval between experience and interview.

In a review of the literature on the effect of drawing and younger children's verbal accounts, Patterson and Hayne (2011) sought to determine whether drawing "continues to facilitate children's reports as they get older" (p. 120). They concluded that "drawing is a highly effective interview technique" (p. 120). In addition, they also examined the effect of drawing on interviewer questions across the age range (Patterson & Hayne, 2011). Their study included 90 children between the ages of 5 and 12. "Age-related changes in children's appraisal of their drawing ability" were explored, and the influence of the appraisals on the effectiveness of the drawing technique was evaluated. Whether "children's increasing self-consciousness about their drawing skills might interfere with their verbal reports" and thus negate the facilitative effect of drawing was considered (Patterson & Hayne, 2011, p. 124). The authors concluded, "Clearly, drawing is not only useful in terms of facilitating children's verbal reports, but it is also an interview tool that children of all ages clearly enjoy" (Patterson & Hayne, 2011, p. 124).

Guidelines That Acknowledge Use of Drawing

Guidelines on conducting investigative interviews with children in England and Wales are outlined in the document, "Achieving Best Evidence in Criminal Proceedings" (Barlow et al., 2011; Home Office, 2007). The document stipulates that it is rarely possible to use only open-ended questions with children and that specific questions are often necessary to cue children's memory further and to obtain sufficient evidence with regard to charging. Furthermore, "[w]hen posing questions, the interviewer should try to make use of information that the child has already provided" (Home Office, 2007, section 2.159).

Barlow et al. (2011) contend that their study paper (discussed earlier) extends this practice to a child's drawings. The guidelines of the Home Office (2007) allow the provision of drawing materials in the interview room. Barlow et al. (2011) state, however, that the document is mute with regard to how the interviewer should incorporate a child's drawings into the interview, most notably in respect of the interviewer's questioning, "no doubt because research has yet to address how this should be managed in legal interviews with children" (p. 486).

The Drawing Effect

Although drawing has been used for assessment of trauma and to treat children with traumatic exposure (Burgess & Hartman, 1993; Burgess et al., 1981; Ceci & Bruck, 1993; Clements et al., 2001; Driessnack, 2005; Gross & Hayne, 1998, 1999; Salmon et al., 2003), there has been a paucity of data "on the effectiveness" of drawing with regard to recall of memorable events (Bruck et al., 2000, p. 170). It has been put forth that "most forensic investigators and therapists who use drawing to facilitate young children's understanding and recall of traumatic events assume that it does" (Bruck et al., 2000, p. 171), meaning that effect exists with regard to the use of drawing in relation to the recall of memorable events.

In an effort to understand how drawing enhances children's abilities to communicate about past experiences, research on the effect of drawing has been conducted (Gross & Hayne, 1998, 1999; Patterson & Hayne, 2011; Salmon et al., 2003). In some studies, findings revealed that drawing increased the amount of verbal information that children reported (Paterson & Hayne, 2011; Salmon et al., 2003). Researchers also determined that the actual means through which drawing facilitates children's accounts is unclear (Patterson & Hayne, 2011; Thomas & Jolley, 1998), "as there has been relatively little published experimental work testing these claims" and "evaluation on their respective merits remains speculative" (Jolley, 2010, p. 236) despite various explanations as to why drawing might facilitate recall.

Earlier research studies considered this dilemma. Reasons or mechanisms that may account for why drawing is effective have been examined by researchers who have evaluated the use of drawing as discussed previously (Butler et al., 1995; Gross & Hayne, 1998, 1999). Various explanations have been offered for the facilitation factor associated with drawing and the enhancement of recall and detail of material (Gross et al., 2009). As such, it has been noted that researchers who previously evaluated the use of drawing have shifted from "the practical issue of whether drawing works to the more theoretical issue of why it might work" (Gross et al., 2009, p. 967). Understanding the theory behind the concept might provide information as to when "the drawing technique" might be effective (Gross et al., 2009). "The answer to this theoretically motivated question might, in turn, help us to predict the range of practical situations in which the drawing technique is likely to be effective" (Gross Hayne & Drury, 2009, p. 967). Moreover, "it is theoretically interesting to know what it is about drawing that facilitates recall within these circumstances" (Jolley, 2010, p. 236).

Underlying Mechanisms That May Account for the Drawing Effect

In an attempt to understand why drawing helps children recall information, researchers have studied the use of drawing within forensic investigative interviews through field and laboratory studies to identify possible mechanisms that account for the enhanced recall and facilitative effect of drawing (Patterson & Hayne, 2011; Pipe et al., 2004). As has been stated, the facilitative effect as well as the underlying mechanisms that account for the facilitative effect of drawing are unclear. Lamb et al. (2008) state with regard to this issue, "To date, the mechanisms by which providing drawings in interviews facilitates children's ability to recount experiences have not been conclusively established" (p. 46). According to some engaged in this work, "to gain any useful information from a drawing, the relevant active mechanism needs to be identified" (Thomas & Jolley, 1998, p. 133).

Although studies tend to be supportive of the use of drawing within interviews for clinical and forensic purposes, researchers contend that the underlying mechanisms by which drawing works within such contexts is unclear and unknown (Gross & Hayne, 1998, p. 174). Indeed, the "mechanism" by which drawing facilitates children's reports has been referred to as "elusive" (Gross et al., 2009, p. 967). "Given so many different mechanisms that could be in operation, inspection of drawings on their own seems unlikely to lead to reliable conclusions" (Thomas & Jolley, 1998, p. 133).

Still, possible mechanisms that may account for why drawing is effective have been articulated (Gross et al., 2009; Gross & Hayne, 1998). These "mechanisms either independently or in combination may offer an explanation regarding "the recall facilitation from drawing" (Davison & Thomas, 2001, p. 157). It has been speculated that drawing may be effective for keeping children focused for a longer amount of time as compared to a tell condition (Butler et al., 1995; Jolley, 2010) because drawing "may act as a retrieval cue". Moreover, some studies have demonstrated that children's drawing skill is related to the amount of information reported (Gross et al., 2009). Yet in deference to art therapy, artistic skill or level is not a factor.

Another mechanism involves the positive effect on the behavior of the interviewer (Gross et al., 2009; Jolley, 2010). When a child draws in an interview, the interviewer has been shown to use twice the amount of facilitative utterances such as "uh-huh" or "really" (rather than asking direct or focused questions and possibly leading a child). Facilitative utterances have been considered as a means of building rapport during the interview. They are also used to maintain the conversation without directing the child, as well as providing social support. Correspondingly, the more times facilitative utterances were used by interviewers in response to a draw and tell condition, the more information children reported that was consistently accurate (Gross et al., 2009; Salmon et al., 2003; Wesson & Salmon, 2001), and young children tended to narrate as they drew (Butler et al., 1995; Gross & Hayne, 1998, 1999; Gross Hayne & Drury, 2009).

Gross and Hayne (1998) deduced from their respective research studies that the effect of drawing may be attributed to four different things. They identified reduction in the perception of social demands of the interview, given that drawing may provide social support in both clinical and legal contexts. They also determined that memory retrieval may be facilitated by drawing because children may be self-generating retrieval cues through drawing. The data demonstrated that as drawing skill increased, so did the amount of information provided by children. They elaborated by saying that drawings with better representational qualities may be a means of enhancing retrieval cues. They found as well that even young children with far less developed artistic or developmental drawing skill were able to retrieve cues from their graphic representations. They expressed that these youngsters were able to identify and interpret their graphic depictions even after a delay and despite the lack of identified representational elements. They stated, "Although these drawings appear to be void of meaning from an adult perspective, this is not the case for the child who produced them" (Gross & Hayne, 1998, p. 175). Wakefield and Underwager (1998) addressed this concern:

> Unfortunately, during early developmental stages when children are difficult to communicate with, adults who want to elicit information from children may attempt to use images and symbols in an effort to break through the limitations. But the child may not have the capacity to use one object to represent another. If adults are not familiar with this developmental process, they may miss opportunities to accurately understand children and may then introduce unnecessary error into the interaction.
>
> (Wakefield & Underwager, 1998, p. 176)

Gross and Hayne (1998) also attributed the effect of drawing to the idea that drawings helped facilitate organization of narratives by children, since children in the draw condition provided very descriptive details about the experienced event as compared to the tell-only group. Lastly, they provided that drawing may account for the facilitative factor, given that the interviews with the draw component were longer in duration.

All in all, the authors/researchers determined that there was a "significant relation" between children's drawings and the amount of information children reported during interviews (Gross & Hayne, 1998, pp. 175–176). Fundamentally, they allowed, this work is contributory to a small but growing body of research that "indicates that drawing facilitates children's abilities to talk about the past" (Gross & Hayne, 1998, p. 176).

In comparison to Gross and Hayne's study of 1998, Davison and Thomas (2001) allowed that "talking while drawing an item might lead to some types of information being more readily reported" (p. 174). Davison and Thomas (2001) asked children to recall specific items (item recall), whereas in Gross and Hayne's studies "children's memory reports encompassed many different aspects of real-life events" (Davison & Thomas, 2001, p. 173). As with the study of Gross and Hayne in 1999, facilitation of recall was reliant upon drawing in Davison and Thomas's study (2001). Even with the latter in which drawing was thought to function as another retrieval cue, recall was not enhanced. In contradiction to previous studies, Davison and Thomas (2001) found that "drawing acted as an additional demand" on the children's "processing resources" (p. 173). They attributed the lack of recall to "the demands of making a drawing", which "somehow interfered" with verbal recall (Davison & Thomas, 2001, p. 173).

Thomas and Jolley (1998) conducted their own experiment to address the "possible mechanisms which could operate to influence the characteristics of children's drawing" (p. 127). They also reviewed "the evidence that such mechanisms operate to allow meaningful psychological evaluations of children from their drawings" (p. 127). They challenged the significance of interpreting drawings made by children in their study. They identified that the challenge lies in the belief that a particular element may be interpreted differently based upon a host of different reasons or circumstances. In addition, variances in interpretation may be a reflection of different processes incumbent in the creation of the picture. They characterized their findings in the following manner:

> Drawings are inaccurate and unreliable as personality or state assessments but can be influenced by children's emotional attitudes towards the topics depicted. The form of that expression, however, may be personal and idiosyncratic. Analogue studies of these effects undertaken with non-clinical samples under controlled conditions have produced mixed results. At best the reported effects are small.
>
> (Thomas & Jolley, 1998, p. 127)

> Children's drawings on their own are too complexly determined and inherently ambiguous to be reliable sole indicators of the emotional experiences of the children who drew them. Further research is needed to establish the extent to which such drawings can usefully facilitate assessment of children by other means or provide useful support as one of several converging lines of evidence.
>
> (Thomas & Jolley, 1998, p. 127)

Other explanations in response to ascertainment of what the drawing effect is and how the underlying mechanisms work with regard to facilitating recall and contributing to enhanced details within an interview context have been examined. Some studies have suggested that children may use drawings to organize and detail a story (Butler et al., 1995; Salmon et al., 2003). Butler et al. (1995) offer that a child with expressive communicative impairments may benefit from the use of drawing to supplement their verbal accounts. Without the addition of a drawing strategy, Butler et al. (1995) contend that children may be limited by their own expressive communicative capabilities to fully describe their experiences. Additionally, their research found that children who draw report more information than children who do not use a drawing strategy. Also, their research revealed that an increase in fantasy-based material was not identified when drawing was incorporated (Butler et al., 1995). Overall, despite being labeled as elusive, underlying mechanisms associated with a drawing effect have been identified in the relevant literature and appear to be receiving support as possible explanations for the facilitative effect of drawing within investigative interviews of children (Jolley, 2010).

Variables Attributed to the Effect of Drawing

The effect of drawing may be attributed to different variables. One such variable has been identified as the reduction in the perception of social demands associated with the interview process. As such, drawing may provide social support in both clinical and legal contexts (Gross & Hayne, 1998). The focus is directed at a child-centered approach rather than an interviewer-led process in which the expectation is a question-and-answer format. Another effect identified pertains to memory retrieval. Drawing may facilitate memory retrieval due to cues that are self-generated, promoting recall of experience.

Another variable offered is that drawing helps facilitate organization of narratives, as young children tend to narrate as they draw (Gross & Hayne, 1998; Gross et al., 2009). Gross and Hayne (1998) found a significant relationship between children's drawings and the amount of information reported during the interview process. As drawing skill increased, so did the amount of information according to their findings. Increased verbalization provided by children is thus another variable that may account for the facilitative factor of drawing (Gross & Hayne, 1998).

Brown (2011) identified two ways in which drawings have been used "in assessing children's experiences" (p. 235). The "draw and talk" method, which she explains as a method that provides children "with the opportunity to draw while recounting their experiences, with only their verbal responses being of interest" (i.e., the content of the drawing is not evaluated) (Brown, 2011, p. 235). Brown (2011) explains that "[t]he facilitative effects of allowing children to draw while talking are thought to be derived from a number of possible mechanisms" (p. 235). She offered that "drawing allows children to generate their own retrieval mechanisms" (p. 235). She explained the mechanisms as follows:

> Drawing allows children to generate their own retrieval cues . . . , by reminding them of additional event-related details as they construct their drawings. Drawing may also serve to make the interview context more comfortable by giving the children a focus other than the interviewer. Finally, interviews that include drawings tend to be longer than verbal interviews also, which may extend the opportunity for recall and reporting.
>
> (Brown, 2011, p. 235)

Studies examining the use of drawings to enhance children's reports of personally experienced events (Gross & Hayne, 1998; Salmon et al., 2003; Wesson & Salmon, 2001) have shown that, under ideal circumstances (i.e., when asking children about true events using non-suggestive questioning), drawing while talking yields an increase in the amount of information recalled, without compromising accuracy.

Structured Narratives

Drawing may help structure narratives, enabling children to recall and report information (Butler et al., 1995; Wesson & Salmon, 2001). Rather than being distracted or anxious talking to an investigator, the child is free to depict his or her experience and provide a narration in a manner that makes the process less intrusive, invasive and offensive (Salmon et al., 2003). It has been posited that children generate their own retrieval cues via drawing, which in turn prompts enhanced recall and reporting of more information (Butler et al., 1995; Gross et al., 2009; Macleod et al., 2013).

Decrease in Stress and Social Demands

Researchers have determined that drawing may account for a decrease in stress by shifting the emphasis from the interview process. With the emphasis directed at the child's drawing, the process is child centered and child friendly, which may account for increased discussion or narration by the child with regard to the drawing (Driessnack, 2005; Patterson & Hayne, 2011; Pipe & Salmon, 2009). Drawing may allow children to be removed from the intense emotional nature of the interview context (Cohen-Liebman, 1999; Thomas & Jolley, 1998). This is attributed to the minimization of stress, which results in reduced anxiety. Thus, drawing may provide children with a focus other than on the interviewer and the context of the interview, such as elicitation of information or fact-finding (Cohen-Liebman, 1999; Thomas & Jolley, 1998).

Increased Verbalization

Researchers have postulated that drawing may be effective for keeping children focused for a longer amount of time as compared to a tell-only condition (Butler et al., 1995; Gross & Hayne, 1998, 1999). Also, drawing "may act as a retrieval cue", which implies different understanding with some researchers explaining this as meaning that children's drawing skill is related to the amount of information reported (Butler et al., 1995; Gross et al., 2009; Patterson & Hayne, 2011; Wesson & Salmon, 2001). As such, remembrance of information and recall of material is enhanced. Young children, according to some researchers, encode more information about an event than they report, and they may have difficulty retrieving that information without specific cues (Patterson & Hayne, 2011). When children draw about an event, the amount of information articulated or verbalized has been demonstrated to increase (Patterson & Hayne, 2011; Salmon et al., 2003).

Representational Quality of Drawings

Retrieval cues stemming from drawing may assist with recall through a positive correlation between representational quality and the amount of information recalled (Butler et al., 1995; Davison & Thomas, 2001; Gross & Hayne, 1998, 1999; Wesson & Salmon, 2001). Gross et al. (2006) assessed whether or not the use of drawing "facilitated" "memory performance". In all, 64 children participated, with an equal split between the two groups: ages three to four and ages five to six. The study sequence was 1) memory event, 2) interview and 3) random assignment to either draw (experimental) or tell (control) group. The results of the study revealed that the older children reported more information than the younger children, yet overall, the children in both conditions provided more information than children who participated in the tell or control groups. Yet upon age analysis, it was found that the younger children in the drawing condition did not provide more information than the control group. The older experimental group did, however, report twice the information provided by the same age control group. As reported by Gross et al. (2006), this study demonstrated that "children's verbal performance during the interview was related to the representational quality of the drawings" (p. 121). The more realistic the drawing, the more information that was provided by the subjects. If children included more representational features or elements within a drawing, then they have more material to comment on, given their general knowledge about something, according to the study authors. Thus, they concluded that representational quality of drawing functions as a cuing mechanism (Gross et al., 2009).

Educational Perspective on What a Child Communicates Through Drawing

From an educational perspective, Cox (2005) advocated that emphasis should focus on the process rather than on representational quality when trying to ascertain what a child communicates through drawing. The process is akin to what happens when a child draws, with interest directed to the catalyst that gave rise to the imagery rather than on developmental elements. For Cox (2005), the lack of realism is not a deficit or indicative of an inability for a child to render what he or she knows. "When by contrast, the process itself becomes the focus, different kinds of representational purposes become apparent which may not necessarily be evident in the drawing itself" (Cox, 2005, p. 120).

Prior Knowledge of an Event Versus Schematic Knowledge

Gross et al. (2009) examined whether or not amount of information reported was enhanced when children did not have prior knowledge about an event (Gross et al., 2009). They found that drawing did enhance the amount of information provided when they interviewed 56 children between the ages of five and six about an experienced event after a one- to two-day delay and after a seven-month delay. The findings were counter to a study conducted by Davison and Thomas (2001) in which they determined that details included in children's drawings when interviewed about an event may be reflective of general knowledge about a situation or a concept instead of being reflective of episodic memory. Gross et al. (2009) provided that, if true, then Davison and Thomas's findings would in effect limit when a drawing strategy might be prudent within experimental and field situations. Episodic detail contributes to the assessment and understanding of the child's experience, and drawing has been demonstrated to enhance reporting of such material (Macleod et al., 2013, p. 571).

Davison and Thomas (2001) sought to "elucidate the means by which drawing facilitated recall in young children" and "to establish whether drawing an external representation of recalled items would cue recall of additional things" (Davison & Thomas, 2001, p. 157). Their overall results found that under some drawing conditions, children's recall is not facilitated and is instead impaired (Davison & Thomas, 2001). The lack of recall facilitation attributed to drawing in Davison and Thomas's experiments was related to the kind of event to be recalled. They determined that recall benefits from drawing may depend on the nature of the memory event and the way it was encoded (Davison & Thomas, 2001). According to Davison and Thomas (2001), these "mechanisms either independently or in combination may offer an explanation regarding the recall facilitation from drawing" (Davison & Thomas, 2001, p. 157).

Additionally, Davison and Thomas (2001) stated that "any cueing benefit from drawing was negated by interference from the extra demand on cognitive processes imposed by the task of actually executing a drawing" (p. 162). Davison and Thomas (2001) explored the "possibility of competition between drawing and verbal recall" (p. 162). They referred to drawing as "a demanding activity, requiring coordination and planning" (Davison & Thomas, 2001, p. 162). They speculated that carrying out both drawing and uncued verbal recall at the same time might result in a mutual interference, resulting in less information being verbalized or depicted (Davison & Thomas, 2001).

> The pattern of results observed here supports our suggestion that drawing concurrently with verbal recall can result in diminished recall in children ages 5 and 6 years. These children recalled more information when they verbally recalled alone than when they either drew and verbally recalled or when they drew without concurrent verbalization. Removing the demands of concurrent verbalization when drawing did not improve recall. These findings suggest that drawing did not act as a useful memory support, albeit one impeded by concurrent verbalization, but instead reduced recall.
>
> (Davison & Thomas, 2001, p. 165)

In contradiction to previous studies reported, Davison and Thomas found that "drawing acted as an additional demand" on the children's "processing resources" (p. 173), meaning that children were distracted by having to attune to more than one activity (drawing and recall of specific items). These authors attributed the main difference between their experiments and those of other researchers to the design. Their experiment entailed recall of specific items, whereas in other studies "children's memory reports encompassed many different aspects of real-life events" (Davison & Thomas, 2001, p. 173).

In comparison to Gross and Hayne's study of 1998, Davison and Thomas (2001) allowed that recall facilitated information pertaining to objects and descriptions rather than people and actions or settings and that "talking while drawing an item might lead to some types of information being more readily reported" (p. 174). As with the study of Gross and Hayne in 1999, facilitation of recall was reliant upon drawing in that children interviewed in the draw and tell after the interval (one year) reported more information than children who were in the tell condition and/or were given their original drawings to look at. Even as with the latter in which drawing was thought to function as another retrieval cue, recall was not enhanced by merely looking at the drawing. Recall was enhanced when children were given the opportunity to draw and tell even after the time delay (Davison & Thomas, 2001; Gross & Hayne, 1999).

Davison and Thomas (2001) concluded from their research, and in consideration of the Gross and Hayne studies (1998, 1999), that "it seems as if the act of drawing is necessary to produce recall facilitation, perhaps because drawing naturally leads to the reporting of certain aspects of the event, which were not present in the encoding task" (p. 174). They referenced a study by Salmon and Pipe (2000) in which drawing was considered not amenable to facilitating recall. Salmon and Pipe offered that unlike a prop, drawing does not cue children and is reliant upon children being responsive to the task (Davison & Thomas, 2001, p. 174). Based upon the earlier studies in combination with their findings, Davison and Thomas (2001) concluded that "when children spontaneously recall very little from an event, drawing may be of limited use" (p. 174). They determined that their findings make sense with the explanation that if a child does not draw much, then there is not much to prompt or support verbal recall of additional information (Davison & Thomas, 2001).

Drawing as a Function of Recall

Research on drawing as a function of recall or as a means of eliciting or stimulating recall has been demonstrated to both facilitate and hinder recall. Through comparison of various memory tasks in different experiments, Davison and Thomas (2001) allowed that understanding the underlying mechanism of drawing as a means of facilitating recall might be established. They offered the following conclusions: Information has to be remembered by children in order for drawing to be useful (Salmon & Pipe, 2000); direct questioning had a correlation to information recalled (Butler et al., 1995); only certain elements of an event may be recalled (Gross & Hayne, 1998, 1999); and finally, drawing in and of itself was not enough to facilitate recall (Davison & Thomas, 2001).

Overall Davison and Thomas (2001) concluded that "[i]t seems that the effects of drawing are very much dependent on the nature of the memory event and the type of information to be recalled" because "drawing encourages the reporting of schematic information" (Davison & Thomas, 2001, p. 176). Gross et al. (2009) refuted Davison and Thomas's findings, contending that children may in effect be reporting schemas (and scripts) which they defined as "prototypical representations of event information" (Davison & Thomas, 2001, p. 175), leading to generic representation rather than event-specific information. In essence, children may be providing information about things they have knowledge about and that are known to them.

Davison and Thomas (2001) advocated that "in most of the previously published reports of drawing facilitating recall, it is not possible to distinguish whether 'correct' details that children reported arose from general schema knowledge or from a specific event memory" (p. 175). They stated that it is important to understand whether drawing facilitates recall in and of itself or if recall is related to schemas or scripts.

Jolley (2010) weighed in on this discussion by allowing that the ability to differentiate whether information is evoked from recall of the event or a byproduct of generic or script knowledge is not possible (Jolley, 2010). Jolley provided alternative explanations for the negative findings (associated with Davison and Thomas's study of 2001) with regard to drawing as a memory aid. Jolley offered as one possible explanation that drawing "facilitates recall of event-based memories but not for singular and isolated items" (p. 230). His explanation was that since children depict narrative scenes, a drawing may prompt memory of an event, including an emotional response; however, items not aligned with the narrative may not be recalled or reported (Jolley, 2010). His second alternative explanation was that a mundane or routine event, detail or an item to be recalled from a laboratory experiment may not provoke a response given the commonality or the lack of remarkability. Such elements may not stimulate a personal or memorable memory inasmuch that the child may be prompted to disclose this information. Jolley (2010) concurred with Davison and Thomas (2001) that drawing, instead of contributing to memory recall, taxed the cognitive properties of the children in the study and mitigated recall of the items to be remembered in the simulated experiment.

Salmon and Pipe (2000) explained this by allowing that the lack of interest may account for the lack of recall. Jolley summed up this argument by saying,

> For most children drawing is a pleasurable activity because it allows them to draw the things and events that interest them. Thus, the interaction of the enjoyment experienced in drawing and a captivating event may lead to drawing being a more useful recall tool for special events than for a mundane and typical experience.
>
> (Jolley, 2010, p. 230)

Gross et al. (2009) stated that many studies that examined the effect of drawing when children reported on past experienced events do involve script-based knowledge. To test this hypothesis, Gross et al. (2009) designed a study in which children were interviewed about an event of which they had no prior knowledge. Their results found that through the use of drawing, children provided enhanced amounts of information (Gross et al., 2009). They stated,

> Although the mechanism by which drawing facilitates children's reports remains somewhat elusive, the data reported here rule out the possibility that drawing only works because children can exploit their semantic knowledge of similar events rather than rely primarily on their episodic memory for a particular past event. They concluded that when children directed their own recall what they learned and what they recalled differed.
>
> (Gross et al., 2009, p. 967)

Gross et al. (2009) attempted to address if drawing facilitated recall of factual information and whether or not children retained that information after a delay. Their study explored the general content of the event and was designed to assess what children learned from a trip to a museum (Gross et al., 2009). This study, in conjunction with others of a similar nature (Butler et al., 1995; Gross & Hayne, 1998, 1999; Patterson & Hayne, 2011; Salmon et al., 2003; Wesson & Salmon, 2001), is indicative of "a growing body of research showing that under some circumstances, drawing facilitated children's reports when they were interviewed about a wide range of experiences" (Gross et al., 2009, p. 966). The difference with this study was that the design concentrated on recall of factual information rather than on children's narrative reporting of events or autobiographical material and the effect of drawing on these scenarios (Gross et al., 2009). In this study, drawing facilitated the subjects' ability to recall and report not only narrative information but factual or educational information as well (Gross et al., 2009). From the study, it was determined that to better understand what children learn from an experience, it may be best to ask open-ended questions in conjunction with drawing (Gross et al., 2009).

Interviewer Minimal Responses

Theoretical and practical implications for interviewing children about their past experiences have been reported in the literature (Patterson & Hayne, 2011). Previous explanations were directed at the effect of drawing, whereas the findings of Patterson and Hayne (2011) show that "drawing works primarily because it alters the interviewers' questions by prompting more open-ended queries or minimal responses. The best predictor of the number of clauses that children reported was the number of minimal responses that the interviewer used" (Patterson & Hayne, 2011, p. 124). Thus, minimal responses were determined to be a byproduct of children's responses by the interviewer and considered the driving force behind the drawing effect according to Patterson and Hayne (2011). Ultimately, they concluded that "[w]e are increasingly confident that, even when children are encouraged to report more through drawing, they still stick to the facts and do not confabulate about the target event" (p. 125). Thus, Patterson and Hayne (2011) suggested that drawing may be a useful tool for obtaining information from children of all ages.

Recall of Information When the Event Is Videotaped

Jolley (2010) described a newer method of assessing the facilitative effect of drawing with regard to recall. He offered that in order to address issues previously identified as promoting mixed findings, video supplants some of these dilemmas. Video offers children an opportunity to witness an event that is "interesting" but not "easily related to children's generic and script knowledge" (Jolley, 2010, p. 230). Jolley explained that this design integrates advantages while limiting disadvantages from staged events and item recall.

In an experiment, two 10-minute educational videos were presented to 60 five- and six-year-old children. Each clip incorporated designated criteria, including novel events, to manage script and general knowledge. Jolley and colleagues determined that each clip was "interesting and entertaining" (Jolley, 2010, p. 231). Video was determined to enable the participants to experience the same event in the same manner, more so than an actual event. This was controlled for by compiling a categorical list of items and features contained in each video segment, including verbalizations and actions (Jolley, 2010). Three conditions were used to interview children one day after viewing the videos: draw and tell, draw then telling (in which the participants described or recalled the videos only after finishing their drawings) and tell only. The second condition was designed to maintain separation of "the cognitive demands of drawing and telling" (Jolley, 2010, p. 232). The findings were consistent with Gross and Hayne's (1998) findings with regard to recall of objects and descriptions (Jolley, 2010).

Jolley (2010) identified two other studies that utilized video in a similar manner: one an unpublished doctoral thesis (Rowlands, 2003) and the other study was presented both as a poster and paper in Britain (Rowlands and Cox, 2002, 2003 as cited in Jolley, 2010). These studies by Rowlands and Cox evaluated what Jolley termed the "video approach" to investigate "drawings as a tool for event memory" (p. 233). Jolley reported that the findings in these explorations were consistent with his video approach study. The video clip was intended to provide an analogous scenario to what a child might have to recall as an event eyewitness.

Jolley advocated for more experimental studies to test the "reliability of these preliminary findings from video studies" (p. 233). He offered that these studies "provide important support for the use of drawings as aids to children's recall" (Jolley, 2010, p. 233). Jolley (2010), like other researchers, acknowledged that drawing is a self-generated cue that ultimately facilitates the retrieval of additional details about an event (Gross & Hayne, 1998, 1999). Lamb et al. (2008) contend that

> [d]espite impressive evidence about the extent to which drawing facilitates the
> retrieval of information by children about events they have experienced, we do not

know whether the same benefits would occur when the events involved sexual abuse and the interviews were conducted for forensic purposes.

(p. 162)

Field Studies and Recent Research

Recent research has been conducted to explore the benefit of drawing as a retrieval source within forensic contexts. Relative to the recall and reporting of experienced events, Katz and Hershkowitz (2010) studied the effects of drawing on children's accounts of sexual abuse in a field study. They introduced the use of drawing only after children had described abusive events in response to open-ended questions using the NICHD protocol (Katz & Hershkowitz, 2010). Thus, drawing was utilized not as a primary resource in the interview process, but rather after a verbal process had been completed. Despite the fact that their study utilized drawing as a secondary retrieval process, their findings suggested that event drawing enhanced children's forensic statements in child abuse investigations (Katz & Hershkowitz, 2010). Moreover, the beneficial aspects of drawing within investigative interviews and as an intervention that enhanced children's reporting of experienced events was addressed in a different study by Katz et al. (2014).

In their study, Katz and Hershkowitz (2010) examined the use of free drawing during forensic interviews. The study considered whether "free drawing of an abusive event in association with open-ended questioning helped children retrieve additional information about the event" (Katz & Hershkowitz, 2010, p. 173). They evaluated if drawing helped children report larger proportions of information. They also considered the nature of the information collected in terms of forensic relevance and content categories, including disclosure of information pertaining to people, actions, time and location (Katz & Hershkowitz, 2010). The findings from Katz & Hershkowitz's (2010) study, the first to evaluate children's free drawings in a real-time design, revealed that the opportunity to draw, followed by open-ended questioning, produced richer reports about forensically relevant information related to experienced events (Katz & Hershkowitz, 2010). In the field study, free drawing "of the alleged sexual abuse incidents was combined into the NICHD protocol instructions" in interviews with young children (Lamb et al., 2008, p. 161). Drawing, however, was introduced only after children had described abusive events in response to open-ended questions conducted in association with a standardized protocol (Katz & Hershkowitz, 2010).

As described by Brown (2011), the field study conducted by Katz and Hershkowitz (2010) "demonstrated increases in information reported about alleged abuse when children were given the opportunity to draw a picture of their experience *after an exhaustive verbal interview*" (Brown, 2011, p. 235). The study was designed to explore the effects or "richness of the accounts" of "event drawing" during investigative interviews of children. The researchers interviewed alleged child victims of sexual abuse between the ages of 4 and 14. Children were first interviewed with open-ended invitations in a verbal process (NICHD). After questioning was exhausted, the children were randomly assigned to one of two interview conditions: with or without event drawing. Children in the drawing group disclosed more free recall information or gave richer accounts than children in the comparison group.

Brown (2011) explained with regard to the findings that "[w]hen children were asked to recount their experience again (after an exhaustive verbal account), with the drawing present, they reported more information than those who had not drawn, although the accuracy of this information could not be established" (p. 235). The study considered whether drawing by a child prior to having the child provide a narrative account impacted recall (Katz & Hershkowitz, 2010). This was after first completing a verbal process, then the drawing assignment, then reinterview using the designated verbal protocol (without further reference to the drawing).

Katz and Hershkowitz (2010) concluded that "the effect of drawing was evident regardless of age, gender, type of abuse, and time delay" (p. 171). The findings suggested that event drawing enhanced children's forensic statements in child abuse investigations (Katz & Hershkowitz, 2010). "The goal of this study was to determine whether drawing during an interview dominated by open-ended questions (NICHD) might facilitate the retrieval of information in forensic contexts" (Katz & Hershkowitz, 2010, p. 172).

In the study, the children were first interviewed according to the NICHD, a structured protocol, then given a short interlude to make a drawing or rest depending upon the assigned interview condition. The children were then reinterviewed to determine if the drawing strategy in between the two verbal interviews enhanced the richness of the content subsequently reported. In reviewing the results, Gentle et al. (2014) concluded that the research study may lend credence to drawing prior to a verbal account, as the drawing may increase or enhance what a child recalls during an investigative interview. Gentle et al. (2014) allowed that the research conducted by Katz and Hershkowitz (2010) demonstrated that drawing within the study design enhanced accuracy and amount of information recalled.

Despite findings that drawing promoted accuracy and an increased amount of salient information or a richer account, there is debate as to whether or not drawing protects against or promotes suggestibility (Gentle et al., 2014). However, according to Gentle et al. (2014), when asking children to draw about a remembered event, it is not known if without being given suggestible information if children will incorporate nonexistent details into their verbal accounts. Whether this "also increases the reporting of incorrect information when they are later asked suggestive questions" is unclear (Gentle et al., 2014, p. 160).

Gentle et al. (2014) compared memory techniques to assess the impact upon children's recall and ability to resist suggestive questions. It was determined that drawing the context of the event to be remembered would enhance recall because of the self-generation or personally relevant retrieval cues (Gentle et al., 2014). The process was intended to help children re-experience contextual information encoded during the experienced event being recalled. In the study, 141 children participated. Of that number, 70 were between the ages of five and six and 71 were between the ages of eight and nine. In an analysis of the complex set of statistics, the reinstatement techniques did not affect how children responded to free recall. Older children provided more details about the "to be remembered" event than the younger children and were less suggestible (Gentle et al., 2014). The study revealed that interview condition had no effect on response regardless of free recall and open-ended prompts. Similar levels of accuracy and completeness were noted across conditions (Gentle et al., 2014).

Gentle et al. (2014) found contrary results to the findings of the study conducted by Katz and Hershkowitz (2010). Accordingly, they offered that perhaps the memory set was not effectively probed through the free recall and open-ended prompts (Gentle et al., 2014). They provided that the protective properties of drawing with regard to suggestive questioning "may lie in the effectiveness of reinstating the context via drawing instead of mentality", meaning that utilizing a drawing to aid in responding to a prompt designed to elicit a narrow response may aid the child to be more "effortlessly directive in their memory search and thus more accurate" (Gentle et al., 2014, p. 165). Also,

Gentle and colleagues concluded, "It is possible that asking children to self-generate retrieval cues through drawing at the beginning of the investigative process might be used to protect the child from changing testimony on the face of repeated questions if they were allowed to refer to their drawing" (Gentle et al., 2014, p. 166). Finally, Gentle and colleagues called for future research to clarify "the extent of this easily implemented, potentially protective exercise" (Gentle et al., 2014, p. 166).

In a more recent study by Katz et al. (2014) the beneficial aspects of drawing within investigative interviews and as interventions that enhance children's reporting of experienced events were explored (Katz et al., 2014). Drawing within investigative interviews and as an intervention to enhance children's reporting of experienced events was determined to be confirmed by the study findings (Katz et al., 2014). They found that event drawing "can enhance children's forensic statements in child abuse investigations" (Katz & Hershkowitz, 2010, p. 172). As a result, these researchers advocated for research and interventions that enhance children's reporting of experienced events. It has been determined that information or details that are engendered in response to free recall (memory prompts) are more likely to be accurate than those that are engendered by recognition (memory prompts).

Drawing as a Self-Report Tool for Emotional Experiences

Katz and Hamama (2013) explored the ways in which drawing facilitates children's narratives in investigative interviews as a self-report tool. They determined that drawing is a "natural, accessible language that children can use for emotional expression" (Katz & Hamama, 2013, p. 877). Through studying children's narratives before, during and after an investigative interview, they assessed the way in which drawing "aided children's retrieval processes" (Katz & Hamama, 2013, p. 877). Their study identified the "contribution of using drawing when interviewing children about experiences of trauma" (Katz & Hamama, 2013, p. 877).

Research has shown that drawing increases the amount of information that children report about some emotional experiences, according to recent studies by Macleod (2013) and colleagues. They investigated the clinical and forensic relevance of what children report while drawing. Sixty children ages 5 to 6 and 11 to 12 were interviewed about prior experiences and accompanying emotional states (happy, angry, proud and worried). The results revealed that drawing and telling increased the amount of forensically relevant, episodic details; however, clinically relevant details pertaining to thoughts and emotions were not enhanced when drawing was incorporated into the interview (Macleod et al., 2013).

Overall, despite being labeled as elusive, underlying mechanisms associated with a drawing effect have been identified in the relevant literature and appear to be receiving support as possible explanations for the facilitative effect of drawing within investigative interviews of children (Jolley, 2010).

Drawing Assessments and Projective Drawing Techniques

Diagnostic procedures and assessments emerged in the 20th century, including projective drawing techniques in which formal procedures and standardized methods for interpretation were conceptualized (Rubin, 1999; Vick, 2003). Standardized projective drawing assessments such as the house-tree-person or human figure drawings were used to provide evaluative information for psychological assessment and testing as well as to determine treatment. These psychological tests were used to offer insight regarding the projection of internal experience into an external form (Vick, 2003). Projective techniques have been considered useful in obtaining information that derives from the unconscious (Rubin, 1999). This material is inaccessible without a direct method to uncover it (Rubin, 1999). When included as part of a battery of tests, drawings have been utilized to gain understanding about the personality and psychodynamics of a person (Rubin, 1999).

As a means of understanding intelligence and psychological well-being, drawings have been used in psychological and clinical assessments to obtain information from individuals (Buck, 1970; Dileo, 1973; Goodenough, 1926; Kellogg, 1969; Koppitz, 1968, 1984; Machover, 1980; Thomas & Jolley, 1998). Projective drawing techniques have been used for interpretative and analytical purposes. Drawings have also been used as interpretative mechanisms for understanding children from educational and psychiatric perspectives (Driessnack, 2005). Within clinical applications, drawings have been deemed beneficial for helping facilitate communication about thoughts, emotions and memories that may be difficult to discuss (Butler et al., 1995; Gross & Hayne, 1998).

Projective Techniques and Art Therapy

Assessment and projective techniques from an art therapy perspective differ from the intentions of the psychological community in that "the making and viewing of the art have inherent therapeutic potential for the client" (Vick, 2003, p. 7). Moreover, the expressiveness of the materials is a factor that is considered within the realm of art therapy and has implications for a less formalized process (Vick, 2003). In addition, the client is encouraged to interpret their own work rather than have the artwork formally assessed according to a standardized protocol. As Vick (2003) stated, "Even today, the notion that artwork in some way reflects the psychic experience of the artist is a fundamental concept in art therapy" (Vick, 2003, p. 7). Subject matter and formal elements of pictorial content are evaluated in an effort to understand a patient or client through artwork (Rubin, 1999).

Art Therapy

Art therapy is defined as a mental health profession that is predicated upon an intersubjective relationship, the art-making process, the meaning that the artwork acquires within the relationship and the applications of that meaning to the broader context of an individual's life (Robbins, 2000; Wadeson, 2010). The American Art Therapy Association's (AATA) website offers the following definition:

> Art therapy is a mental health profession in which clients, facilitated by the art therapist, use art media, the creative process, and the resulting artwork to explore their feelings, reconcile emotional conflicts, foster self-awareness, manage behavior and addictions, develop social skills, improve reality orientation, reduce anxiety, and increase self-esteem. A goal in art therapy is to improve or restore a client's functioning and his or her sense of personal well-being. Art therapy practice requires knowledge of visual art (drawing, painting, sculpture, and other art forms) and the

creative process, as well as of human development, psychological, and counseling theories and techniques.

(www.arttherapy.org, 2015)

Art therapy encompasses a continuum between two schools of thought: "art as therapy" and "art psychotherapy". Art as therapy emphasizes the innate healing power of making art, and the product is emphasized. Art as therapy is focused on the healing potential inherent in art making (Kramer, 1993). In art psychotherapy art is used as a healing tool within the framework of verbal psychotherapy and is associated with process (Junge & Asawa, 1994; Rubin, 2001; Wadeson, 2010). The client-created imagery is symbolic in nature. It provides an external representation of internal material. Art psychotherapy emphasizes the process of art therapy and the belief that an individual's thoughts and feelings are derived from the unconscious. Projections reach expression in images rather than in words since projections are emblematic of the self or the creator (Naumburg, 1987).

Within a therapeutic application, art therapy may provide a means of reconciling emotional conflicts, developing social skills, managing behavior, solving problems, reducing anxiety and increasing self-esteem (arttherapy.org, 2013). Understanding the meaning of artwork in art therapy often draws from principles from psychodynamic theory and psychoanalytic theory in which drawings are thought to represent unconscious processes as represented by symbolism. According to Dunn-Snow (2015), the history of art therapy "is steeped in psychoanalytical theory, but today art therapists embrace all theories of education, psychology, and counseling" (p. 80). Thus, diversity underlies the identified dichotomy, art as therapy and art psychotherapy. This contributes to variability within the field given the array of theoretical underpinnings and approaches that currently exist within the field. Inherent struggles with professional identity and a definitive theoretical framework (Acosta, 2001; Huss, 2009) do exist.

Art therapists have embraced and proffer various theoretical structures to provide a holistic panoptic frame to "encompass the richness, effectiveness and wholeness" of the profession (Huss, 2009, p. 154). As Huss (2009) explains, "[A]rt's inherent ability to layer multifaceted levels of meaning – its multiplicity – makes it a medium capable of encompassing multiple levels of theory simultaneously" (p. 155). "Contemporary art therapy flows along a continuum of numerous approaches and has become so much more nuanced than the original perspectives" (Gussak & Rosal, 2016, p. 1).

Inherent Advantages Associated With Art Therapy

Six inherent advantages have been associated with art expression. These advantages were identified by Harriet Wadeson (2010) and are considered innate to the practice of art therapy. These advantages embrace the underlying attributes that define art expression and resonate with the practice of art therapy regardless of which school of thought one might inculcate within one's scope of practice. Each advantage contributes to the underlying effectiveness of art expression and art therapy however, in deference to the evolution and progressive development of the modality, intrinsic benefit is multifarious and extends beyond Wadeson's original thesis. The six advantages that underlie art therapy as identified by Wadeson have been defined as imagery, decrease defenses, objectification, permanence, spatial matrix and physical and creative energy. The advantages are defined in the following manner (as excerpted from Wadeson, 2010 in brief):

- **Imagery**: We think in images, rather than in words. Images are less threatening than words.

- **Decreased Defenses**: Visual expression provides distance and allows for uncovering of material that may be repressed.
- **Objectification**: Artwork is a tangible or concrete product that is generated by the client, rendering it an objective expression. Drawing or artwork provides information that concretely reflects one's experience in an objective manner.
- **Permanence**: Artwork makes concrete the behavior, thoughts and feelings of a client at a particular point in time. The tangible nature of the artwork allows for review of the material as needed.
- **Spatial Matrix**: Graphic representation allows for information to be presented on several levels. Unlike verbal communication, artwork is not limited to a linear configuration.
- **Creative and Physical Energy**: The very act of creating allows for a release of physical and creative energy. Participation is invoked by the process.

Dynamic Relationship and Art Therapy

Art therapy encompasses a dynamic relationship between opposing concepts (Gilroy & McNeilly, 2000). Some of these tensions, according to Gilroy and McNeilly (2000), include art and therapy, images and speech, subjectivity and objectivity, doing and thinking (p. 8). Art therapy has also been characterized as dialectical given the interplay between verbal expression and imagery (Burt, 2012). It is through this dialectic that learning and transformation occur (Moon, 2001). For some art therapists the power of the artistic process is of most value where the potential to create art acts as an emotional container for experiences that might otherwise provoke distress (Burt, 2012). Yet for other art therapists, "it is the relationship between themselves and the client or group that provides the most valuable experience" (Bird, 2012, p. 272). For some, the "dual heritage" of art and psychodynamics provides the underlying basis for art therapy (Case & Dalley, 2014, p. 3). Still others have advocated that a synthesis of these viewpoints underlies art therapy (Ulman, 1992). Many art therapists subscribe to this interplay in their work (Gussak, 2013).

Depending upon the orientation of the art therapist, either the art-making process or the therapeutic relationship within the context of creating are fundamental components of the modality (Case & Dalley, 2014). The therapeutic relationship has been described as encompassing artwork, the client and the art therapist (Gussak & Rosal, 2016). The art making and the intrinsic and inherent nature of the various mediums promote a relational interactive engagement between client and facilitator (art therapist).

According to British art therapist, David Edwards (2004), there is a dynamic interplay in the practice of art therapy or a triangular composition. The relationship between the art/image, the client and the therapist is interactive (Chapman, 2014; Huss, 2009). Chapman (2014) states, "The symbolic and metaphorical content of the image is not found; it is revealed through the interactive process between client, therapist, and image" (p. 114). According to Huss (2009) this is the "differentiating factor" that distinguishes art therapy from verbal therapy (p. 155). Within this triangular relationship greater or lesser emphasis may be placed on each axis, for example, the client and their artwork or between the client and the art therapist (Edwards, 2004, p. 2).

The importance accorded to these respective positions is central to the whole question of where healing or therapeutic change in art therapy takes place. That is to say, whether this is due primarily to the creative process itself, to the nature of the relationship established between client and therapist or, according to Edwards, as many UK art therapists acknowledge, "a combination of these factors" (Edwards, 2004, p. 2).

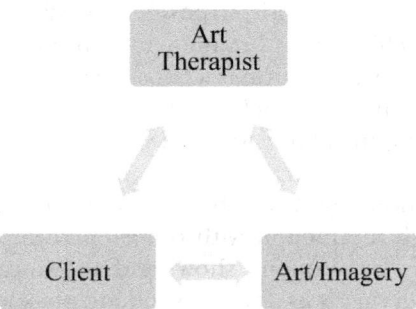

Figure 5.1 Dynamic interplay or triangular composition ascribed to art therapy, which encompasses the art therapist, the client and the art/imagery.

Meaning Making

Understanding or making meaning of images has been addressed in art therapy as well as by various disciplines and professions, including teaching (Soundy, 2012), art education (Cox, 2005), philosophy (Karlholm, 2009), aesthetics (Arieti, 1976), nursing (Clements et al., 2001; Driessnack, 2005) and semiotics (Hopperstad, 2008), as well as others. From an educational perspective, meaning making (of drawings) has been characterized as a dynamic process that is predicated upon a dialogical interaction between child and instructor (Soundy, 2012).

Art therapists incorporate many skills to understand and derive meaning from a client's artwork, including critical thinking skills and art psychotherapeutic skills (Curtis, 2011). Making meaning of art or images has been described as "a dynamic practice that can be described by three processes: cyclical, relational and personal" (Curtis, 2011, p. 9). According to McNiff, "By and large our profession (art therapy) has used art as a way to understand what an individual is experiencing" (McNiff, 1994, p. 255).

Integration of art and language through various techniques is intrinsic to art therapy. Morrell refers to verbal assessment of visual or imagery as "processing the art" (Morrell, 2011, p. 25). "Processing in this way, in the context of a therapeutic relationship, distinguishes art therapy from art-making" (Morrell, 2011, p. 25). In art therapy "art and language are integrated for psychological exploration and therapeutic gain" (Morrell, 2011, p. 25). Morrel discussed how art therapists use language to process art (Morrell, 2011). Through examination of the literature, Morrel related that different authors/art therapists (such as Wadeson, Rubin and Gantt) have offered different ideas for theoretical development based upon their own orientations.

Morrell examined the relationship of art and language with regard to a theory of art therapy. She identified different methods and applications regarding the integration of art and language by various practitioners. She included in her discussion the work of art therapists, including Naumburg, Kramer, Betensky, McNiff and Allen. She provided that art itself may be considered a "language or mode of communication" (Morrell, 2011, p. 26). She stated, "The unsayables – the symbols, not the signs, of the internal experience – can be profoundly explored and altered through the process and product of art" (Morrell, 2011, p. 28).

Cox (2005), an art educator, considered the process of drawing rather than the pictorial content in addressing meaning making. In her naturalistic observations of children, she theorized that children's drawings are purposefully directed rather than developmentally determined (Cox, 2005). The way a child chooses to depict whatever they select to draw has "meaning and purpose" (Cox, 2005, p. 120). Cox considered drawing to be a part of children's "broader, intentional, meaning making activity" (p. 115). She stated that "representation is a constructive, self-directed, intentional process of thinking in action, through which children bring shape and order to their experience, rather than a developing ability to make visual reference to objects in the world" (Cox, 2005, p. 115).

From realism to intentionality, Cox observed that children provided information about their marks through interaction with other children or in conversations either with one's self or with another student, showing that "we can gain a different view of children's drawing by observing it as a process, taking place over time in a specific context" (Cox, 2005, p. 120). The child offers clarification and explanation to give meaning to his or her art productions:

> Talk and drawing interact with each other as parallel and mutually transformative processes. Sometimes talk feeds into the drawing with the verbalized intention being transformed into drawing. Sometimes the drawing feeds into talk: the drawing intention is transformed into talk. Sometimes these processes are apparently concurrent.
>
> (Cox, 2005, p. 123)

Verbalization is the means for grasping the meaning of the drawing and the purpose. What children verbalize while drawing enhances the meaning of the image (Hopperstad, 2008; Soundy, 2012). Cox (2005) described drawing as a language in which children have control, given their intentionality. When drawing, there is a "process of decoding and encoding mark and meaning" (Cox, p. 123).

Betensky (1987) examined intentionality in her phenomenological perspective of art therapy. She addressed the role of the unconscious in the "emergence of meaning" yielding different possibilities and ways of seeing. Karlholm, a philosopher, suggested that beyond the content and form of the drawing there is a "deeper level of intentionality" "whereby the drawn marks are treated as symptoms or traces of what produced them" (Karlholm, 2009, p. 93). He stated that we bring the drawing into being because experience of the drawing is beyond a visual and extends to imagination and projection (p. 93).

Imagery

Arnheim (1994) is credited with saying that expressive language is not necessarily verbal and verbal language is not the only way to make meaning of experience. Arnheim developed "a theory of pictorial composition" (McNiff, 1994, p. 246), and he is credited with the "translation of meaning into the language of the senses" (McNiff, 1994, p. 246). In addition to art therapy, the fields of psychology and art education were impacted by Arnheim's philosophies (Franklin, 1994). Arnheim offered the following sentiment:

> Although immensely useful, language, as I have endeavored to show, derives only secondarily from the concepts evolved by the senses, as they cope with their surroundings, both natural and social. All thinking I maintain relies on perceptual imagery.
>
> (Arnheim, 1994, p. 246)

Imagery functions as a bridge between the "inner and outer world of the client as well as between the client and the therapist" (Case & Dalley, 2014, p. 13). McConeghey (1994) states that "[i]t is crucial to derive our work directly from the image and to always return to the image" (p. 291). According to Acosta (2001), who based her ideas on the work of Arnheim, language has been considered limiting and superficial with regard to describing art (p. 96).

The manner in which art therapy uses imagery and how information is derived from the art therapy process is an ever-expanding area of exploration (Acosta, 2001; Lusebrink, 2014). Despite acceptance of the beneficial elements afforded, understanding of the underling processes involved is still under investigation. Although there is potential in how information is processed and expressed via drawing, empirical data, including art therapy research, is needed to establish concrete evidence of such (Lusebrink, 2014).

Imagery, Preverbal Cognition and Encoding of Trauma

Preverbal cognition encompasses different ways of knowing (Leclerc, 2006, 2012), which is intrinsic to the process of information gathering. Acquisition of information at a preverbal level is derived through kinesthetic, sensory and imaginal means (Lusebrink, 1990). The use of imagery allows for other channels of communication, given that imagery is rooted in preverbal forms of expression. Thus, images can add preverbal forms of cognition or ways of knowing (Harris-Williams, 2010; Hinz, 2009; Lusebrink, 1990; Naumburg, 1987; Robbins & Sibley, 1976). A child may be able to access or uncover information through drawing because imagery taps into preverbal ways of knowing and allows for retelling in a manner that is developmentally congruent. The use of imagery provides a means of gaining access to preverbal memory, which corresponds to the encoding of traumatic memory (Lusebrink, 1990).

Knowledge about the brain coupled with an understanding of the processes that underlie trauma have paved the way for the development of new possibilities for evaluation and intervention based upon neuroscience (Steele & Malchiodi, 2012). Van der Kolk (2014) identified pathways such as talking and interpersonal connecting as a means to help trauma survivors move past their traumatic experiences due to neuroplasticity. "We have learned that trauma is not just an event that took place sometime in the past; it is also the imprint left by that experience on mind, brain, and body" (van der Kolk, 2014, p. 21). Nonverbal sensory-based experiences "allow children to rework their traumatic memories and their trauma related sensations, images and feelings (Steele & Kuban, 2013, p. 4). According to McNamee (2004), "Our culture has privileged the linguistically focused left side over the more nonverbal, creative right side" (p. 136). A "bottom-up" or nonverbal approach rather than a "top-down" or cognitive approach to working with traumatic memory is supported by neuroscience, according to researchers in various fields (Gantt & Tripp, 2016; McNamee, 2004; van der Kolk, 2014).

Art Therapy and Trauma

Van der Kolk acknowledged the benefits of the "expressive therapies" to "circumvent speechlessness that comes with terror" and as such "may be one reason they are used as trauma treatments in cultures around the world" (van der Kolk, 2014, pp. 242–243). Although he did not specify art therapy, he allowed that there are "thousands of art, music and dance therapists" who work with individuals that have experienced various traumas (van der Kolk, 2014, p. 242). Despite assertions of effectiveness, van der Kolk

(2014) stated that very little is known about how expressive therapies work, and he granted that there are challenges to establish empirical or scientific value.

Art therapy has been ascribed to both right and left hemispheres (McNamee, 2004). Due to the interplay between the unconscious and linguistic functionalities of the different brain hemispheres in art therapy, Chapman asserts that art therapy is effective "in fostering bilateral integration" (Chapman, 2014, p. 126). According to Chapman (2014), "The art media, besides being the facilitator of expression, allows for the creation of symbols and metaphors beyond the limitations of language" (p. 114). Through making the symbolic conscious via the verbal elaboration, understanding and awareness emerge.

It is the process of understanding the latent (symbolic) meaning behind the manifest (overt) content or the formal elements (consisting of the collection of lines, shapes, colors, etc.) that relates to the art therapy process. This invokes both the right brain accessing the unconscious and merging it with the more cerebral functions of the left brain such as cognition and language. King (2016a) stated that "[t]he externalization of preverbal internal feeling states is central to the work of the art therapist and can now be further articulated with scientific findings" (p. 81). King (2016a) asserts "developments in neuroscience are helping to provide a psychobiological context to explain the nature of human experience and expression" (King, 2016a, p. 81).

Trauma is identified as "a predominantly sensory process for many children and adolescents that cannot be altered by cognitive interventions alone" (Steele & Malchiodi, 2012) since information is initially processed at a sensory level. Children often suppress the sensorial nature of their experience, which is often encoded in images. To disclose information regarding trauma such as sexual abuse, art mediates the re-experiencing of the trauma in a safe and protected manner (Gantt & Tripp, 2016).

Trauma and Preverbal or Sensory Knowledge

Steele and Kuban (2013) described trauma as "not a primarily cognitive experience but a series of subjective experiences that do not respond well to our use of reason, logic or talk-based interventions" (p. xvi). To help children who have experienced trauma, interventions must match how a child perceives and experiences the trauma (Steele & Kuban, 2013). In effect, interventions must appeal to a "sensory level rather than primarily to the cognitive level", since trauma has been determined to be associated with the midbrain or limbic region, considered the "feeling" brain, which is devoid of "reason, logic or language" (Steele & Kuban, 2013, p. 4). The mid-brain is responsive to sensory-based activities rather than verbal prompts since trauma is "experienced, stored and remembered within the sensory, not cognitive context" (Steele & Kuban, 2013, p. 7). Thus, the accessibility to make sense of an event and respond accordingly is not feasible (Steele & Kuban, 2013). Trauma mitigates upper brain cognitive functions, rendering them difficult to access (Steele & Kuban, 2013).

Different types of memory demonstrate that trauma is not cognitively based. Trauma has been associated with implicit memory, which is affiliated with the right hemisphere, which lacks cognitive functions such as language or reason (Steele & Kuban, 2013). Implicit memory is sensory based since logic and reason are not considered available. Explicit memory is associated with the left hemisphere and is synonymous with cognitive processes and language. Information processing and reasoning are additional factors to consider (Steele & Kuban, 2013).

The encoding of traumatic memory occurs at a preverbal or sensory level (Steele & Kuban, 2013; Steele & Malchiodi, 2012). Traumatic memories are stored in "iconic and sensory forms" (Steele & Malchiodi, 2012, p. 3). They are maintained in the various sensoriums such as taste, touch, etc. (Steele & Kuban, 2013). As such, they are "experienced and remembered through images and sensations" (Steele & Malchiodi, 2012, p. 3). According to Steele and Kuban (2013), at times, especially with regard to trauma, there simply are "no words to accurately describe or communicate what is being experienced" (p. 7). In the absence of language capability, children need opportunities "to communicate what it is like without words" (Steele & Kuban, 2013, p. 7).

> When memory cannot be linked linguistically, in a contextual framework, it remains at a symbolic level and therefore there are no words to describe it. To retrieve that memory, it must be externalized in its symbolic, perceptual iconic form.
>
> (Steele, 2003, p. 142)

Trauma is more readily able to be expressed via images, given the nature of encoding. "The trauma experience is more easily communicated through imagery" (Steele & Kuban, 2013, p. 10). According to Chapman (2014), "Engaging in a visual dialogue with the symbolic and metaphorical content of the image sustains right hemisphere access" (p. 115). This activates an affective response which corresponds to an emotional reaction. This process precedes what has been referred to as "knowing" since "the meaning of the image finds its way into consciousness" (Chapman, 2014, p. 115). This knowing is not always subject to verbal articulation or conscious elaboration (Leclerc, 2012). Meaning is derived from "unconscious transmissions which are constituted through a process of elaboration" (Leclerc, 2012, p. 371). This may be at a nonverbal or an unconscious level, which is the platform for the creation of meaning (Leclerc, 2006). From the art aspect of art therapy, there are many different kinds of knowing since there are different ways of seeing (Junge & Linesch, 1993, p. 62).

Images provide preverbal forms of cognition or ways of knowing not accessible through traditional language (Harris-Williams, 2010; Hinz, 2009; Leclerc, 2006, 2012; Lusebrink, 1990; Naumburg, 1987; Robbins & Sibley, 1976). As noted, the use of imagery provides a means of gaining access to preverbal memory, which corresponds to the encoding of traumatic memory. Traumatic memories are thought to be stored in image form, rendering art therapy an appropriate or effective method for uncovering them, given the use of imagery (Wadeson, 2016). Based upon Damasio's model concerning imagery, recognition and memory, Lusebrink (2014) explains imagery in the following way:

> Images are formed in memory through a person's multiple interactions with an object or entity. These interactions involve sensorimotor patterns associated with viewing, touching, and manipulating the object; previously acquired memories that are pertinent to the object; and emotions and feelings related to the object.
>
> (Lusebrink, 2014, p. 88)

Betensky (1995) identified sensory and formal qualities of art as intrinsic to meaning. The art maintains the underlying emotion, and it is through the mutual exploration between therapist and client that awareness with regard to the imagery happens. Tinnin (1990) spoke about consciousness and the nonverbal mind. He provided that emotional memories are not accessed by the conscious mind given the lack of verbal encoding. In essence, he said that the conscious or verbal mind "sensors feelings when converting them into words" (p. 9). It is through the process of art making that emotional memory can be reached (Tinnin, 1990). This correlates with the psychodynamic premise that through art making, censorship is bypassed (McNiff, 1994; Tinnin, 1990).

Drawing as a Means to Access Traumatic Memory

Drawing has been shown to overcome the inherent limitations of verbal interviews (Steele & Kuban, 2013, p. 68). Steele and Kuban (2013) use what they term structured drawing "to access the sensations and iconic and implicit trauma memories stored in the right brain" (Steele & Kuban, p. 68). "This approach gives us a much more comprehensive view of the child than question and answer interviewing and history gathering" (Steele & Kuban, 2013, p. 68). The intervention process they developed involves multiple sensory-based activities, which "brings the trauma or sensory memories to life in a safe, contained context so they can be regulated, reordered and reframed" (Steele & Kuban, 2013, p. 8).

Art provides a means of accessing unconscious content and facilitates expression (Chapman, 2014). Traumatic experiences are stored implicitly and ironically, without language or context (Steele & Kuban, 2013). Drawing provides the opportunity for children to externalize those "iconic meanings into a contextual format that makes it easier to then give them meaning" and "reorder . . . those memories in ways that can be managed" (Steele & Kuban, 2013, p. 70). Alternatively, enabling information to be extracted at this level, without going through linguistic filters, may reduce its vulnerability to misinterpretation (Williams et al., 2002).

Forensic Art Therapy

Art therapy, when combined with forensic protocols, yields a distinct and complex investigative method (Cohen-Liebman, 1999, 2003). The relationship component within a forensic art therapy investigative interview process is critical to the procurement of fact-finding. Interviewer and child are co-investigators working together to discover and explore facts (Cohen-Liebman, 2016). Information is uncovered through imagery created in a dialogical process in which verbalization is concomitant. Enabling a child to find the images and the words to communicate his or her experience fosters a meaning-making experience rather than an aesthetic one (Cohen-Liebman, 2016).

Forensic art therapy or FAT emerged from the integration of standard art therapy principles and practices with a forensic application. This juxtaposition constituted an innovative and unique mode of practice that extended the parameters of the field of art therapy beyond evaluation/diagnoses and intervention/treatment (Cohen-Liebman, 1999, 2002, 2003; Gussak & Cohen-Liebman, 2001). FAT is a fact-finding endeavor, intended to assist in the resolution of legal matters in dispute. It is investigative in nature, rather than interventive or evaluative (Cohen-Liebman, 1999, 2002, 2003; Gussak & Cohen-Liebman, 2001). FAT is a specialized field of art therapy requiring modification of standard art therapy practice to meet the needs of the legal system (Cohen-Liebman, 1999).

FAT is sensitive to the parameters of clinical interviewing yet adheres to forensic principles in order to be acceptable in a legal context. Investigative interviews that derive from FAT are based on a scientific framework, while subscribing to an art therapy paradigm (Cohen-Liebman, 2016). Fact-finding, the primary objective of an investigative interview, improves when approached within a format that is commensurate with a child's developmental level and interactive patterns (Cohen-Liebman, 1999; Melinder et al., 2010). "The use of a standard forensic interview protocol provides a more systematic means of data gathering in a manner that is consistent with the evidentiary needs of scientific information" (Gould, 1998, p. 400). FAT has the capacity to meet the respective goals of the law, while protecting the rights of the child and safeguarding emotional wellbeing.

FAT interviews are conducted in a developmentally sensitive, forensically defensible, culturally aware manner. Goals of these processes include maximizing information gathering and minimizing repetitive interviews toward eliminating secondary victimization. In a FAT interview, free drawing is incorporated in the capacity of an open-ended prompt to facilitate fact-finding and elicit a narrative response. Information gathered from the use of drawing as a primary resource within an investigative interview contributes to the acquisition of knowledge through a fact-finding process. This assists in understanding the experience of a victim or witness and ultimately may impact investigation as well as intervention.

Drawing as an Open-Ended Prompt in FAT

FAT incorporates nondirected or free drawing within the investigative interview format. Drawing functions in the primary capacity of an open-ended prompt to facilitate free recall of experience, including traumatic events. Telling or fact-finding is facilitated via drawing. The use of free drawing provides a method of obtaining information in an investigative interview with a child that corresponds with a child's maturational spheres, including cognitive, social and emotional (Cohen-Liebman, 1999). In addition, drawing provides distancing, which may enable a child to express imaginally what cannot be said or explained until pictorially depicted. Without the constraints of formal language, a child may express his or her experience in a more tangible way (Cohen-Liebman, 1999, 2016).

Drawing provides a nonverbal means of expression that affords distance from the event and may stimulate recall of additional material, since traumatic memory is often stored at a sensory level or a precognition level (Steele & Malchiodi, 2012). A child experiences and encodes a multiplicity of information that linguistically is explained one element at a time. A child can depict information that extends beyond a verbal (linear) configuration, resulting in a pictorial matrix (Wadeson, 2010) that may contain details and idiosyncratic information. As Wadeson has conveyed, "Sometimes this form of expression more nearly duplicates experience" (Wadeson, 2010, p. 13).

Dialogical Process

Drawing as an open-ended prompt within a relational context is a means to enhanced disclosure (Cohen-Liebman, 2016). Within FAT, evidentiary disclosure is predicated on the use of drawing as a primary resource in an investigative interview that is art therapy-based. Disclosure in this context is identified as a "fundamentally dialogical process" (Jensen et al., 2005). The interactive relationship or dialogical process is supported by drawing, which often precipitates verbalization and often stimulates verbal elaboration by a child (Kelley, 1984; Cohen-Liebman, 1999, 2003).

Interviews happen in a relationship that has a corresponding influence on the process. The interview relationship creates an intersubjective matrix that is safe and supportive. The child-centered milieu encompasses the interviewer and the child. Consistent with the relationship and the dialogical interaction, information and understanding occur.

This dynamic process is circular rather than linear. Information may emerge from a preverbal level through kinesthetic, sensory and imaginal means (Lusebrink, 1990). Leclerc (2012) states that there is a "knowingness" that evolves from an experiential process, which is relative to the dialogical process. This includes the interviewer, the child and imagery or drawing (which is the primary mode of artistic expression incorporated within the interview).

This is consistent with art therapy practice in which the associations of the artist (child) are elicited in order to understand the context as well as the content of a drawing. The creative process facilitates recall, enabling a child to express his or her experience pictorially and elaborate verbally. Information is uncovered through imagery coupled with verbal expression. Verbalization is often motivated by the creation of nondirected drawing within the investigative interview. Speech may evolve visually or pictorially before manifesting verbally.

Fact-finding emerges as information is disclosed via the artwork in tandem with a child's verbalizations and narrative (Cohen-Liebman, 2016). The creator's intentions are communicated in association with the artwork. Pictorial disclosure within an investigative interview may contribute to verbal communication. Drawing may provide collateral information. Demonstrative evidence may be disclosed, which might contribute to investigation and may potentially impact outcomes with regard to investigation, prosecution and intervention. Idiosyncratic details that emerge lend credence to a child's disclosure and assist in facilitating additional fact-finding (Cohen-Liebman, 2003). Free drawing as an open-ended prompt in an art therapy investigative interview context has been described as circumventing barriers to disclosure and contributing to self-expression (Cohen-Liebman, 1999, 2003). Empirical evaluation is advocated on the use of free drawing within this context.

Drawing and Forensic Interviewing

Strategies to enhance children's abilities to retrieve, recall and describe experienced events in investigative interviews continue to be explored (Everson & Boat, 2002; Faller, 2014; Olafson, 2012; Patterson & Hayne, 2011). One such strategy is the use of drawing. Researchers have studied the use of drawing and its effectiveness in assisting children to communicate and recall information in various contexts from clinical assessment to investigative interviewing in an effort to decipher what drawings do and, more importantly, how drawings work. Studies have been conducted and continue to be implemented to determine whether drawing facilitates enhanced recall and reporting of experience in interviews.

> Researchers who have investigated this topic for many years put forth in 2009 that their primary concern has shifted from "the practical issue of whether drawing works to the more theoretical issue of why it might work" (Gross et al., 2009, p. 967).

According to Pipe et al. (2004), "a dynamic interchange" is taking place "between researchers exploring questions of applied relevance and those with a more theoretical focus" (p. 457). This is attributed to a confluence in experimental, analogue and forensic field research (Lamb & Thierry, 2005; Pipe et al., 2004). Practical applications have resulted given the emergence of research findings and trends that have implications for forensic investigative interviewing. Drawing has been identified as the most consistent means to facilitate communication to procure information from children in a child-centered manner (Driessnack, 2006).

Several studies have demonstrated that drawing promotes or facilitates communication by children, especially with regard to topics difficult to describe (Gross & Hayne, 1998; Gross et al., 2006; Salmon et al., 2003; Wesson & Salmon, 2001). The focus in research has addressed understanding what a child has experienced via adult observations and interpretations according to Driessnack (2006) as opposed to asking a child about their experiences and allowing them to relay information in a manner that is ego syntonic.

> It is only recently that children's drawings are being revisited as a potential facilitative method for communication in investigative interviews shifting the focus from what a child draws to what the child says about what they draw.
>
> (Driessnack, 2005, p. 420)

Research indicates that when a child draws during an interview, communication is facilitated and accuracy of information about an experienced event is not compromised by the use of a drawing strategy (Driessnack, 2005; Gross et al., 2006). When children are interviewed, the brevity of their verbal responses may actually relate more to their ability to retrieve information than to their knowledge or understanding of an event or concept (Driessnack, 2005). By giving children a means for expression that is self-motivated and determined, active rather than passive participation is promoted (Driessnack, 2005). "Children will tell us what they are up to and what they are about if we set the stage and listen" (Driessnack, 2005, p. 422). This "child centered disclosure" is what underlies what and how children communicate their experience (Clements et al., 2001). "One of the most compelling implications for health care researchers and practitioners is the emergence of children's drawings as facilitators of communication in the interview process" (Driessnack, 2006, p. 430).

Drawing, Sensory Stimulation, Memory and Art Therapy

From an art therapy perspective, an investigative interview that incorporates the use of an open-ended prompt in the form of drawing may provide a resource for communicating one's story in an accurate and reliable way due to the intrinsic benefits associated with imaginal expression. Memory and its contingency upon sensory stimulation are intrinsic to an art therapy–based interview process. The use of imagery provides a means of gaining access to preverbal memory, which corresponds to the encoding of traumatic memory (Hinz, 2009; Lusebrink, 1990). Preverbal cognition encompasses different ways of knowing (Leclerc, 2006, 2012), which is intrinsic to the process of information gathering. Thus, a child may be able to access or uncover information through drawing in an investigative interview because imagery taps into preverbal ways of knowing and allows for retelling in a manner that is developmentally congruent. Images can add the preverbal forms of cognition or ways of knowing that include the sensorial and embodied experiences not accessible through traditional language (Harris-Williams, 2010; Hinz, 2009; Lusebrink, 1990; Naumburg, 1987; Robbins & Sibley, 1976).

Literature Summation

Literature from the domains of investigative interviewing, art therapy and trauma were explored. The review of the literature is consistent with the material that underlies the study of the CIG. Literature associated with the exploration and understanding of drawing within an art therapy investigative interview process in the context of an open-ended prompt was identified. Moreover, relevant literature pertaining to the use of drawing as a means to facilitate fact-finding and enhance disclosure was examined. In addition, underlying mechanisms ascribed to the drawing effect that have been identified in the literature were considered. The collated material represents the integration of a diverse array of topics that underlie the study. This constellation of material was presented and juxtaposed to establish the basis for an art therapy investigative interview process predicated upon the use of free drawing in a primary capacity.

The use of an open invitational drawing process to stimulate memory and facilitate disclosure through recall and retrieval of information within an art therapy–based investigative interview is a new area of study which included exploration of the CIG. The three central principles of the CIG: an open invitational drawing process; the dialogic and relational process; and the encoding, storage and recall of (traumatic) memory in image form provided the impetus for exploring an art therapy–based investigative interview process, and the underlying mechanisms associated with the drawing effect. It is hoped that the data collected in this research may contribute to understanding the use of drawing in a primary capacity as an open-ended prompt in investigative interviewing and the relevance of an art therapy–based process.

Exploration of the causal mechanisms that underlie the drawing effect in tandem with an art therapy–based process may contribute to a basis for the inclusion of drawing as a primary resource in investigative interviews of children. In addition, acceptance and understanding of an art therapy–based investigative interview process for children may provide an alternative to traditional verbal techniques for the facilitation of information gathering and fact-finding with regard to experienced events.

As a means to safeguard the emotional well-being of child victims and witnesses who are interviewed about experienced events, the risks associated with revealing a traumatic event may be lessened through the use of drawing in a primary context. The sensory-based nature of certain crimes coupled with the understanding that trauma is encoded on a preverbal level suggest that victims of sexual abuse and other forms of interpersonal violence may be responsive to recall and disclosure of information through imaginal expression in tandem with verbal associations.

> The precise mechanism for the facilitation of recall by drawing has yet to be established but "examining this and other novel uses for pictures seems more promising than further research based on the conception of a drawing as a projective test of personality.
>
> (Thomas & Jolley, 1998, p. 137)

Rationale for Use of Bullying for the Analogue

Before discussing the study proper, a section pertaining to the literature on bullying follows. Since bullying is the analogous topic to be explored within the context of an experienced event, the next section will consider the concept of school-based bullying. A definition, background information and the mechanics and dynamics associated with bullying will be considered through review of the literature. Comparisons between bullying and child sexual abuse will be presented in an attempt to demonstrate the linkage between these two societal ills in an effort to situate the analogue design. Parallels between bullying and child sexual abuse will be presented with regard to the following domains: relational, perpetration and behavioral. In addition, patterns of victimization and disclosure surrounding bullying and child sexual abuse will be discussed.

Review of the Literature on School Based Bullying

Bullying among school-aged children is not a recent or new phenomenon. Bullying is a serious problem for school youth (Hong et al., 2012) that spans the globe and occurs in both developing and developed countries (Chan & Wong, 2015; Cook et al., 2009; Kanetsuna & Smith, 2002; Liang et al., 2007; Smith et al., 2002; Tsaousis, 2016). The idea of "peer bullying" was first introduced in the late 1960s and early 1970s in Sweden (Olweus, 1993, 2013).

Bullying is a common and pervasive social and public health problem (Shetgiri, 2013) that is typical in schools today, with one out of every three children experiencing some type of bullying during their school years (Shetgiri, 2013). Research within the past two decades confirms that bullying is prevalent within elementary and secondary grades (Haynie et al., 2001; Holt et al., 2007b; Nansel et al., 2001; Smith et al., 2002; Tsaousis, 2016) and is ubiquitous across the elementary and secondary school years (Haynie et al., 2001; Nansel et al., 2001). Research findings have shown that between 10% and 15% of students in grades three through six experience peer victimization at least once a week (Harachi et al., 1999; Nansel et al., 2001). Bullying prevalence and victimization are estimated to range from 15% to 50% according to Shetgiri (2013). Variations in the incidence of bullying among studies may be attributable to variability in how bullying is identified, including the type of bullying examined (Shetgiri, 2013).

Definition of Bullying

According to Olweus (2013), "Bullying is aggressive behavior with certain special characteristics such as an asymmetric power relationship and some repetitiveness" (p. 757). Bullying is identified as having the following three criteria: 1) aggressive behavior or intentional "harm doing" 2) which is carried out "repeatedly and over time" 3) in an interpersonal relationship characterized by an imbalance of power (Olweus, 1994, 2013; Shetgiri, 2013; Tsaousis, 2016). Bullying behavior often occurs without apparent provocation. A power differential, either implicit or explicit, accompanies the behavior (Olweus, 1993, 1994, 2013; Nansel et al., 2001; Shetgiri, 2013; Smith et al., 2002).

According to Olweus (1993, 1994, 2013), bullying is proactive and intentional, which separates it from typical or normal peer interactions. Bullying is associated with negative outcomes for both bullies and victims (Olweus, 2013; Tsaousis, 2016). Bullying may involve a single perpetrator or multiple perpetrators, and it is directed at another child or adolescent who is considered vulnerable and unable to protect or defend themselves (Espelage & Swearer, 2003; Shields & Cicchetti, 2001). Antibullying interventions are predominantly school-based and demonstrate variable results (Browne & Finkelhor, 1986; Shetgiri, 2013). Cyberbullying is beyond the scope of this review; however, it is an emerging problem, which may be more difficult than traditional bullying to identify and intercede.

Background

The most common definition of bullying was established by Olweus. Olweus described bullying as frequent and systematic harassment (Espelage et al., 2010). A native of Scandinavia, Olweus's research was initially confined to that country; however, interest and study expanded in the 1980s and early 1990s. Given that empirical studies were limited at the time, Olweus advocated that in the future methodological diversity would contribute to the exploration of the phenomena under more "varied contextual and cultural conditions" (Olweus, 1994, p. 1187).

Bullying was first referred to as "mobbing" (Olweus, 2013; Smith et al., 2002). The term was used to describe the phenomena, which was derived in the context of racial discrimination and was taken from a Swedish book on aggression written by the ethologist Konrad Lorenz (Olweus, 2013). According to Olweus (2013), the word mobbing is used "to describe a collective attack by a group of animals on an animal of another species, which is usually larger and a natural enemy of the group" (p. 753). The term was also concomitant with a group "ganging up" against "a deviating individual" according to Olweus (2013).

Olweus, who was interested in aggression research, is credited with conducting the first systematic research project on bullying by peers (Olweus, 1994; Shetgiri, 2013). His results were published as a book in Swedish in 1973. In 1978, the book was expanded and was available in the United States under the title *Aggression in the Schools: Bullies and Whipping Boys* (Olweus, 1993, 2013). Olweus described the purpose of his research as an attempt to provide an introduction to peer harassment in schools and to seek empirical answers to help explain the myriad of issues and concerns associated with the concept that was under-researched at the time (Olweus, 1993, 2013).

Olweus developed the first program against bully/victim problems to be evaluated in systematic research (1994) with the intended goal to reduce problems and prevent more. Olweus's research was included in the development of a questionnaire as a method for assessing bully/victim problems for students in response to a government-initiated campaign against bullying that emanated in Norway in 1983 (Olweus, 2013). The Olweus Bully/Victim Questionnaire has been revamped (as of 2007) and is used as a measure throughout the world to gather data from students (Smith et al., 2002). Olweus's bullying prevention program was the first whole-school, multidisciplinary, school-based intervention program that was evaluated (Shetgiri, 2013). Contextually, interventions are directed at the entire school rather than focusing exclusively on bullies and victims (Shetgiri, 2013).

The use of the Olweus questionnaire in various countries provides a means of comparing frequency and structural characteristics of the problem in different societies (Smith et al., 2002). Olweus's questionnaire has been utilized across the globe to collect data about bullying and related victimization, resulting in prevalence findings that confirm the existence and pervasiveness of the problem in other countries (Olweus, 1994). This information is helpful in determining interventions to reduce occurrence; however, difficulties arise with terminology since bullying does not always translate easily (Smith et al., 2002). This may impact research endeavors given the emphasis on comparability and interpretation for accuracy.

The international dimension in the study of bullying is complicated, some researchers contend, due to difficulties with commonality in terminology of correspondents to the word bullying (Smith et al., 2002). The English word bully does not translate verbatim into every language and culture; however, derivatives and corresponding definitions are applicable (Olweus, 2013). The lack of clarity with regard to the operationalization of the term makes bullying an overarching term that is used to describe the phenomena generally, while "bullying perpetration" and "peer victimization" relate to different aspects of bullying (Tsaousis, 2016). Bullying perpetration refers to aggression toward someone else, while peer victimization is a reference to aggressive, violent or abusive acts perpetrated by another. These terms are used to differentiate experiences that correlate to the various forms of behavior (Tsaousis, 2016).

Dynamics and Mechanics of Bullying

Bullying is defined as "verbal, physical, or social forms of aggression inflicted by an individual or a group of individuals and directed against a child or adolescent who is not able to defend himself or herself", and the aggression is "proactive, intentional, and repeated" (Olweus, 1999, p. 168). Typically, bullying is characterized into three types: verbal, physical and social or relational. Direct bullying consists of physical and verbal aggression, and indirect bullying involves relational aggression (Drennan et al., 2011). Direct bullying/victimization includes open attacks on a victim, while indirect bullying/victimization manifests in social isolation and intentional exclusion (Drennan et al., 2011; Olweus, 1994). Indirect bullying is considered by some researchers to be covert and may include gossiping, rumor mongering and social exclusion (Smith et al., 2002). It may be considered within the realm of social bullying, which is directed at undermining social and or interpersonal relationships (Smith et al., 2002). While the first two types are explanatory, the third is directed at harming someone's reputation.

Bullying behavior encompasses a range of activities that exist on a continuum from less threatening to more threatening. Bullying consists of three types of participants: the bully or the aggressor, the victim and what is referred to as the bully-victim – individuals who perpetrate and are victims of bullying (Shetgiri, 2013). The latter have been determined to have the highest rates of victimization (Holt et al., 2007b). These children are construed as victimized, rendering them powerless, which may contribute to their inability to protect themselves, which in turn may perpetuate victimization by others (Hong et al., 2012). Bullies, victims and bully-victims are at risk for negative short- and long-term consequences such as depression, anxiety, low self-esteem and delinquency (Shetgiri, 2013).

Olweus (1994) differentiates between types of victims as well as bullies. He describes victims as anxious with low self-esteem and exhibiting tendencies to withdraw and self-isolate. He characterizes these children as passive or submissive victims. These children tend to state that they are insecure and will not retaliate if provoked or bullied. In contrast, he identifies provocative victims as the ones who are not only anxious but aggressive and reactionary as well. In their meta-analytic work, Hawker and Boulton (2000) showed that victimized children display significantly higher levels of psychological problems, including depression, loneliness and anxiety. Trends in bullying demonstrate an increase in childhood, with peak occurrence coinciding with early adolescence, followed by a slight decline in late adolescence (Nansel et al., 2001; Tsaousis, 2016). In later years, research appears to indicate that overt or direct physical bullying declines, while other indirect or relational bullying appears to increase (Espelage et al., 2004).

Bullies may be aggressive or passive in that they may not lead but may follow others in provoking and victimizing others. Bullying involves more than just perpetrator(s) and victim. Bullying progresses along a continuum, with participants assuming a role such as bully, victim or bully-victim and bystander (Espelage et al., 2010; Espelage et al., 2000; Nansel et al., 2001). Graham (2010) provides that the myth of the bully and victim has to be debunked in that there are variants that accompany school-based incidents. She advocates as well that bullying provides teachers with teachable moments and opportunities to facilitate dialogue and conversation about tolerance and diversity.

School-Based Bullying

Bullying is a topic that has generated regulation and policy within educational frameworks in recent years (Holt et al., 2007a). Accordingly, research has revealed that between 10% and 15% of students in grades three through six are experiencing peer victimization or bullying weekly (Nansel et al., 2001; Tsaousis, 2016). Several authors report that serious consequences for both bullies and victims result and impact school achievement, social skills and psychological well-being (Hawker & Boulton, 2000; Juvonen et al., 2003; Pepler et al., 2008).

A concentrated movement to manage and reduce incidences of bullying within schools has been embraced by policy makers, educators and researchers attempting to stave off this issue. In the United States, the 2014–2015 School Crime Supplement (National Center for Education Statistics and Bureau of Justice Statistics) indicates that, nationwide, about 21% of students between the ages of 12 and 18 experienced bullying. According to the Centers for Disease Control and Prevention in 2015, nationwide, 20% of students in grades 9 to 12 reported being bullied on school property (stopbullying.gov, 2015).

States have passed antibullying legislation (Limber & Small, 2003) as a means of quelling this problem. The first antibullying legislation was passed in Georgia in 1999 (stopbullying.gov). In the United States, antibullying laws exist only at the state level as there are no antibullying laws at the federal level (Shetgiri, 2013). Although antibullying laws require school districts to adopt antibullying policies, they vary by state, including the level of detail. Some states have minimal requirements, while other states demonstrate very complex laws. All include a state definition for bullying, as well as standards for reporting and investigation. Punitive measures for bullying and intimidation are also outlined.

In an effort to remediate bullying within school districts, initiatives and resolutions to address the problem have been crafted and implemented in states. States have developed programs and resources for the implementation of a framework and structure directed at reporting, investigation and prevention. States have created guidelines, including program and curriculum strategies, to address current incidents and to prevent future happenings at every grade level. In the state of New Jersey, the Department of Education has addressed these issues at the state and district levels. New Jersey adopted the Anti-Bullying Bill of Rights Act in 2011. This bill was signed into law as a means of "strengthening procedures for preventing, reporting, investigating and responding to incidents of harassment, intimidation and bullying (HIB) of students that occur on school grounds and off school grounds under specified circumstances". Under the Anti-Bullying Bill of Rights Act (ABR), the New Jersey Department of Education (NJDOE) was required to issue guidance for use by parents, students and school staff in resolving complaints concerning HIB and for the implementation of the ABR (N.J.S.A. 18A:37–24) (Cerf et al., 2011).

Linkage Between Bullying and Other Forms of Victimization and Lack of Research

What sets bullying apart from other forms of abuse is the context in which it occurs and the relationship characteristics of the interacting parties (Olweus, 1994, 2013). According to Olweus (1994), his definition demarcates bullying as a form of abuse. Research devoted to bullying is a burgeoning arena; however, there is a paucity of exploration directed at the associations and possible links between bullying and other forms of victimization, including child maltreatment and child sexual abuse (Hebert et al., 2016; Holt et al., 2007a). According to Holt et al. (2007a), research is needed to discern potential connections between bullying and other forms of victimization and "to disentangle the unique effects of bullying involvement from influences of other forms of victimization that children experience" (p. 345). This sentiment is echoed by Hong et al. (2012), who state that there is a complex and interrelated relationship between abuse, neglect and bullying. A call for research devoted to exploring the relationship between child abuse and bullying/victimization is advocated (Hong et al., 2012) as a means of unraveling the complexity of the linkage between these forms of maltreatment in an effort to develop appropriate and purposeful measures. Such study will help to inform intervention and prevention programs (Hebert et al., 2016; Holt et al., 2007a).

Hong et al. (2012) reviewed several studies that confirm the connection of child maltreatment, including sexual abuse, with bullying. Within their broader review of the literature, they determined that maltreated children are more likely to be victimized or bullied outside of the family. They cite studies by Bolger and Patterson (2001), Knutson and Schartz (1997) and Shields & Cicchetti (2001).

Hong et al. (2012) propose that there is a gap in the literature on mediating and moderating factors associated with bullying and child abuse, which may be attributed to the independent development of literature in these domains. Child abuse has been identified as a risk factor for victimization from bullying (Shetgiri, 2013). Hong et al. (2012) have identified mediators and moderators that may impact victimization. They discerned that there is a growing body of literature indicative of a relationship between maltreatment and bullying. In their review of the literature, they identified four mediators, or explanatory factors, and three moderators, or mitigators. Mediators were defined as "emotional dysregulation, depression, anger and social skills deficits" and moderators as "relationship such as parent-child, peer and teacher" (p. 167). Moderators enhance or reduce, while mediators explain the association. Information about these domains impacts design and development of intervention and prevention programs.

Graham et al. (2006) have identified that little is known about youth who are both victimized and aggressive. They suggest that an explanation for this empirical void may be due to these areas being researched separately rather than concomitantly, resulting in separate research literatures – at least in American scholarship. European studies have conducted large-scale studies of bully/victim problems since the 1970s. The literature demonstrates a complementarity between aggression and victimization. "A dyadic interchange between perpetrator and target" has been a focal point (Graham et al., 2006).

Hong et al. (2012) comment that until such time that the realities of human subject research are considered, the link between child maltreatment and bullying cannot be completely understood or explored unless referrals are provided to subjects within the research protocol. As researchers, Hong et al. (2012) appeal to school-based researchers to collaborate with institutional review boards (IRBs) with regard to asking directly about maltreatment experiences. They assert that these questions cannot be asked "because they have been required by their IRB to report the abuse to school administrators which impedes research and promotes ethical considerations" (p. 178). All in all, their research provides a "blueprint for researchers in understanding the pathways from maltreatment to bullying perpetration and victimization in school that explain or inhibit this association, which has major implications for research and practice" (Hong et al., 2012, p. 180). The identification of factors that connect maltreatment to bullying will benefit interventions to break the cycle of victimization (Hong et al., 2012). Exploration of the association between child maltreatment and school-based bullying is gaining awareness as evident in examination of the literature (Hong et al., 2012; Shields & Cicchetti, 2001) and may eventually contribute to minimization of the cycle of victimization.

In a recent Canadian study, the direct and indirect links between sexual abuse and cyberbullying, as well as traditional forms of bullying, in adolescents were considered. The Canadian study sought to examine and identify connections between cyberbullying and child sexual abuse (Hebert, 2016, p. 624). The study found that twice as many girls who were sexually abused experienced cyberbullying. The findings reveal that child sexual abuse is a significant risk factor for youth to experience cyberbullying or other forms of bullying. The researchers found a correlation between vulnerability and revictimization in the study (Hebert et al., 2016). Results revealed that child sexual abuse victims were more vulnerable to poly-victimization with regard to both cyberbullying and other types of bullying (Hebert et al., 2016). Cyberbullying is defined as "an aggressive, deliberate, and repeated behavior inflicted by an individual to another through the use of computers, cell phones, and other electronic devices".

Research is also directed at exploring poly-victimization in children between the ages of 2 and 17 in which participants experienced four or more different kinds of victimization (Espelage et al., 2010; Finkelhor et al., 2009). Finkelhor et al. (2009) studied "the complex and diverse patterns of developmental vulnerability to different kinds of victimization at different ages in the face of improving prevention and intervention polices" (p. 711). They explain that this is difficult to study, given that "childhood victimization is categorized by various subtopics including bullying and sexual abuse with limited study aimed at assessing risk associated with victimization in a systematic and comparative manner" (p. 712). Holt and colleagues in their respective research as cited (2007a, 2007b) found that more victimization was reported in other domains regardless of the role within the bully cycle, meaning they were found to be victims of other forms of maltreatment, whether bullies or victims or a combination. Bully-victims were classified as high risk for other forms of victimization given the results. These researchers also found that bullies, while mainly engaging in aggressive behaviors towards others at school, reported being victims within their own home or within the community. Their research also revealed that other types of victimization may contribute to engagement in bully-type behaviors.

The other domains considered in relation to bully and victimization were identified as more conventional crimes such as child maltreatment, sexual victimization and witnessing or indirect victimization (Holt et al., 2007b). Ultimately, the study determined that there is a need to broaden understanding of the bully and victimization cycle and to consider the need for more comprehensive bullying assessment that considers the potential that bullies and bully-victims may be hiding victimization. Determining if victimization has played a role in the bully's or the bully-victim's behavior thus merits consideration.

Bullying and victimization may overlap, and this information is important for schools to address in considering how to be effective in handling bullying situations and prevention. In a study conducted by Shields and Cicchetti (2001), bullying was prevalent among abused children who were victims of commission (physical or sexual abuse). Maltreatment also placed children at risk for victimization by peers. Gender did not moderate these findings, in that maltreated boys and girls appeared to be at similar risk for bullying and victimization (Shields & Cicchetti, 2001).

Finkelhor et al. (2007) advocate for researchers to consider a range of victimizations, rather than focus on single forms due to the negative effects associated with maltreatment and victimization. They state that there are inherent problems associated with limiting study to singular patterns rather than consideration of poly-victimization, given the resulting impact upon children. Examination from a wider perspective may reveal if certain forms of victimology raise the potential for other forms of victimization. Moreover, Browne and Finkelhor (1986) have identified that children who have been subjected to abuse may develop a sense of powerlessness when coupled with the inability to self-protect, which may inadvertently set them up to become targets of aggression by peers or bully perpetrators. Victims come to the assumption and exhibit the expectation that harm is due to them given their presentation, which is in effect a byproduct of their abuse narrative (Browne & Finkelhor, 1986).

Study Connection

The study to be described originally was conceptualized as a field study; however, the forensic nature of the interview process was a deterrent, and the design was mitigated by ethical and legal concerns. As such, a real-time study was unachievable. Additionally, the need to minimize risk to participants resulted in the development of an analogue study. Minimization of risk was a high priority in designing the analogue and the overall study. Bullying, which has been identified as a contemporary societal issue that impacts school-aged children, shares themes and demonstrates parallels with child sexual abuse. As such, bullying was deemed to be an analogous topic to address the study question. Within the realm of the analogue design, bullying provided study participants with a simulated experienced event that did not promote victimization or traumatic response. Participants were not exposed to bullying in a real-world scenario, nor did they engage in related behavior(s) and they were not exposed to physical or mental harm; rather, antibullying strategies were considered within the context of the study design. The underlying rationale for the use of an analogue study surrounding bullying will be explained. A gap that emerged was the call for research initiatives exploring the linkage between bullying and child maltreatment or victimization.

Parallels Identified in Bullying and Child Sexual Abuse

Olweus (2013) has defined bullying as a specific type of aggressive behavior. Bullying has four main characteristics: 1) it is an intentional behavior (2) which could cause harm, (3) involves a power imbalance and (4) occurs over time (Olweus, 2013). Child sexual abuse is considered a complex event that children are ill prepared to describe (Everson & Boat, 2002).

Bullying and Child Sexual Abuse

- both are pervasive public health problems that are underreported
- both share commonalities such as an intentional behavior/activity and a power imbalance
- a continuum of progression is fundamental to both types of victimization
- disclosure patterns resemble each other and may be accidental or purposeful
- recantation is probable
- resultant psychological and physical damage may occur as a result of the interaction that is unwarranted and unprovoked in both
- victimization of school-aged children, whether through child sexual abuse or bullying, contributes to hopelessness and powerlessness (Olweus, 2013)

Bullying shares with child sexual abuse recognition as a pervasive public health problem that is underreported (National Sexual Violence Resource Center, 2012). The definition of bullying and the definition of child sexual abuse include similar dynamics. Both share commonalities, such as an intentional behavior/activity and a power imbalance. A continuum of progression is ascribed to both types of victimization. Respective continuums include behaviors, interactions and activities. Disclosure patterns resemble each other and may be accidental or purposeful. Recantation is probable given the circumstances under which disclosure occurs. Participants assume similar roles and include bullies or aggressors, victims and often bystanders, which in child sexual abuse may be construed as perpetrators or perpetrators by omission. Psychological and physical damage may occur as the result of the interaction in both child sexual abuse and bullying. Victimization of school-aged children, whether through child sexual abuse or bullying, contributes to hopelessness and powerlessness (Olweus, 2013). Residual traumata may manifest given the types of behaviors and interactions resultant to bullying or child sexual abuse.

Parallels Between Child Sexual Abuse and Bullying

- parallel relational aspects
  - perpetrator may not be unknown to victim
  - relationship not capricious
  - power differential either real or implied
  - victim feels helpless and hopeless
- behavioral parallels
  - unwarranted harassment/intimidation/contact
  - follows a continuum from less threatening/intimate to more
    - overt/covert
    - direct/indirect
  - disclosure may be accidental or purposeful
  - recantation may follow
- victimization variances
  - attributed to context and type of abuse
  - psychological and maybe physical impact
  - social, behavioral and school/educational impact
- comparable investigative measures for experienced event
  - use of the "b" word (bullying) provokes immediate response within a school setting
  - with child sexual abuse investigative process initiated once report is received
  - both types of victimization invoke an investigative interview to elicit information from victims and often witnesses or (with bullying) bystanders

---

Content Analysis

The literature review concludes with the topic of content analysis including definition, description and information pertinent to the collection and analysis of the study data. The way in which content analysis was used and the model that emerged are explained. The use of content analysis with regard to art therapy research is examined as well.

Content analysis is a systematic, replicable technique for textual analysis in which content categories are identified through coding (Stemler, 2001). The technique of content analysis is not restricted to the domain of textual analysis but may be applied to other areas such as coding student drawings (Wheelock et al., 2000). In order to allow for replication, data must be durable in nature. Originally intended as a quantitative methodology for communication or textual data, qualitative content analysis was expanded interdisciplinarily in the mid-20th century and broadened to encompass other forms of media. Through this differentiation, qualitative content analysis expanded into different models of communication, including nonverbal (Wheelock et al., 2000).

A qualitative procedure for content analysis preserves quantitative content analysis (Mayring, 2000). Two approaches are central to this approach of analysis: inductive category development and deductive category application. A criterion of definition is formulated which emerges from the research question. This will determine what aspects of the textual material are to be considered. From this process, categories are identified, revised and reduced to central themes. "The qualitative step of analysis consists in a methodological controlled assignment of the category to a passage of text" (Mayring, 2000, p. 2). The premise is to provide "explicit definitions, examples and coding rules" (Mayring, 2000, p. 3) for each category, including the determination of how each passage within the text or other form of communicative text is to be coded within a category. Once the categories are determined and identified, a coding agenda brings them together: category, definition, examples and coding rules are placed in a matrix or chart configuration. Mayring (2000) explains that these columns or topics are determined in conjunction with the material obtained and in accordance with theory within a step-by-step process and are subject to revision within the process of analysis. Content analysis is applicable when the research question is not open-ended or variable. Content analysis is a method that may be used with either qualitative or quantitative data, and it may be either inductive or deductive depending upon the aim of the study (Elo & Kyngäs, 2008; Mayring, 2000).

Content analysis as a research method is a systematic and objective means of describing and quantifying phenomena that is content-sensitive (Krippendorff, 2013). It affords flexibility with regard to research design, and it offers a way to understand and make meaning out of various forms of communication (Elo & Kyngäs, 2008). Qualitative content analysis enables a systematic means of identifying categories or themes in an effort to make sense or meaning of the text/image being analyzed (Graneheim & Lundman, 2004; Mayring, 2000). Content analysis allows for the distillation of "words into fewer content related categories" in an effort to consolidate text with shared meaning (Elo & Kyngäs, 2008, p. 108). According to Krippendorff (2013), content analysis is a research method for making replicable and valid inferences from data to context.

The purpose of content analysis is to provide "knowledge, new insights, a representation of facts and a practical guide to action" (Elo & Kyngäs, 2008, p. 108). Elo and Kyngäs (2008) explain that the aim of content analysis is to "attain a condensed and broad description of the phenomenon, and the outcome of the analysis is concepts or categories describing the phenomenon" (p. 108), perhaps leading to the development of a model or conceptualized map of categories or themes.

Approaches to Content Analysis

The exploration of the literation on qualitative content analysis reveals that different researchers adhere to different stages/phases or steps in the gathering and analysis of data. Analogous to investigative interviewing with respect to the incorporation of stages wherein interviewers utilize phase-specific models, with some utilizing more and others fewer (stages or phases) elicitation or cultivation of information is central. Phase-specific processes associated with content analysis provide a map that encompasses stages from gathering data to meaning making of information to reporting. Relative to this study, four different approaches to content analysis are considered. The models that were reviewed were Elo and Kyngäs (2008), Graneheim and Lundman (2004), Henning et al. (2004) and Thyme et al. (2013).

Elo and Kyngäs (2008) identified a three-phase model for the progression of the steps of content analysis. This model provided an understanding of the method of content analysis, which encompassed three phases related to data: preparation, organization and reporting. Their three-phase process encapsulated a six-phase stage model utilized by Henning et al. (2004), which addressed gathering, coding and analyzing data. Thyme et al. (2013) adhered to and adapted Graneheim and Lundman's (2004) model for educational and nursing research that is consistent with the previous two models. Emanating from Graneheim and Lundman (2004), Thyme et al's. (2013) model delineated a conceptual frame that addresses manifest and latent content. This conceptual basis inspired Thyme et al. (2013) to apply their approach to content analysis to psychodynamic art psychotherapy, which considers manifest and latent material. By combining and blending the various elements from these distinct yet intertwined frameworks, a concept model emerged for this study that enabled the organization, sorting and analysis of the findings.

Elo and Kyngäs, 2008

With regard to their three-phase model, Elo and Kyngäs (2008) discuss that there are no rules for data; however, the intent is to determine how to categorize or make content categories out of the text under analysis. In the first or preparation phase, the unit to be analyzed is determined. In the second or organizing phase, the goal is to make sense of the data via immersion. Through an inductive approach, the data are coded through open coding and through categorizing. Codes are then collapsed, and categories emerge. This occurs via a classification process of the data through comparison of similarities and dissimilarities to condense and reduce the data in an effort to understand and foster a sense of what the data mean. Coding and categorization lead to construction of an unconstrained matrix in which flexibility and movement promote understanding and highlight relationships, giving rise to emergent themes and patterns. In the reporting phase the results are "formed through a process comprising a number of phases" (Elo & Kyngäs, 2008, p. 113). This is often one of the most demanding phases of content analysis because of the challenges implicit in conveying the researcher's "actions and insights" (Elo & Kyngäs, 2008, p. 113).

Graneheim and Lundman, 2004

Qualitative content analysis evolved from the quantitative use of the method. Qualitative use of content analysis has been used in nursing and educational research; however, differences of opinion exist in the literature with regard to defining and naming concepts associated with content analysis (defined as manifest and latent content, unit of analysis, meaning unit, condensation, abstraction, code and category) as well as procedures and interpretation and conceptual ideology (Graneheim & Lundman, 2004, p. 106). Some of these issues are due to the ontological beliefs of the researchers. As such, "a text always involves multiple meanings and there is always some degree of interpretation when approaching a text" according to Graneheim and Lundman (2004, p. 106). The unit of analysis, which is fundamental to qualitative content analysis, included both verbal and pictorial or imaginal units in this study. Graneheim and Lundman (2004) proposed that "the most suitable" unit of analysis is the interview itself given that it constitutes a whole that is manageable as the basis for the meaning unit. They described this as "the constellation of words or statements" that share a central meaning (p. 106). Different researchers use different terminology to describe this concept, which is considered the same as codes, themes and categories.

Qualitative Comparative Exploratory Analogue

Qualitative research has been defined as including the following four aspects (Merriam, 2009) which were applicable to the study design and research question: 1) research that focuses on meaning and understanding; 2) the researcher is the primary instrument through which data are collected and analyzed; 3) inductive research approach; and 4) research that provides a rich description of the phenomenon under investigation. According to qualitative researchers Denzin and Lincoln (2000), qualitative research involves interpretive practices in which interviews are representations garnered from naturalistic milieus. "Qualitative researchers study things in their natural settings, attempting to make sense of, or to interpret, phenomena in terms of the meanings people bring to them" (Denzin & Lincoln, 2000, p. 3). Qualitative research provides a systematic means to gather new insights by assessing the research phenomena under investigation and answering the research question (De Wet, 2010).

According to Henning et al. (2004), qualitative research is typically conducted from an interpretative paradigm, although with different philosophical underpinnings. Kohlbacher (2006) explained that an interpretive approach to social knowledge encompasses an emergent meaning making process. For this study, an interpretative framework provided the underlying basis given the focus on "experience and interpretation" (De Wet, 2010). "Interpretive research is concerned with meaning and it seeks to understand people's definitions and understanding of situations" (De Wet, 2010, p. 191). The interpretive paradigm "seeks to produce descriptive analysis that emphasizes deep, interpretative understanding of social phenomenon", according to Henning (De Wet, 2010, p. 191).

Although qualitative studies may differ with regard to design, the goal is "an in-depth understanding" according to Thyme et al. (2013). The application of qualitative content analysis within the context of art psychotherapy was drawn upon for this study. The use of content analysis was researched by Thyme et al. (2013) wherein a research method from one type of research was applied to another. They used a model from nursing (Graneheim & Lundman, 2004) and then transferred that to art psychotherapy, providing a frame to guide the analysis of drawings within this study. This approach will be discussed shortly and the relevance and application within the scope of the study will be explained.

Content Analysis and Art Psychotherapy

Qualitative content analysis in art psychotherapy research was discussed by Thyme et al. (2013). They determined and identified that the type of design that is used to explore the use of art within a therapeutic context is dependent upon the type of therapeutic process. They delineated three types: art therapy, art psychotherapy and analytical art psychotherapy. Although research in this area is in a nascent state, Thyme et al. (2013) identified three forms of therapeutic artwork reviewed across different fields: art therapy, art-based methods in health research and creative arts. They determined that researchers engaged in studying these areas come from various professions and utilize both quantitative and qualitative as well as mixed methods research (Thyme et al., 2013). The art psychotherapeutic process was credited as being examined through the use of qualitative content analysis (Egberg-Thyme et al., 2008; Howells & Zelnik, 2009) because of the broad and in-depth understanding the method provided (Thyme et al., 2013). Content analysis was considered to be "in line with the psychodynamic practice" and congruent with art psychotherapy (Thyme et al., 2013, p. 102).

Thyme et al. (2013) constructed a method of analyzing drawings and the words that accompany them or preceded them through use of Graneheim and Lundman's (2004) model of qualitative content analysis. In doing so, they determined that "words and pictures cannot be regarded as autonomous and free from their context" (Thyme et al., 2013, p. 103). Furthermore, they allowed that "[i]t is not possible to interpret a single word or picture without accounting for these two aspects of context" (p. 103). They reported that this method of qualitative content analysis has seldom been used as a means for analysis of art psychotherapy. Through the inductive use of the research method coupled with their own identification of a deductive approach related to art psychotherapy, they were able to move back and forth between the manifest messages and the latent meanings, as stated by Graneheim & Lundman (2004).

This combined methodological approach provided a means of exploring "various phenomenon in pictures" (colors and elements) and the "clarifying words and emotions connected to the art-making process and to systematize them" (Thyme et al., 2013, p. 104). Drawing upon the method put forth by Graneheim and Lundman (2004), a framework or "a sensible guide provided a structure for the pictures and the words connected to the pictures" (Thyme et al., 2013, p. 104). Thyme et al. (2013) essentially described "transferring a method from one field to another, from nursing research to art psychotherapy research, to enlarge the use of qualitative content analysis and to build bridges between different contexts" (Thyme et al., p. 106), which was applicable and prudent in this context.

Manifest and Latent Content

Manifest and latent content were considered through the analytical process of qualitative content analysis in this study for both text and drawings. According to Graneheim and Lundman (2004), manifest content provided a means of condensing the text without reducing or altering the meaning of the text, while latent content provided a means of understanding the underlying meaning of textual material (or the manifest content). Thus, interpreting the text through qualitative content analysis allowed for different levels of interpretation, and it provided a wide-ranging in-depth understanding (Thyme et al., 2013) of the imaginal material as well.

Interpretation of both manifest and latent content will vary according to Graneheim and Lundman (2004) with regard to depth and abstraction.

> According to Graneheim and Lundman (2004), qualitative content analysis can be performed with various degrees of interpretation and with various focuses. In each text or picture, there are manifest messages to be described and latent meanings to be interpreted. This means that the epistemological basis of qualitative content analysis can be referred to various scientific approaches (Thyme et al., 2013, p. 102).

Thyme et al. (2013) applied and described the use of qualitative content analysis within a psychodynamic art psychotherapy context in which the verbal associations that preceded and accompanied art making were analyzed. In doing so, they coded and categorized elements, resulting in subthemes as well as the identification of an overarching theme. Thyme et al. (2013) concluded that qualitative content analysis is "a meaningful method for analyzing pictures and words from psychodynamic art psychotherapy sessions, keeping the manifest messages and the latent meanings in the pictures intact" (p. 101).

Basis for Empirical Study

In conclusion, several themes emerged from review of the various literature segments. Collectively, identified themes and gaps materialized that were deemed worthy of empirical study and underlie the focus which contributed to the conceptualization of the research. Additionally, topics and themes to be explored internally within this study as well as externally (within the scope of other research projects) were identified and are noted in the following chart. Ultimately, it is hoped that the various gaps and areas of study that directed and factored into this exploration will contribute to the literature and study pertaining to the use of free drawing as an open-ended prompt within investigative interviewing as well as the use of an art therapy–based investigative interview process. The data collected in this research were an attempt to address the use of free drawing within an art therapy–based investigative interview process and to explore the effects and associated mechanisms ascribed to drawing within this context from an art therapy perspective.

Empirical Study is Advocated with Regard to . . .

Enhancing self-report	Evaluation of the use of drawing	The efficacy of free drawing within interviews	Drawing as a means of memory retrieval	Bullying and child sexual abuse	Art therapy	Art therapy research
Empirically sound and forensically relevant research regarding interventions that enhance children's self-report and thus their testimony has been and continues to be advocated	Increasingly, researchers have identified the need for empirical evaluation of the use of drawing within the process of forensic interviews	The call for empirically sound and forensically relevant research regarding the efficacy of free drawing within investigative interviews	How drawing has "aided children's retrieval process" has been explored and continues to be a current area of inquiry	Research devoted to bullying is a burgeoning arena; however, there is a paucity of exploration directed at the associations and possible links between bullying and other forms of victimization, including child maltreatment and child sexual abuse	The manner in which art therapy uses imagery and derives information from the art therapy process is an ever-expanding area of exploration	Understanding of the underlying processes involved in art therapy is still under investigation, and although there is potential in how information is processed and expressed via drawing, more empirical data and art therapy research are needed to substantiate
Katz et al., 2014	Everson & Boat, 2002; Faller, 1993, 2007; Katz et al., 2014; Lamb et al., 2007; Macleod et al., 2013; Olafson, 2012	Driessnack, 2005; Everson & Boat, 2002; Jolley, 2010; Macleod et al., 2013; Olafson, 2012; Patterson & Hayne, 2011; Pipe et al., 2004	Katz et al., 2014, p. 877	Holt et al., 2007a, 2007b; Hong et al., 2012, Shetgiri, 2013	Acosta, 2001; Lusebrink, 2014	Lusebrink, 2014

Methodology and Design

A qualitative comparative analogue design was used to retrieve data that were rich and descriptive. The rationale for using the design was to explore how drawing facilitates witnessed or experienced events within an investigative interview as compared to an investigative interview without drawing. Due to the limitations associated with conducting a field or real-time study wherein the participants would be victims or witnesses to a traumatic event such as sexual abuse, the analogue focused on antibullying strategies.

Research Question and Rationale

The intention of the study was to provide a systematic investigation of drawing as an open-ended prompt in the CIG, a forensic art therapy investigative interview process. The research question for this study was: *How does drawing facilitate disclosure of experienced events of school-aged children in an art therapy–based investigative interview process when compared to a verbal investigative interview process?* The CIG was both the instrument and object of investigation in this study.

The study was originally conceptualized to compare the CIG (investigative interview with drawing) to a verbal investigative interview process without drawing in a forensic setting. However, legal and ethical issues associated with conducting real-time forensic interviews to explore allegations of sexual abuse with school-aged children was prohibitory and an experimental design of this nature or a field study was not conducted. Consequently, an analogue or laboratory study was designed. As has been noted, analogue studies are commonly used in investigative interview research because of the implicit challenges in conducting real-time studies (Lamb & Thierry, 2005).

An analogue study provides a laboratory scenario within a seemingly controlled setting. In this study, 12 children were assigned to one of two interview conditions after watching two short animated videos about antibullying strategies. The videos about bullying provided the analogous condition of an experienced event for the study. The analogue aspect of the design allowed for a descriptive comparison of the participants' response to witnessing and reporting on an event through one of two interview conditions: with drawing and without drawing.

Unlike in vivo forensic interviews, the laboratory study ensures authenticity in that the variables or conditions of the event are known to the participants and the researcher. This knowledge helps in ascertaining if the information/material that a child discloses actually happened, which contributes to understanding the veracity of the information disclosed regardless of the interview condition. Thus, the analogue or simulated laboratory study provided an opportunity for comparison of information disclosed with and without the use of drawing with a normative participant school aged population as will be explained.

Contributing to the rationale for exploring a forensic interview process predicated upon art therapy and the use of free drawing was that methods for extracting viable information from child victims of sexual abuse remain a focal point of research and study (Everson & Boat, 2002; Olafson, 2012; Wakefield & Underwager, 1998). Recent findings suggest a trend in both analogue and real-time studies directed at assessing whether drawing enhances forensically relevant information disclosed by children in an investigative interview about experienced events (Macleod et al., 2013). Investigative interviews are predominantly conducted as conversational verbal processes (Carnes, 2000; Hoffman, 2005; Macleod et al., 2013). Due to developmental limitations and the nature of traumatic memory, children in an interview condition are often unable to provide a clear and detailed verbal account (Lippert et al., 2009; Melinder et al., 2010).

The rationale for this design was to systematically investigate the CIG, which foundationally,

- provides a child-friendly means for recalling and communicating experienced events using nondirected or free drawing
- is conducted within a relational context in which children can disclose experienced events in a developmentally congruent manner
- offers a common language and a guideline for investigative interviews of children

Additionally, the rationale addressed,

- the systematic investigation of the CIG, a forensic art therapy process
- the comparison of recall and disclosure of evidence under two conditions: verbal and verbal with a drawing strategy
- a forum to explore the theoretical principles that underlie the CIG

Finally, the drawing effect and associated underlying mechanisms from an art therapy perspective were examined.

As such, the gaps in the literature that contributed to the rationale for conducting this study included:

- the debatable acceptance that currently surrounds the use of drawing in investigative interviews of school-aged children
- the identified need for research in forensic interviewing approaches for children
- the lack of systematic study of the CIG
- the need to explore the medium of drawing as a primary component in investigative interviews
- the elusiveness of the drawing effect and the underlying mechanisms attributed to it

Participants

Participants were recruited through announcement as well as through snowballing after approval from the university IRB (institutional review board). A normative participant sample was recruited to gather baseline data. Children of all ethnic, racial, socio-economic and religious backgrounds were eligible. Resultant enrollment consisted of 12 children between the ages of seven and ten years old: 6 male and 6 female. Inclusion criteria deemed participants had to reside within geographical proximity of the study sites due to the need for in-person contact. Artistic ability was not required for study participation since it was not a factor in the study.

This age group was selected because children are thought to be dealing with similar developmental issues given the psychosexual phase of latency, which encompasses ages 6 to 11. The participants were elementary school students in third through fifth grade who received educational instruction in regular school settings. For this study, participants had to meet the following two criteria. First, the children were not identified as having special needs or mental illness. Second, and relative to the first criteria, the participants did not require special educational services such as an individualized education plan, (IEP) or a 504 accommodation plan. The rationale for these exclusion criteria was twofold. First, this study used a normative participant sample to examine the research question and to collect baseline data; second, the normative criteria minimized risks to participants given that accommodations that may have been addressed in an IEP or a 504 plan were not available to assist or support participants.

Risks

This was a minimal-risk study. As such, the risk to participants was low. The videos to be shown were publicly available for educational purposes. Although unlikely, there was a possibility that a child may have experienced minimal anxiety if he or she was uncomfortable with the material presented in the videos. It is also possible that a child may have become anxious during the interview when asked to describe or draw what they witnessed in the videos. It was also possible that witnessing the videos and/or participating in the interview may have triggered a recollection or memory that was unpleasant for a child and may not have been previously disclosed.

Investigational Procedure

Following parental consent and child assent, participants were assigned a PIN number correspondent with enrollment, which garnered assignment to one of two interview conditions: CIG with drawing and CIG without drawing. The CIG juxtaposes forensic application with art therapy principles and practices. It is a FAT investigative interview process that was used both as the focus of study and the method to gather data for this study.

Each child watched two short animated videos on a laptop computer featuring McGruff, the Crime Dog, with the investigator. McGruff is an anthropomorphic character who was created in the early 1980s for the National Crime Prevention Council to promote personal safety and crime awareness. McGruff is used by law enforcement and educational agencies to address antiviolence platforms. The videos provided the analogous condition of an experienced event (bullying). The short clips addressed antibullying strategies.

Instrumentation: The Common Interview Guideline

CIG

The CIG is an investigative/forensic art therapy interview guideline
Three central principles form the basis of the CIG
  1. an open invitational drawing process
  2. a dialogical and relational process
  3. the encoding, storage and recall of memory in image form (including traumatic)

The CIG encompasses five phases that are fluid
  1. rapport building
  2. developmental screening/skills assessment
  3. anatomy identification
  4. fact-finding
  5. closure

In accordance with the analogue design, the anatomy identification phase was omitted for the study.

The CIG is an interview guideline that is comprised of phases that are fluid and flexible. It is not a linear process. The interviewer moves in and out of the phases as necessary, accommodating the child by following the child's lead, albeit while staying in control of the process. Although the phases, rapport building, developmental assessment, fact-finding and closure, are presented here in a seemingly linear fashion, they are dynamic and not static; thus the process is active and emergent.

The CIG is not a scripted interview process. Rather, it is semi-structured and predicated upon open-ended questions. The CIG incorporates free or nondirected drawing as an integral part of the interview process in the capacity of an open-ended prompt. Drawing is used to facilitate free recall and elicit event-specific information in a nonthreatening manner. Artistic skill or talent is not a prerequisite.

Although the CIG has existed and been utilized as an investigative interview procedure for more than 20 years, it had not been empirically tested prior to this study. Data were collected to determine how nondirected drawing, when used in a primary capacity in an art therapy–based investigative interview process, influenced verbal communication, memory recall and evidentiary disclosure.

The children in the study were assigned to one of two conditions: CIG with drawing or CIG without drawing. Because this study was an analogue or laboratory study rather than a field study or a real-time forensic interview with sexually abused children, the CIG was modified. The anatomy identification phase of the interview guideline was omitted and the CIG was amended for this study to consist of four rather than five phases given the analogue design. The CIG is not a step-wise process, meaning that phases are not structured and the process is not intended to follow a prescribed order. The phases are fluid and not static. Phases may evolve concomitantly or occur simultaneously or be independent. They may also merge and blend.

The guideline was developed to provide multidisciplinary team members with a common language and a consistent method for investigating allegations of child sexual abuse. A multidisciplinary team is composed of individuals from a host of disciplines that represent a myriad of backgrounds, experience and expertise. Representatives from diverse fields and disciplines, including law enforcement, mental health, medicine, prosecution and social services, work together and blend their respective skills (Cohen-Liebman, 1999). It is the combination and integration of these diverse resources that contribute to comprehensive investigations by the systems that intervene. An interview format that addresses the respective needs of each discipline is essential. The disciplines that comprise the multidisciplinary team have distinct and specific investigative needs that are pertinent to their respective purview (burden of proof). Often, desired information is essential to more than one, if not all, of the respective disciplines. A CIG is essential for three reasons: to improve the fact-finding process, eliminate secondary victimization by minimizing repetitive interviews and the process is known to each discipline and affords consistency.

Each phase of the interview guideline is designed to refute the argument of suggestibility. This means that the interviewer is not leading the child to say or give a particular response, nor is the interviewer suggesting a given response. Each element incorporated into the interview process, whether with or without drawing, is included for a specific reason and is conceived with the idea that everything within the process must be legally defensible in a court of law.

The phases for CIG with and CIG without drawing are briefly explained as well as the integration of drawing within each phase (in-depth description was addressed earlier in the text). Children assigned to the nondrawing condition were interviewed with a verbal format. Free drawing was not incorporated, and as such, the CIG without drawing is a verbal process. The four phases that were incorporated within each condition (with and without drawing), although not necessarily sequential, include rapport building, developmental assessment, fact-finding and closure.

Rapport Building – Rapport building begins at the commencement of the process and concludes at the end of the process. It is not limited to a particular segment of the process; rather, rapport is built and sustained throughout the process. Comfort is promoted with the interviewer, as well as with the process. Empowerment through various measures, including the promotion of dialogue/exchange of information, is encouraged (Cohen-Liebman, 1999).

- promote comfort and trust
- activate participation
- address standard operating procedure

  - in conjunction with child's developmental level and presentation

- familiarize child with setting, task, etc.
- introduce self (interviewer) and explain role
- understand child's understanding of process

  - clarify misperceptions as to impetus for interview

- address surroundings, including observers and location of them
- explain documentation/memorialization
- empower via choice
- promote dialogue/participation
- encourage child to challenge interviewer

  - permission to correct or disagree with interviewer
- importance of accuracy

  - enhanced when grounded in experience/application
  - practice via role play and through exploration of real-world scenario(s)
  - instruct child to say "I do not know" rather than guess
  - avoid words play/pretend and make-believe

- give permission to decline to answer

  - emotional distress may preclude response or engagement

    - depending upon topic of discussion or disclosure of information

  - child may deny, recant or minimize
  - sensitivity to child's ability to discuss aspects of experience

    - information may be embarrassing, painful or fearful for child to verbalize
    - balance child's distress with ability to tolerate self-expression

Developmental Assessment – Developmental assessment assists the interviewer in comprehending the child's level of functioning. This information is used by the interviewer in an effort to adapt language, concepts and tasks in order to accommodate a child's abilities and promote rapport. In order to engage the child and facilitate the fact-finding process, the interviewer has to communicate in a developmentally congruent manner. The interviewer assesses the child's cognitive level, social skills and emotional state, as well as linguistic skills, expressive-receptive capability and concept formation (Cohen-Liebman, 1999). During this phase, competency is assessed as is congruency of concepts. These concepts include but are not limited to truth versus lie and real versus pretend (Cohen-Liebman, 1999).

- assists interviewer in comprehension of child's level of functioning and dynamic processes

- enables interviewer to modify and adapt language and patterns of interaction

    - congruency of communication and interaction/engagement

- interviewer's developmentally congruent and sensitive response
- accommodate child's level of presentation and capabilities

    - avoid disconnect in perception/comprehension

- assess maturational spheres

    - cognitive level
    - social skills
    - linguistic
    - emotional
    - artistic
    - psychosexual
    - expressive (words used by the speaker)
    - receptive (words understood by the listener)

- concept formation
- choice of words, syntax will mirror child's patterns
- responsive listening

    - repeat back to child to reduce misunderstanding/miscommunication

- confirmation of what child has articulated
- congruency of concepts

    - truth versus lie
    - real versus not real

        - even if child is unclear, a child can still provide information that is accurate and cogent

- explore concepts

    - address separately to establish level of functioning and comprehension

- provide concrete examples rather than request a definition

    - prepositions
    - colors
    - numbers
    - practice and role play
    - assess errors of commission (add something)
    - omission – leave something out

Fact-Finding – The interviewer facilitates fact-finding in an effort to elicit information from the child, including specific facts and corroboration of information disclosed. The interviewer attempts to elicit situational and contextual details relative to the experienced/witnessed event, including what, when, where, how and who.

- fact-finding process
- question continuum

    - reverse continuum – general to specific

- open-ended to more focused/directed/structured
- questions versus type of response
- opportunities for free recall
- elicit narrative
- minimization of interviewer influence (reinforcement behaviors/nonverbal behaviors)
- contextual information

  - what, when, where, how, who

- situational information
- collateral information

  - details

- charge enhancements

  - coercion/threats/bribes/rewards/promises/secrecy
  - pornography/sexual aids/media/exposure

- explore alternative explanations
- explore developmentally incongruent information/knowledge
- assess idiosyncratic details
- consider motivational factors within the context of the interview if appropriate
- corroboration of facts/details/information
- assess competency and credibility

Closure – The child's participation and effort are acknowledged. If the interview proved to be stress provoking for the child or if the child is unable to manage their emotional response, the child may need to regroup before leaving the interview room. The process is intended to be concluded on a positive note rather than on a negative.

- thank the child for participation and for effort

  - inquire as to whether or not there is anything else the child may want to share
  - Are there any additional things or questions you might like to ask?
  - Is there anything else I should know about what we have been discussing?
  - Is there anything I did not ask that you wish to share?

- leave the door open for possible reinterview
- bridge to what happens next – concretely or literally
- address concerns or fears or issues honestly
- avoid false hopes
- respond truthfully but generally
- address personal safety (within a developmental context)
- allow for regrouping if necessary
- conclude on a positive note
- do not end interview negatively or allow child to leave in distress
- if appropriate, provide contact information for child/adolescent

  - this may be a contact for someone else involved in the case such as an officer

Common Interview Guideline Component Phases

CIG and Drawing

Key Elements	*Integration of Drawing*

RAPPORT BUILDING

Engage
promote comfort, trust
activate participation
Empower
provide choice (seat selection/choice
 of media) = control
Encourage
challenge authority correct, disagree
Address standard operating procedure
clarify misperceptions
emphasize accuracy
assess suggestibility

Function
open-ended prompt
primary resource
ice breaker
free or nondirected
develop comfort
promote trust
Engagement
verbally, nonverbally
establish rapport
Media
stimulate participation, active and passive
promote conversation
choice = empowerment/control
stimulus to explore topics
bridge to fact-finding
Forensic Aspects
emphasize accuracy
assess suggestibility

DEVELOPMENTAL SCREENING/SKILLS ASSESSMENT

Assess skill level
Communication skills
Patterns of interaction
Modify and adapt communication,
 interaction and patterns of
 engagement
Developmental spheres and concepts
Spatial relationships
prepositions
basic skills – color identification and
counting
developmentally congruent tasks
Comprehension of concepts
Congruency of concepts
truth/lie, real/pretend, right/wrong,
good/bad, comfortable/not
 comfortable
Practice and role play
Assess competency
Assess suggestibility

Assess
 maturational spheres: cognitive, social/emotional,
 linguistic, psychosexual, artistic developmental
 levels correlating with developmental capabilities
identify strengths and weaknesses
focus and attention
expressive/receptive capabilities
mastery or paucity of developmentally congruent tasks
adaptation of interactive patterns
meet child at his or her level
parallel not disjointed interactions
refute argument of suggestibility by demonstrating
 child's comprehension, skill set and skill level

FACT-FINDING

Question continuum
open-ended, general to specific
nonleading to more focused
reverse continuum of questioning
Details
contextual, situational, idiosyncratic
who, what, when, where, how
Fact-finding
specific facts
corroboration of information/details

drawing as open-ended prompt
additional or previously unknown information
information may be disclosed via drawing
may lead to verbalization or a narrative
depict what child may not be able to express
 verbally until disclosed pictorially or imaginally
details
situational
idiosyncratic, specific to personal
experience (indirect/direct, overt/covert)

Common Interview Guideline Component Phases

CIG and Drawing

Key Elements	Integration of Drawing
Collateral material	contextual
charge enhancements	map scenes
Explore alternative hypothesis for allegations	disclosure drawings
	facts
Assess credibility	**charge enhancements**
Address competency	threats, bribes, use of force, accoutrements, coercion, rewards, promises, media, pornography, exposure photography
	facilitate disclosure
	clarification
	memory stimulus/trigger
	confirmation of verbalizations
	stimulate recall

	CLOSURE
Thank for participation/effort	**Review**
not for information	**Revisit**
Leave door open for possible reinterview	**Clarify**
Address personal safety issues	**Confirm**
Address concerns and questions realistically	**Bridge** to what happens next
	allow for re-constitution before leaving
Avoid false hopes and promises	end on a positive note
Bridge to next steps – may be literal	take away drawing created after conclusion of
End positively	process – to support child with closure/next steps

Forensic Relevance

Investigative interviews, including the CIG, adhere to legal strictures, and as such, forensic relevancy is considered in evaluating information elicited from these processes. Forensic relevance as was discussed in the literature review refers to information and the manner in which it is disclosed relative to an experienced event. Types of memory are considered with regard to how a child stores and recalls information. Whether or not information is episodic (referring to a personal experienced event) or script (generalized knowledge) is considered and evaluated with regard to determining credibility.

Forensic relevance encompasses information or facts. These facts may pertain to core or peripheral information and may include material related to people, places and activities. Episodic memory (event specific) versus script memory (generalized knowledge) are also considered with regard to assessing whether or not information communicated is forensically relevant. Episodic details contribute to the assessment and understanding of a particular experience. In a forensic process, information or details regarding an event are needed in an effort to determine event-specific information, including who, what, where, how and when. Drawing has been demonstrated to enhance reporting of such material (Macleod et al., 2013).

In a forensic process, credibility and competency are variables that are also considered. Forensic relevance increases and is enhanced with the quantity and the quality of the information disclosed by a child within an investigative process. In addition, facts or details, including central, peripheral, contextual and idiosyncratic, are considered. Accuracy and inaccuracy also factor into a child's statements about an experienced event. All of these elements are critical components associated with forensic relevance. These aspects contribute to the assessment of forensic relevancy in an investigative interview process. Moreover, consideration of this information distinguishes a fact-finding process (investigative) from a clinical process. The CIG is unique in that it blends these factors with fundamental underlying tenets associated with art therapy, including the relationship or dialogical component (between the child and the interviewer), the creative process (art making) and the child's associations resulting in a forensically oriented but (emotionally) supportive process.

Data Collection

Data were gathered from three sources: 1) face-to-face semi-structured interviews utilizing the CIG either with drawing or without; 2) the drawings made by the participants assigned to the drawing condition (imaginal data); 3) reflective notes or memos created by the researcher (Cohen-Liebman). Each interview was audio-taped and transcribed verbatim by the investigator resulting in the procurement of textual data.

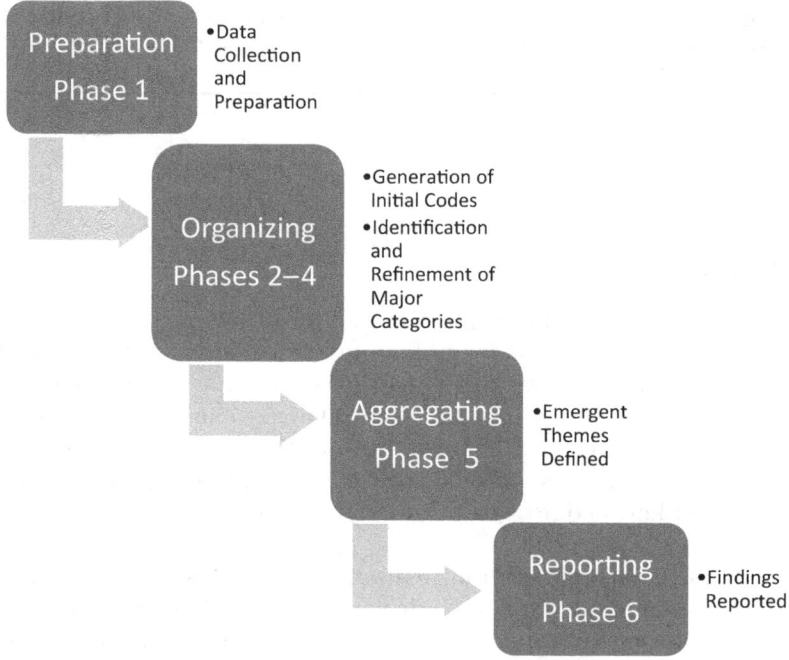

Figure 5.2 Meshed model for qualitative content analysis derived from Elo and Kyngäs (2008), Henning et al. (2004), Graneheim and Lundman (2004) and Thyme et al. (2013).

Content analysis was used to organize, code, aggregate and analyze textual and imaginal data, enabling a systematic means of identifying categories and themes. This provided a way to make sense or meaning of the textual/imaginal data (Graneheim & Lundman, 2004; Mayring, 2000). A meshed model for qualitative content analysis was derived from an amalgamation of models (Elo & Kangäs, 2008; Thyme et al., 2013; Henning et al., 2004; Graneheim & Lundman, 2004). By combining and blending the various elements from these frameworks, a concept model emerged providing the organization, sorting and analysis of the findings.

Dedoose, an electronic data management and cross platform application for analyzing qualitative and mixed-methods research (Gerbic & Stacey, 2005), assisted in the identification and acquisition of meaningful insights through highlighting units of analysis, including words, phrases and text passages, as well as graphic data through frequency codes. Codes and categories were checked to ensure they captured patterns and themes.

Reading and review of the data, including interview transcripts (textual data), drawings (graphic or imaginal data) and reflective notes (made by the investigator), were repeated in an effort to identify codes and categories, which contributed to the generation of emergent patterns and trends, themes and relationships between concepts (Shams et al., 2017). The process of analysis was complex and involved multiple reviews, resulting in the identification of two levels of content: manifest and latent.

As noted by Shams et al. (2017) with respect to Graneheim and Lundman (2004), review of the transcripts helped with the recognition of patterns or relationships among concepts or excerpts extracted from the primary units of analysis (the interviews). This enabled the identification of "hidden themes and patterns" (Shams et al., 2017, p. 2) as they emerged from the data. The steps utilized for qualitative content analysis that factored into the study and were excerpted from Shams et al. (2017) are based upon the work of Graneheim and Lundman (2004). The associated activity of each step is identified.

Steps	Activity
Start Point	The interviews were transcribed.
Step 1	The texts were read through several times to get a sense of the whole.
Step 2	Meaning units were extracted from the text.
Step 3	An abstraction of the meaning units into codes was created.
Step 4	The various codes were read and re-read and compared against each other. Based on these readings and a reflective process, the codes were sorted out into subcategories.
Step 5	The subcategories were compared with each other and with the original text to create mutually exclusive categories.
Step 6	An independent analysis of the textual data was performed and cross checked, resulting in a consensus about categorization.

The analyzed units for this study consisted of the verbal statements from the 12 participants as well as the visual depictions made by half of them. Once the unit of analysis (interviews and imaginal data) was determined, then meaning units were identified. For this study, these included textual data such as sentences, phrases or utterances in which "aspects related to each other through content and context were identified" (Graneheim & Lundman, 2004; Thyme et al., 2013). The label of the particular meaning unit became the code. For instance, for the drawings in the study there were two codes:

manifest content and latent content. After codes were identified, categories emerged. Thyme et al. (2013) described categories as "a group of codes that share a commonality on a manifest level" (p. 103).

Categories are a fundamental aspect of the process of content analysis and refer to "a descriptive level of content and can thus be seen as an expression of the manifest content of the text" (Graneheim & Lundman, 2004, p. 107). Themes were derived from categories and are described as "a recurrent thread of underlying meaning running through codes and categories which can be seen as an expression of the latent meaning of a text" (Thyme et al., 2013, p. 103). Themes can be subdivided. According to Graneheim and Lundman (2004), a theme is considered "to be a thread of an underlying meaning through, condensed meaning units, codes or categories, on an interpretative level" (p. 107).

For clarity, terms associated with content analysis as they related to this study and as described are identified:

- **Unit of Analysis** – 12 interviews, 6 with drawing and 6 without.
- **Meaning Units** – Passages/phrases/text from the interviews and individual drawings. Meaning units (transcripts and drawings) helped with the recognition of patterns or relationships among concepts extracted from the primary units of analysis (the interviews).
- **Codes** – Identified through comparison of "differences between and similarities within codes and categories" (Graneheim & Lundman, p. 111). Differences and similarities in the textual content resulted in identification of main categories and subcategories. These categories revealed the manifest content of the textual data. Textual data were reduced to remove irrelevant material or meaning units through condensation, a process of shortening the textual unit while still engaging the core of the relevance according to Graneheim and Lundman (2004). This occurred after reading and reviewing the transcripts in an effort to focus the textual analysis on material that was related to the research question. Once this was completed and codes were cross checked, aggregation and abstraction were conducted, leading to dominant codes/categories and themes. Coding allowed for meaning units to be understood with regard to the context. Codes were cross checked, and categories were reduced further and collapsed. Discussion of textual passages and corresponding codes contributed to consensus with regard to code affirmation as well as the discovery of additional codes/categories.
- **Categories** – Refer to "a descriptive level of content" and provided an "expression of the manifest content of the text" (Graneheim & Lundman, 2004).
- **Themes** – Derived from categories and are described as "a recurrent thread of underlying meaning running through codes and categories that are seen as an expression of the latent meaning of a text" (Thyme et al., 2013, p. 103) and can be subdivided. According to Graneheim and Lundman (2004), a theme is considered "to be a thread of an underlying meaning through, condensed meaning units, codes or categories, on an interpretative level" (p. 107).
- **Manifest Content** – Refers to the textual content and is reported in categories.
- **Latent Content** – Refers to the underlying meaning of the text (textual content) and is identified through the use of themes, which are "seen as expressions of the latent content that is, what the text is talking about" (Graneheim & Lundman, 2004, p. 111).

Dedoose

A cross platform application for analyzing qualitative and mixed-methods research, including textual and graphic data, to integrate and identify emergent patterns and trends.

Dedoose, a flexible, web-based subscription tool, was used to find meaningful insights through highlighting and coding text as well as imaginal data. Dedoose was originally designed for mixed-methods research by UCLA affiliates and is operated by SocioCultural Research Consultants (SCRC). It is considered an alternative to qualitative data analysis software and has been used for social science research. It is described as "[a] cross-platform application for analyzing qualitative and mixed methods research with text, photos, audio, videos, spreadsheet data and more" (www.Dedoose.com, 2017). Qualitative data analysis software programs offer a means of managing and ordering data associated with content analysis and afford new levels of analysis (Gerbic & Stacey, 2005).

Dedoose was used in this study to assist in the identification and acquisition of meaningful insights through highlighting units of analysis, which included words, phrases and or textual passages as well as imaginal data. Dedoose provided a platform for managing data "in a seamless manner". Similar to other computer-assisted software, Dedoose allowed for "browsing and exploration of themes as the ongoing analysis of transcripts continued" (Sullivan & Sheehan, 2016, p. 79.) Once coded, the text contributed to the identification of categories resulting in subthemes and overarching themes. For this study, the use of Dedoose assisted in analysis of the text by allowing for coding and categorizing textual and imaginal passages. This process involved reading/reviewing and re-reading/re-reviewing each transcript, which resulted additionally in the identification of two levels of content that emerged through this process: manifest and latent. Themes and patterns, as well as relationships between concepts, emerged from the interview transcripts (Shams et al., 2017).

Cross checking contributed to the process of coding and categorical itemization. The occasioned merging of codes, including both parent and child, contributed to the collapse of some codes. The aggregation led to the identification of overarching emergent categories and reduced the number of codes that ultimately converged into themes.

Data Analysis

Data analysis commenced after verbal and pictorial data were generated, collected and transcribed. The data were analyzed using content analysis (Elo & Kyngäs, 2008; Graneheim & Lundman, 2004; Henning et al., 2004; Thyme et al., 2013), which provided a structure for identifying codes, categories and themes. Themes were identified and synthesized, including textual and graphic data, in relation to the four phases of each interview process, allowing for the systematic organization of overarching themes.

Dedoose was used to integrate the data and identify emergent patterns and trends. A matrix of parent and subcodes was extracted from Dedoose following the coding of the original transcriptions. Through open and axial coding of the interview transcriptions, parent and subcodes were identified, leading to emergence of categories.

Working with categories was not restrictive in this sense. Systematic analysis was sought in this study, and the qualitative procedures were methodologically controlled (Mayring, 2000).

The imaginal data, along with the pre- and post-associations made by the children, were considered along with the memos written by the investigator. This process provided a method for understanding the pictorial data within the context of the research question and the instrument of study: the CIG. The unique blending of qualitative content analysis with art psychotherapy based upon the work of Thyme et al. (2013) provided a structural frame regarding how to approach the use of imaginal and textual data for this study. It guided the relationship between the participant's associations and the graphic depictions.

The codes or categories represented the manifest content of the data (Graneheim & Lundman, 2004) and contributed to the identification of overarching themes (the latent content) through a systematic comparison of the two conditions of the study: CIG with drawing and CIG without drawing. In an effort to compare the drawing condition to the nondrawing condition, the underlying mechanisms associated with the drawing effect were also considered. This provided a method for understanding the data within the context of the research question, as well as the instrument of study, the CIG.

Data, both textual and imaginal, was generated after participants watched two short animated videos about bullying with the investigator. Following the viewing of the two animated videos, the 12 study participants were interviewed about the content via the CIG either with or without drawing. Each interview was audio-taped and later transcribed verbatim by the investigator, resulting in the procurement of textual data. Through open coding, themes were identified (Schreier, 2012). Once the full transcripts were reviewed, irrelevant or extraneous material was bracketed and reduced. Parent codes and subcodes were identified, and the reduced transcripts were coded via Dedoose in an emergent process. Once a coding framework was devised, related codes were grouped together. Categories were selected and placed within the code frame. Codes and categories were checked to ensure that they captured the patterns and themes emerging from the data and to determine if they resonated with the research question.

Coding of the data led to construction of an unconstrained matrix that enabled flexibility and movement within categorization. Reading and review of the data, including interview transcripts (textual data), drawings (graphic or imaginal data) and reflective notes, were repeated in an effort to identify codes and categories, which contributed to the generation of themes. The process of analysis was complex and involved multiple reviews of the textual and graphic data. "A back-and-forth strategy" (Graneheim & Lundman, 2004, p. 103) and a process of review consisting of analysis involving "the whole and parts of the text" (p. 107) constituted the manner in which parent and child codes were determined and themes emerged. Phases of analysis for this study were derived from meshing various models of content analysis, as was previously described.

For clarity, terms associated with content analysis as they relate to the study (which were identified earlier) are reviewed here. The unit of analysis for the study consisted of 12 interviews: 6 with drawing and 6 without. Meaning units or codes helped with the identification of patterns or relationships and included passages, phrases or words as well as imagery. This in turn led to identification of main categories and subcategories.

Categories revealed the manifest content of the textual and graphic data. The method involved condensation, a process of shortening the textual unit while still engaging the core of the relevance (Graneheim & Lundman, 2004). This involved the reduction of data in an effort to remove irrelevant material or meaning units. This occurred after reading and reviewing the transcripts in an effort to focus the data analysis on material that was related to the research question. Once this was completed and codes were cross checked, aggregation and abstraction were conducted leading to the uncovering of dominant codes, subcategories and categories resulting in emergent themes. A theme was considered "to be a thread of an underlying meaning through, condensed meaning units, codes or categories, on an interpretative level" (Graneheim & Lundman, 2004, p. 107).

The text (textual data) or imagery (imaginal or graphic data) was considered to be the manifest content. The themes that derived from the manifest content (the data) were a reflection of the underlying meaning of the textual or graphic data and were construed as the latent content. The emphasis on manifest versus latent content factored into the study with regard to art therapy, wherein the manifest content is the collection of lines, shapes and colors, or what is visible, while the latent content is the underlying or symbolic meaning that gave rise to the manifest content.

Thyme et al. (2013) applied and described the use of qualitative content analysis within a psychodynamic art psychotherapy context in which the verbal associations that preceded and accompanied art making were analyzed. They concluded that qualitative content analysis is "a meaningful method for analyzing pictures and words from psychodynamic art psychotherapy sessions, keeping the manifest messages and the latent meanings in the pictures intact" (Thyme et al., 2013, p. 101). In summary, codes and categories were indicative of the manifest content of the data, while themes were evocative of the latent content of the data. The process of content analysis as utilized for this study is depicted accordingly.

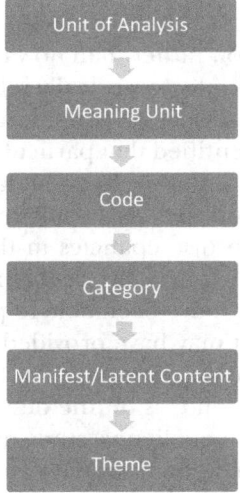

Figure 5.3 Process of content analysis utilized for this study (derived from Graneheim & Lundman, 2004 and Thyme et al., 2013).

In Summary

Verbal and imaginal data were collected from 12 school-aged children to explore how evidentiary disclosure of an experienced or witnessed event was influenced when drawing was incorporated as a primary resource in the capacity of an open-ended prompt in an investigative interview. Content analysis was used to provide a systematic means of assessing how a drawing strategy impacted an interview process when compared to a nondrawing interview process by providing a framework for organizing textual and graphic data. Codes, categories and themes emerged from synthesizing and analyzing the data in relation to the research question as well as the CIG.

Three overarching themes emerged from the data: fact-finding, imagery and relationality. These overarching themes will be identified, described, connected to the data and compared between the two research conditions (drawing and nondrawing interviews). They will also be related to the CIG and situated within the study question, given that the CIG is the instrument and object of study. The categories and codes that underlie and contributed to the themes will be considered as they evolved from the data analysis and with regard to forensic relevance. Comparison of the data that were uncovered between the two research conditions (CIG with drawing and CIG without drawing) is examined. Finally, the mechanisms that underlie the effect of drawing will be considered as they relate to the study findings. How these mechanisms contributed to recall and disclosure in the study will be considered.

Themes and Descriptive Findings

The descriptive qualities or the qualitative findings that emerged were examined in comparison to the quantitative or frequency of occurrence of codes provided via Dedoose. This information is discussed for comparative purposes between the drawing and nondrawing conditions as it relates to the themes and categories. Codes contributed to identification of categories, leading to the emergence of three major or overarching themes which were directly related to the CIG and indicate a correspondence with the process.

To note, the qualitative data yielded rich descriptive findings that were, on occasion, contrary to the quantitative data, as will be discussed. Differences were manifest in the way children described information rather than how many times they said something or through code frequency. For example, forensically relevant information such as facts or details may have been coded as appearing a certain number of times, giving the impression that nondrawing children identified that particular code more times than the drawing children. The drawing children provided qualitative descriptive information that may not have included information such as a name but instead was detailed or descriptive and may have contributed to discrepancies in the findings. Thus, the quant and the qual information may have revealed differences and on occasion conflicting findings. The nondrawing cohort may have been able to provide basic information about a fact; however, the drawing cohort may have provided descriptive qualities in a manner that was confirmatory and revelatory. Although the frequencies of occurrence will be referenced, the emphasis for the study is on the descriptive qualities or the qualitative findings that emerged as this was a qualitative study not mixed methods. Explanation is offered to clarify discrepancies between frequency and descriptive elements.

Theme: Fact-Finding

Fact-finding emerged as an overall theme from the study. Fact-finding as defined in this study was *elicitation of material or gathering of information relative to an experienced event.*

Fact-finding encompassed categories that were related to information gathering, including memory and recall, accuracy/inaccuracy and details. These categories, although distinct, overlapped as well.

The three categories that emerged from the data that were related to fact-finding are commensurate with research regarding investigative interviewing: memory and recall, accuracy/inaccuracy and details. Each of these categories factored into the literature review, given the emphasis on investigative interviewing, which fosters the elicitation of accurate and detailed information about experienced events from children (APSAC, 2002; Barlow et al., 2011; Carnes, 2000; Hoffman, 2005; Lamb & Brown, 2006; Macleod et al., 2013). The codes and categories that gave rise to fact-finding through the process of content analysis were reflective of forensic criteria that are evaluated in an investigative interview. Themes, definitions, categories and codes that emerged are discussed. Fact-finding encompassed the underlying principles affiliated with the CIG.

Fact-Finding Matrix

Theme	Category	Definition	Codes	Question
Fact-Finding	Memory and Recall of Information	The encoding, storage and recall of memory in image form	• who, what, where • person • place • activity • collateral material	How does drawing facilitate disclosure of experienced events of school-aged children in an art therapy–based investigative interview process when compared to a verbal investigative interview process?
	Accuracy/ Inaccuracy		• bully • victim • bystander • main character • supporting characters • setting	How does drawing enhance children's abilities to communicate accurate information pertaining to experienced events in an investigative interview?
	Details		• core vs. peripheral • idiosyncratic • contextual • situational	

Fact-Finding: Memory Recall and Accuracy

The study entailed facilitating elicitation of information as it related to the videos regarding bullying and antibullying strategies. Recall encompassed the ability to recollect information or facts about the videos by the participants. Memory and recall invoked encoding, storage and retrieval (or recall) of information or facts. Information that is considered forensically relevant within investigative interviews such as who (characters), what (activity) and where (setting/location), as well as collateral (additional or supportive) material, was elicited through open-ended questions or prompts.

Children in the drawing condition were invited to make a free drawing or drawings (drawing as an open-ended prompt or nondirected drawing) using the media (art materials) provided during the interview. Drawing was not relegated to a specific phase of the CIG; rather, the children were told that they could make a drawing or drawings while they talked with the investigator about the videos.

Recall was considered with regard to accuracy (whether the information was correct or precise) and inaccuracy (whether information was incorrect, imprecise or mistaken). Whether or not a participant was able to recall information that was accurate versus inaccurate was considered with regard to the particular interview condition. The interview condition, drawing or nondrawing was the descriptor used in deciphering the frequency of the codes (quantitative data) as per Dedoose.

The information from Dedoose revealed that inaccuracy was greater in the nondrawing interviews than in the drawing interviews. Accuracy as well as memory and recall were not as discrepant between the two interviewing conditions. How these terms were coded within the textual and graphic data may account for the findings. Accuracy within an investigative interview process is considered along a continuum, as is inaccuracy. The continuum includes mild, moderate and overt. A child may offer information that is seemingly accurate, but certain criteria may be omitted. For example, a physical description or a descriptive narrative of a character may be provided but the character's name may not be recalled. The material may be considered accurate but lacking in specificity. The frequency information is useful; however, the qualitative descriptions provided substantive data.

Fact-Finding: Accuracy: Strategies

In comparing and contrasting the qualitative or descriptive data with the frequency data, children who drew pictures used words that were consistent with those spoken in the video (episodic), whereas children who did not draw provided bits and pieces of general knowledge (script) about bullying. In addition, the nondrawing cohort tended to juxtapose elements from the videos, thus providing inaccurate responses, which may have contributed to the frequency data. For example, accuracy and inaccuracy were considered with regard to the strategies for handling bullying that were identified in the videos. Strategies for managing bullying were offered in the first video, and viewers were asked to select the correct answer from three choices. Three scenarios were enacted in the first video, and the narrator (McGruff) asked the viewer to make a selection with regard to how his nephew (the victim, Scruff) should handle the situation (bullying). The videos provided time for a response. McGruff described each vignette and offered an explanation why that particular strategy was or was not the best choice. Children in both the drawing and nondrawing condition provided the correct response (they knew what the narrator wanted the response to be from the three choices); however, the strategies that were taught and repeated throughout the videos were not recalled accurately by participants in the nondrawing group, as is reflected in the frequency data. The drawing cohort demonstrated accuracy of recall for the three strategies that were identified and repeated throughout the first video.

The main strategy that was emphasized in the video was "stop, talk and walk". The main character, McGruff, instructed his nephew in the first video, as well as Samantha (the victim) in the second video, how to respond to a bully. Essentially, McGruff explained that when confronted by a bully, a victim or someone who may potentially become a victim should tell the bully to stop bullying and then walk away to avoid further conflict. Children in the drawing condition accurately identified and explained the strategies presented in the videos.

In comparison, the nondrawing group demonstrated a tendency to reword or insert different words into the strategies. The following excerpts illustrate how children in both the drawing condition (odd numbers) and the nondrawing condition (even numbers) explained the identified strategies. P#2 stated that she could not remember it exactly. She offered, "walk, no talk" then she said, "wait, talk and walk". P#4 reported the strategy as "stop, talk, rock", referencing a school-based prevention strategy in which the students are advised to use rock, paper, scissors when trying to solve a conflict. P#6 indicated that he knew there were three strategies discussed in the first video, but he demonstrated difficulty recalling what they were. With regard to stop, talk, walk he stated the following, "walk, talk, rock; walk, stop, talk, rock; paper, scissors, walk, talk", before offering "wait, stop, talk, walk". P#10 reported that the strategy was "stop, talk, ignore".

Frequency Comparison Strategies

Strategies	Drawing	Nondrawing
Stop Talk Walk	65.3	34.7
Tell an Adult	78.8	21.2
Don't Bystand/Lend a Hand	54.5	45.5

Additionally, children in each condition related strategies that were similar but not the exact ones related in the video. P#5 stated, "Don't listen be yourself". P#6 provided, "If someone goes low you go high and do the right thing". P#8 said "Don't fight the bully". P#9 could recall all three strategies demonstrated within the video. P#12 said, "Can't fight. Have to find good things about people not the bad". The latter was a reference to a statement made by McGruff in the second video, which could have been interpreted to be a strategy (the participant merged the videos).

In an investigative process, interviewers typically are advised to consider alternative explanations for core disclosures (central or main ideas) in an effort to establish relevancy and credibility. In this instance, P#12's stated strategy could have been interpreted as a strategy offered by McGruff when he was speaking with the bully girls in the second video; however, this was offered as a pearl of wisdom rather than a specific strategy for addressing bullying.

Accurate information and details related to the strategies are depicted in the drawing by P#11. Her drawing, when juxtaposed with a still shot from the first video, shows her depiction of the strategy "don't bystand lend a hand". Although the drawing appears to be a linear depiction, in truth characters from both videos and strategies are included in the child's drawing. The drawing platform allowed for multiple pieces of information to be communicated at the same time, demonstrating the art therapy advantage identified by Wadeson (2010) known as spatial matrix. Through drawing, P#11 generated self-cues, which appeared to trigger recall of additional information related to the videos and the strategies. Self-generated cues contributed to increased verbalization and pictorial details.

Self-generated cuing was identified as an underlying mechanism contributing to the effect of drawing and accuracy. As the child drew, her narrative appeared to enhance her ability to recall and recollect information. Graphic elaboration seemed to contribute to enhanced verbalization as she demonstrated recall of more information. It was a cyclical process in that drawing seemed to stimulate recall of additional material, while verbalization contributed to enhanced recall both pictorially and verbally. Fact-finding was emergent as information was disclosed in the artwork in tandem with verbal elaboration. This was observed in drawings made by other participants.

In excerpts by the nondrawing children, general statements (script memory) or responses were offered about the strategies presented in the videos rather than details that were associated or congruent with the video content (episodic memory). For example (even numbers were assigned to nondrawing participants, odd numbers were assigned to drawing participants):

P#4   That you shouldn't be a bystander and if you are getting bullied you can just ignore them and think they'll just stop bullying because they're going to come back and bully again.

P#2   They said you should say something like, please stop and if that doesn't work then ignore them and if that doesn't work then tell the teacher.

P#2   McGruff, he says to walk. No talk. Wait, talk and walk.

Fact-Finding: Details: Core, Peripheral and Visual

Another subtheme related to fact-finding was details. Within investigative interviews details consist of core, peripheral, idiosyncratic, contextual, situational and visual. Details support disclosure, given that details provide referential material related to people/characters, actions and settings as well as help to situate and provide contextual information of experienced events. Uniqueness and relevance are also affiliated with details given the range of information communicated. This material spans a continuum that ranges from concrete (manifest) to idiosyncratic (unusual or peculiar in the sense that the detail is personalized in deference to an individual's experience of an event or a situation). How details manifest provides additional information with regard to a child's experience. Often details are considered with regard to determining credibility within a forensic process. Details including situational, contextual and visual (descriptive) provide information associated with an experience or a particular event.

For this study, details were considered to be aspects, elements or features relative to the main video content or threads related to the experienced event. Details were broken into descriptive subcategories, which were identified as core (major or primary), peripheral (minor or secondary), idiosyncratic (unique to the witnessed event as described by the child), contextual (related to the context of the event/experience) and situational (supportive or relative to the surroundings).

Contextual, situational and idiosyncratic details are considered peripheral (minor), while core (major) details are the main trends or ideas related to the experienced event. In this study, core details centered on bullying and the respective information imparted in the videos. Peripheral details for this study included secondary material or supportive information related to the core or central idea(s) or topic.

Frequency Comparison of Occurrence for the Subcategories of Details

Details	Drawing	Nondrawing
Core	56.3	43.8
Peripheral	63.2	36.8
Visual	77.4	22.6

The core (central theme) of the videos surrounded bullying; however, peripheral details or facts such as the number of bullies or victims and their names, as well as personal attributes, in addition to other elements were secondary. In an investigative interview, peripheral or secondary information related to an experienced event may change; however, core material typically remains constant. Facts or details including core, peripheral and idiosyncratic are evaluated and contribute to the establishment of credibility, a hallmark that is assessed in an investigative interview.

The frequency counts (quantitative data) suggest that the children in the drawing cohort disclosed more core, peripheral and visual details about the videos from the coded excerpts than the nondrawing group. Children who drew pictures that were directly related to the content of the videos depicted who, what, where or person, place and thing that was correspondent with the characters and situations depicted in the videos, including details pertaining to antibullying strategies that were presented. Additionally, information pertaining to main and supporting characters (anthropomorphized dogs) was provided, including actions/interactions, settings and the strategies for handling bullying and related situations.

Within an investigative or forensic context, what is disclosed, as well as whether or not the information can be corroborated, impacts assessment of accuracy. A child may be able to describe but not name a perpetrator. A child may be able to provide a physical description, which may support or contribute to additional investigative pursuits or decision making by investigators. Although idiosyncratic details are considered secondary information, these details are often compelling. This type of information may alert investigators or interviewers about personally meaningful information that is unique and specifically related to an experience that might otherwise not be known and hence disclosed. These distinguishing details may in fact yield significant information that may provide confirmation or corroboration of a personally meaningful event in a defining and revelatory manner that concretizes one's experience.

Idiosyncratic material is often unusual, peculiar or particular and not typical or common information; however, it is highly relevant and helps to situate an individual's personal experience. For example, P#6 asked why the characters that were dogs did not live in a dog house. He questioned why the video took place in a human dwelling instead of a doghouse. P#3 also referred to the main character McGruff entering the house via a doggie door which lifted up rather than walking in through a regular door. These details were not reported by all of the children. The children who did acknowledge them recalled from memory these details, since they were unique or remarkable in some way.

Continued exploration and study are advocated in the literature with regard to interview strategies in an effort to improve outcomes with regard to investigation and prosecution (Everson & Boat, 2002; Hiltz & Bauer, 2003). Analogous to an investigative context, the addition or disclosure of information or details whether idiosyncratic or common may be significant for fact-finding, which in turn may impact investigation and/or intervention. Drawing may provide collateral information, including situational and contextual material, that may direct further investigative pursuits or contribute to determination of charge enhancements (Cohen-Liebman, 1999, 2003; Gussak, 2013). A child may report a sensory reference such as seeing or hearing something that may not have been addressed. Sometimes a child may reveal a detail that manifests as a child provides information within the context of the interview that may not have been disclosed previously, such as the content of a television program or the use of force.

Reporting of such distinct details helps to crystalize meaningful and significant aspects of a personal experience. P#9 was able to describe her depiction of McGruff the Crime

Dog in explicit detail. She described McGruff as having his finger pointed up and waving it to emphasize what he was saying. Such details illustrate how distinct or particular information helps to situate an experience and personalize it, demonstrating forensic relevancy.

When data were coded in the study as core, peripheral or visual, details were more frequent in the drawing cohort as compared to the nondrawing cohort. Yet when details were coded individually for the characters in the videos such as main characters (for example, McGruff and Scruff, or secondary characters, including bullies), the frequencies yield different numbers. The quantitative aggregate data of the occurrence of detail categories and subcategories suggest a larger frequency of core, peripheral and visual details in the drawing group; however, when the details about characters are examined individually, comparatively, there was not a large divergence between the two conditions. This may be attributed to how these characters were identified by the children and subsequently coded.

Frequency Comparison of Occurrence for Individual Characters

Characters	Drawing	Nondrawing
Bully Girls	42.4	57.6
Mark	51.7	48.3
McGruff	46.2	53.8
Officer	50.7	49.3
Samantha	43.5	56.5
Scruff	53.9	46.1
Scruff's Friend	56.2	43.8

The responses of twin participants demonstrate how details were coded with regard to memory, recall and accuracy since one was assigned to the drawing cohort and one was not. Their verbalizations and the associations that accompanied the graphic depictions by the drawing twin provide additional illustration of script versus episodic memory and how that translated within the study. Both twins were verbal and communicative, more so after watching the videos. The drawing twin, while speaking about bullying, discussed strategies for handling bullying as described in the video and problem solving in relation to himself. He made two drawings, as he was not satisfied with his initial drawing, one on the front of the paper and one on the back. He identified his first drawing as a trampoline park. He said people were by themselves and just messing around. He then flipped the paper over and started to draw on the opposite side. He said that he was just drawing and could not figure it out. As he drew, he became increasingly animated as he discussed elements of the car in his drawing. He provided an organized and coherent narrative when drawing as he spoke about bullying strategies and prevention. He explained that drawing provided a means of maintaining his focus and his attention, and he expressed how this helps him to stay on target in class. His brother who did not draw (nondrawing condition), talked about bullying and how to stop it. He spoke about issues surrounding bullying, including how the topic is addressed at his school.

The nondrawing twin did not provide salient details regarding the videos and the characters unless the video content was referenced and then he related information tangentially. He was unable to offer concrete details and relate what he recalled from the videos to what he was saying. He spoke in more generalized terms about the topic (bullying) and offered more global thoughts about bullying rather than specifics from the two videos and the respective content in them. He demonstrated script memory rather than episodic memory, given that he discussed the topic in global terms rather than providing information related to the videos. He was difficult to re-engage about the videos, as he was preoccupied with describing the video game from which his Halloween costume derived. Visual details were used by him to describe his Halloween costume, which was what he focused his attention on as well as the corresponding video game. He was unable to generate cues to maintain focus and provide information relative to the experienced event. His associations were not organized, structured or detailed. With regard to forensic relevance, he did not provide core or central details that were related to the videos. He focused on tangential material that was aligned with his own experience and thinking with regard to bullying, which was rooted in general knowledge (script).

Fact-Finding and the Interview Process

Information that is gathered, be it core (central) or peripheral (secondary), as well as idiosyncratic (unique) data, was evaluated within the context of fact-finding. All of the information that is elicited in an investigative interview process is considered and contributes to understanding a child's experience. Through the process, details may be disclosed, such as additional participants or witnesses as well as secondary locations or interactions. Information that was not previously disclosed may emerge. The manner in which information is procured contributes to fact-finding, which is the primary objective of an investigative interview.

In comparing forensically relevant details across the two interview conditions, the drawing group appeared to provide more accurate information or episodic details that were specific to the videos. In comparison, information recalled by the nondrawing group appeared to be more consistent with general knowledge about bullying rather than directly related to the content of the videos. Out of the six children who drew, two made drawings that were directly related to the characters and the video scenes, including bully, victim and bystander, as well as the main character. The other four children made drawings that were related to the topic either indirectly or latently. Bullying was coded as latent in P#1's depiction of sharks and P#3's depiction of triumph over bad or evil as described in relation to his drawing of Simba the Lion King.

Children who did not draw were able to provide details regarding who, what, where and how, but oftentimes without including contextual, situational or collateral material unless asked to do so (in which information was more global in nature than specific to the video content, demonstrating script rather than episodic memory). If a child did communicate information related to the video content, accuracy was not consistent. One participant stated on more than one occasion that she had difficulty remembering things and said as a result she was unable to recall and remember details surrounding the videos and the strategies discussed.

P#9 drew the scene at the end of the second video where Samantha (victim) was trying to ignore the bullies in her ballet class. P#9 explained that the victim was trying to let the bullies know they weren't doing a good job bullying her. She proceeded to draw the girls and Scruff (main character's nephew) in ballet class. As she described what she remembered from the video while she was drawing, she added McGruff (the main character) to her drawing and stated that he was waving his finger and saying, "You shouldn't bully". P#9 said drawing made it easier for her to explain what she remembered and what she was trying to communicate. As she drew, she acted out (kinesthetically) what the characters did, which appeared to stimulate recall of additional details. Drawing provided a means of self-cuing.

P#11 stated with regard to the first video, "He was hurting him" (bully dog to victim dog). "I saw him throw a dodge ball at his head" (bully dog to Scruff). This was a description of what the bully in the first video did to the main character's nephew. By describing the use of the ball, the child provided details that situated the event beyond a mere description of bullying or a generalized or preconceived idea that was script based (rooted in general knowledge). The child provided additional supportive material that was situational as well as contextual in conjunction with her verbalizations. This was demonstrative of episodic memory in that it related directly to the event or episode under discussion.

Investigative interviews are predicated upon the procurement of facts. Although sometimes children may not be able to provide definitive information such as the proper name of a perpetrator (in this analogue the characters), often descriptive material may be revealing and fruitful for investigative purposes. It is interesting to note how children identified characters in their narratives. For example, descriptive identification was provided by the participants when they were unable to identify a character by name

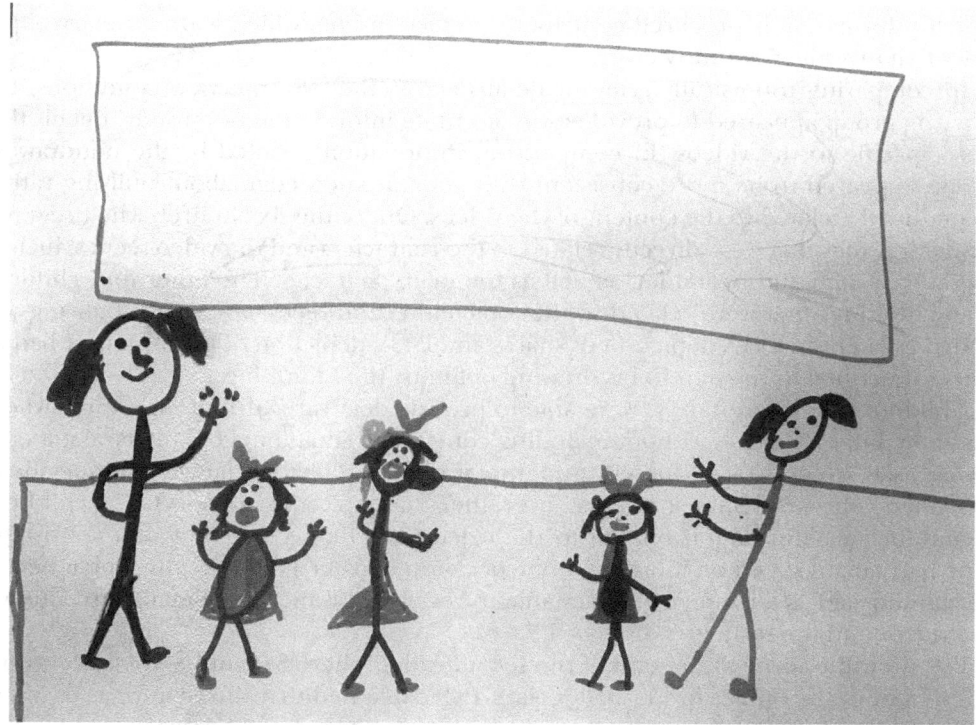

Figure 5.4 Drawing entitled "The Crazy Day of Ballet", featuring a scene from the second video where characters are in a ballet class and McGruff has his finger in the air as he tells them, "You shouldn't bully".

such as McGruff. McGruff was identified by 11 of the 12 children either descriptively or by name. McGruff was characterized in a host of different ways by the children in both conditions. P#2 described him as the one who solves problems or the grandfather. He was the spy dog according to P#3. He was given the title of Crime Detective Dog by P#6, while P#7 called him the Crime Dog. P#8 said he was the uncle. P#9 said he was a crime-solving dog. P#10 explained that she did not remember his name but she described him as a boxer (dog). P#1 did not identify or describe McGruff; however, he made a statement alluding to who McGruff was and what he does while discussing his drawing of sharks. He said that sharks (bullies) could learn from McGruff "not to eat their young". Four participants, two from each condition (P#4, P#5, P#11, P#12), used his name, McGruff, when referring to him. In relation to fact-finding, specific or concrete information such as a name of an individual (for instance, a perpetrator or a witness) may not be disclosed for a myriad of reasons by children in investigative interviews. Rather, facts may be conveyed in a descriptive manner, which contributes to assessment of forensic relevance such as how the children described the main character, McGruff, in the study. Physical description may aid in identification of an individual when a child is unable to provide a name of a particular person.

As noted, however, McGruff was identified in different ways. The descriptions offered by the children provided a myriad of descriptors congruent with McGruff's character, his personality and his physical presentation. Despite the inability to refer to him by his actual name, the descriptors were indicative of who the participants were referencing. In an investigative interview, facts and details are sought in an effort to glean accurate and factual information that is forensically relevant. The information contributes to credibility as well as corroboration of a child's statements. A child may not recall particular information such as a name or a location; however, they may be able to communicate referential material that is consistent with the allegations and congruent with establishing forensic relevancy. This information contributes to understanding the child's experience and facilitates the fact-finding process.

With regard to fact-finding, researchers have determined that it is important to understand whether drawing facilitates recall in and of itself or if recall is related to schemas or scripts when deciphering the information disclosed by a child (Davison & Thomas, 2001). The study findings suggested that the use of drawing as an open-ended prompt helped facilitate recall of episodic memory (event specific). When compared to recall facilitated without drawing (nondrawing condition), information appeared to be reflective of script memory, meaning that what the children reported after viewing the videos was related to schemas or general knowledge rather than the information from the videos about bullying and antibullying strategies.

Given the nature of the investigative process and adherence to forensic standards, the categories that were identified as contributory to fact-finding resonated with how information pertaining to experienced events was conveyed within the interview process. Although discussed independently in the findings section, these categories overlapped. Accuracy (whether the information was correct or precise) and inaccuracy (whether information was incorrect, imprecise or mistaken) were considered with regard to the details communicated by the children. The data analysis revealed that inaccuracy was greater in the nondrawing condition as compared to the drawing condition. In the category of accuracy, memory and recall frequencies or word counts were less discrepant between the two study conditions; however, the nondrawing group demonstrated a slightly higher frequency of occurrence with regard to accuracy and memory/recall. The discrepancy, which is open to interpretation and may be related to the manner in which material was coded, presents differently when the qualitative or descriptive data are considered. For example, this was apparent with regard to how children were able to identify characters. In some instances, the children who drew provided descriptions of characters to designate whom they were referring to rather than the actual name identification. Within the context of investigative interviewing, this poses an interesting conundrum with regard to forensic relevancy and the notion that a forensic process seeks to elicit information that is accurate and detailed (APSAC, 2002; Barlow et al., 2011; Carnes, 2000; Hoffman, 2005; Lamb & Brown, 2006; Macleod et al., 2013; Poole & Lamb, 2009). Information coded for forensic relevance demonstrated that although a child might have been unable to provide a name, an accurate description of the character may have been offered. How accuracy is determined plays a role within the realm of an investigation when identity and relationships (such as between perpetrator and victim) need to be established. Just because a child may not be able to provide the proper name of someone, an accurate and detailed physical description may help establish to whom the child is referring and may impact investigation and other outcomes.

Another category associated with fact-finding was memory and recall. This category is directed at encoding, storage and retrieval (or recall) of information or facts. In the study, recall of information was elicited through open-ended questions or prompts (including drawing). Research studies directed at assessing children's responses to open-ended prompts in addition to focused prompts reveal that free prompts elicited enhanced information and accuracy while decreasing suggestibility (Lamb et al., 2008; Lyon et al., 2012). The literature suggested that the use of open-ended prompts and questions within a forensic investigative interview format is the preferred method to acquire accurate information and evidentiary disclosure from school-aged children (Jolley, 2010; Lamb et al., 2008). Open-ended questions are thought to access free recall memory, which is thought to be more accurate, whereas focused or directed questions activate retrieval processes that may be more prone to error (Lamb et al., 2008, 2011). As such, researchers tend to agree that free recall and spontaneous remarks tend to be accurate responses as opposed to responses to direct inquiries (Hritz et al., 2015).

Accuracy is important with regard to the information or memories elicited (Macleod et al., 2013); however, accuracy is difficult to establish in field studies as compared to analogue studies since variables are unknown. Responses to open-ended questions, however, are likely to be more accurate than responses to focused prompts, as identified by various studies discussed in the literature review (Orbach et al., 2000; Sternberg et al., 1997; Sternberg et al., 2001). The data supported the various contentions from the literature that responses to open-ended questions were more likely to be accurate. This also extended to the use of open-ended prompts in the form of drawing in which accuracy was determined to be qualitatively demonstrated within the study.

The different ways in which the data lent itself to analysis may have contributed to discrepancies in the findings with regard to descriptors (qualitative) versus frequency of occurrence (quantitative). The qualitative data yielded rich descriptive findings. Taken singularly, frequencies may have been recorded or coded such that they indicated that the nondrawing children were providing more accurate information. Differences were manifest in the way children described information rather than how many times they said something (code frequency). The drawing children, however, provided descriptive information that was identified as relevant and accurate despite the lack of specified information such as a proper name. The nondrawing cohort provided basic information that was related to the context (bullying in general), whereas the drawing cohort provided information that was specifically related to the content of the videos. In comparing and contrasting the qualitative or descriptive data with the frequency data (word counts), children who drew pictures used words that were consistent with those spoken in the video (episodic), whereas children who did not draw provided bits and pieces of general knowledge (script) about bullying. In addition, the nondrawing children juxtaposed elements from the two videos, thus providing inaccurate responses. Children in the drawing condition accurately identified and explained the strategies presented in the videos pertaining to intervention and prevention. In comparison, the nondrawing group demonstrated a tendency to reword the strategies or offer personalized points of view about the topic that were unrelated to the video content.

For the study, details were considered to be aspects, elements or features relative to the video content. Details were broken into descriptive subcategories, which were identified as core (major or primary), peripheral (minor or secondary), idiosyncratic (unique to the witnessed event as described by the child), contextual (related to the context of the event/experience), situational (supportive or relative to the surroundings) and visual. In this study, core details were related to the main threads of the video, while peripheral details encompassed secondary material or supportive information related to core or central material.

The frequency counts (quantitative data) suggest that the children in the drawing cohort disclosed more core, peripheral and visual details about the videos from the coded excerpts than the nondrawing group. Children who drew pictures that were directly related to the content of the videos depicted who, what, where or person, place and thing that was correspondent with the characters and situations depicted in the videos (for example, P#9 and P#11), including details pertaining to antibullying strategies that were presented. Additionally, information pertaining to main and supporting characters (anthropomorphized dogs) was provided, including actions/interactions, settings and the strategies for handling bullying and related situations. So, when data were coded as core, peripheral or visual, details were more frequent in the drawing cohort as compared to the nondrawing cohort. Yet when individually coded for certain details such as the characters in the videos, the frequencies yielded different information. The data revealed that children in both of the study conditions provided information about the experienced event; however, inaccuracy was higher in the nondrawing cohort.

Overall, some findings in the study pertaining to accuracy quantitatively may have indicated higher counts in relation to the nondrawing study condition. The findings from a descriptive perspective (qualitative data versus frequency or quantitative information) revealed that the drawing condition provided more specific information or forensically relevant material such as strategies and information including core, peripheral and idiosyncratic details. The need to evaluate how accuracy and inaccuracy are defined and identified within investigative interviewing is suggested, given the findings may have demonstrated ambiguity depending upon the type of data collected and the manner in which information was disclosed. Had word counts not been addressed or quantitative information provided via Dedoose, the findings would have been exclusively rooted in a descriptive format or qualitative context.

Theme: Imagery

For purposes of the study, imagery included pictorial representation (a picture or a drawing in image form) as well as mental visualization (a mental image) or the depiction of something (such as a physical object). Images were used as representational devices (for people, places, things, etc.). Categories that contributed to the identification of imagery as a theme include symbolism and metaphor. Both factored into the use of imagery for the two study conditions (drawing and nondrawing). Manifest and latent content were considered with regard to pictorial depiction, as well as with regard to content analysis, as previously described by Graneheim and Lundman (2004).

Imagery Matrix

Theme	Category	Definition	Codes
Imagery			
	Symbolism	mental images, likenesses of things such that images are used as representational devices for items, elements, like people, places, things, etc.	pop culture heroes association to movies/ television characters
	Metaphor	a figure of speech that implies comparison between two things or a resemblance, albeit not a literal translation	animals people villains
	Visualization	the use of internalized or mental images	imagery
	Manifest Content	collection of lines, shapes, colors, etc. (what is depicted)	representational imagery
	Latent Content	underlying meaning of the manifest content, hidden or symbolic meaning	symbolic meaning

Imagery: Mental Visualization: Popular Culture

Visualization was utilized by children in both of the study conditions. Visualization, whether mental or graphic, seemed to stimulate memory and recall, resulting in verbal elaboration in both cohorts. Recall and memory seemed to be reliant upon mental images, which were either communicated linearly, in verbal description, or through the use of graphic imagery, which allowed for nonlinear disclosure. At times, confirmation of verbal statements was made through graphic depiction. The use of metaphor as well as symbolism was prominent in the graphic depictions and the associations made by both the drawing (P#1, P#3, P#5, P#7, P#9, P#11) and nondrawing cohorts (P#4, P#6, P#10, P#12). Children in both assignments utilized visual images, whether mental or graphic, that demonstrated an association with bullies or iconic figures either from popular culture or other sources such as movies or books.

Within both cohorts of the study, children referenced characters, both animated and not animated, from movies, books and television as examples of bullying or bullies. This in turn contributed to children's abilities to interpret the information from the videos and apply it to their own appreciation of prevention and intervention. References were utilized by the children with regard to known entities or bullies such as Nazis (P #4), characters from the Rocky movies (P#7), Disney characters (P #3) and other iconic and known entities. For example, P#3 explained that Pete from Disney cartoons is basically the bullying friend.

Children in the nondrawing group used mental visualization or mental imagery to describe the videos and associated references to bullying. The children also utilized references to popular culture as a means of assimilating intervention and prevention with regard to bullying. They discussed how various characters managed bullying. For example, P#4 identified Nazis as bullies and explained that in a book he is currently reading, "[T]he Nazis are attacking two people and two 11-year-olds stopped it (their vehicle) with tacks". He continued by saying, "They took a big risk to throw tacks at tires and a lot of them (the Nazis) just stopped the trucks".

An example of the use of drawn imagery to describe bullying and to enhance recall and memory is illustrated through P#9's drawing and her narrative. P#9 said that she uses (mental) imagery to retain and recall information (Image V-5). She demonstrated this by showing how imagery helped her to remember math problems and how to solve them. She discussed that the use of media and drawing helps her to remember information. P#9 stated, "Art is something you can do to get your mind off of stuff and you can go free and wild with whatever you want to draw and you can draw anything". She said that drawing helped her to remember a few things like the main characters from the videos. She titled her drawing "The Crazy Day of Ballet". She explained that drawing helped her to remember more stuff from/about the videos. She explained that she was able to remember more details relating to what happened once she began to draw. This child offered that she has a theory that helps her remember, and she explained it in the following way, "It's like a camera in my brain and I take pictures and memorize stuff and then I remember".

This child spoke to the use of imagery to recall and remember information. She drew and then physically re-created or acted out what she remembered, enabling her to recall more and more details, which were then incorporated pictorially in her drawing. She demonstrated a connection between drawing and recall/memory, which seemed to be sensorial and kinesthetically based. Drawing helped her tap into encoded information, stimulating recall. As she drew, drawing seemed to trigger recovery of memory, which she acknowledged in her associations. Her description resonated with the use of mental imagery or internal visualization, which was externalized in pictorial form. Drawing appeared to promote the uncovering of additional information, which she expressed verbally, demonstrated kinesthetically and conveyed imaginally.

In comparison, children who were in the nondrawing cohort talked and at times would get up and walk around to discharge energy, yet this process did not seem to impact their verbalizations with regard to richer disclosure of information related to the videos. P#6, for example, had difficulty remaining seated and seemed to get distracted. While movement seemed to ground P#9, it provided a means of distilling anxiety and maintaining impulsivity for P#6 as well as P#8, who was easily distracted. He displayed difficulty remaining on task and staying focused.

Imagery: Symbolism and Metaphor

Symbolism and metaphor both factored into the theme of imagery. In the study, reliance upon mental images, or likenesses of things whether pictorial or visual, was apparent. In essence, images were used as representational devices by the participants in both conditions to connote people, places or things. Popular culture provided a means of representation for participants and included heroes or antiheroes (bullies). Associations were made to television and movie characters or personas as being symbolic of good or bad, such as the *Lion King* (P#3). Metaphor for this study was used as a figure of speech, which implied comparison between two things or a resemblance, albeit not a literal translation. For example, this was seen in the use of animals, specifically sharks (P#1), an owl (P#5) and people (Disney characters P#3).

P#3 explored the media while he talked. He initially denied having any idea what he was depicting. He spoke about various figures from popular culture and referenced other visual imagery. He discussed movies that addressed bullying or had bullies in them, including the Back to the Future trilogy. He spoke about each of the bullies in the three films and their various relationships in the three movies. He discussed Disney characters and spoke about Simba. For the latter, he discussed how good triumphs over evil. He offered that his drawing (Image V-6) "kind of looks like Simba the Lion". Although the manifest content (lines, shapes, colors) of his drawing appeared somewhat abstract, the latent content was articulated through his associations. Despite saying he did not know what he was drawing, his verbalizations centered around bullying and bullies from popular culture. He also discussed the implicit messages he derived from the Lion King.

Juxtaposing his drawing with a classic scene from *The Lion King* where Simba is perched on an overhang, the images are similar in composition, although P#3 is an abstraction. As P#3 remarked, "Simba, like the main character in the videos, McGruff, helped problem solve and address bullying". Drawing helped P#3 stay on task and maintain focus. He provided a rich and descriptive narrative. Characters from *The Lion King* were used metaphorically by him as well as symbolically. He discussed details from the videos and translated them into a context that was image based. P#3 stated with regard to his picture, "It looks like when the Lion, when Simba starts singing, I just can't wait to be King and everything just turns rainbow".

Drawing helped P#1 to problem-solve and make meaning through the use of metaphor, as gleaned from his drawing and accompanying associations. While talking about bullying,

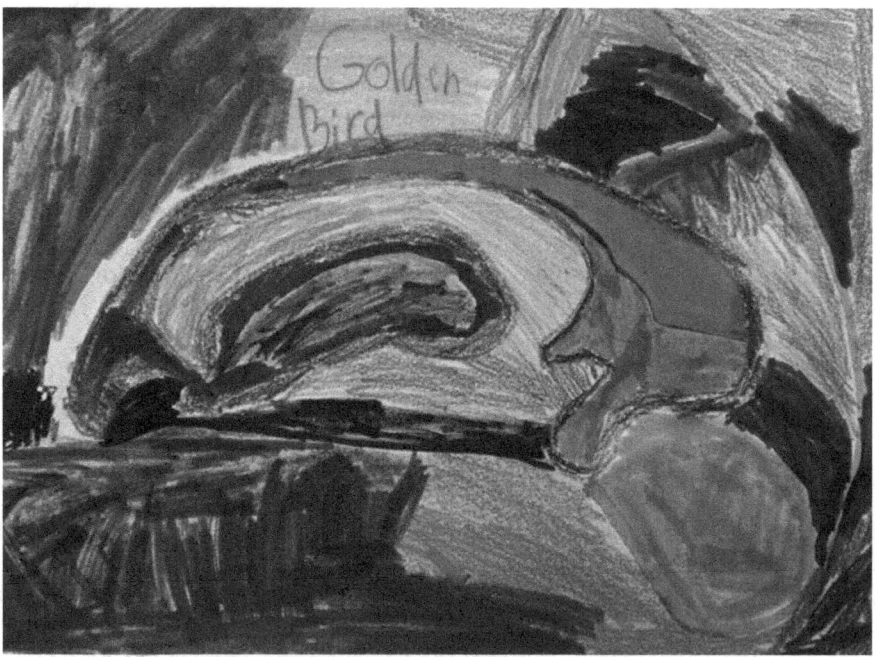

Figure 5.5 P#3's drawing entitled "Golden Bird" which depicts Simba, the Lion King. The child used the Disney character metaphorically and symbolically to discuss the messages pertaining to antibullying strategies from the videos.

he drew a shark with a fish in its mouth (Figure 5.6). He continued to draw and made what he identified as a family of sharks. Although he spoke about sharks as his thing to draw when he does not know what to draw, he discussed how sharks eat their young while discussing the theme of bullying. He connected the video content to his drawing and the drawing to the video content. P#1 stated, "When sharks are born, they have to watch out because their parents like to eat them. Their mother likes to eat them. It's almost like their mom shark is a bully. Sharks could learn from McGruff not to eat their young".

The latent or symbolic content of his drawing was indicative of the topic under discussion (bullying). He spoke about his need to fill up sketch books and make drawings when he is bored. Although initially reluctant to explain why he sketches, he did offer that sketching makes him happy, speaking to the use of imagery and mental visualization. He explained that sketching keeps him from acting out on his impulses. He provided the correct strategy (as requested by the main character in deference to the choices presented) for bullying as offered in the first video. He spoke about the characters in the videos and the theme of bullying as he communicated his knowledge about sharks. He provided a rich narrative that accompanied his drawing. He titled his drawing, "The Weird Seas". He described it as a happy picture that included mama (big shark in the middle) little brother and dad (eating), as well as a little sister and a big brother.

The children who drew pictures as well as the nondrawing children relied upon imagery with regard to identifying bullying and defining it. Imagery, whether mentally visualized or graphically depicted, provided a method for expressing and communicating for the children the experienced event (the videos and bullying, including strategies, messages and behavioral interactions). Imagery appeared to aid with recall and recovery of encoded/stored memory.

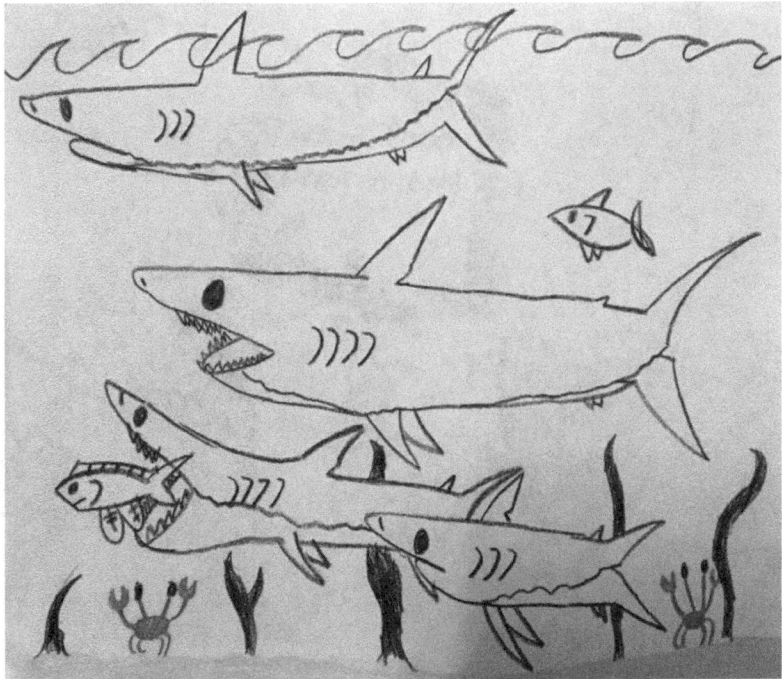

Figure 5.6 Drawing of a family of sharks by P#1, which was related to the video content through metaphor, symbolism and latent content.

Imagery: Manifest and Latent Content

The concepts of manifest and latent factored into the study with regard to imagery as well as the coding process. Content analysis, as described by Graneheim and Lundman (2004), conceptually addresses two levels of meaning through the process of categorizing: overt, or the manifest content, and the covert or latent content which is indicative of the symbolic or underlying meaning (affiliated with the manifest content). Imagery also exists on two levels: manifest and latent. The manifest content is the overt or visible content, while the latent content is covert, or the underlying (symbolic) meaning of the manifest content. As was discussed, Thyme et al. (2013) blended qualitative content analysis with art psychotherapy. Their model provided a frame of reference for the use of imaginal and textual data for this study that included the relationship between the participant's associations and their graphic depictions. Thyme et al. (2013) concluded that qualitative content analysis is "a meaningful method for analyzing pictures and words from psychodynamic art psychotherapy, keeping the manifest messages and the latent meanings in the pictures intact" (p. 101).

Children who drew tended to situate information (fact-finding) within the story lines of the videos. Manifest content revealed themes related directly to the videos in some drawings, with latent identification discernible in others. Dedoose provided a snapshot with regard to how manifest and latent content were coded within the study. The data revealed higher frequencies in the drawing condition than in the nondrawing condition. The latent content was indicative of the topic of bullying (P#1, P#3, P#7) in some of the drawings as noted.

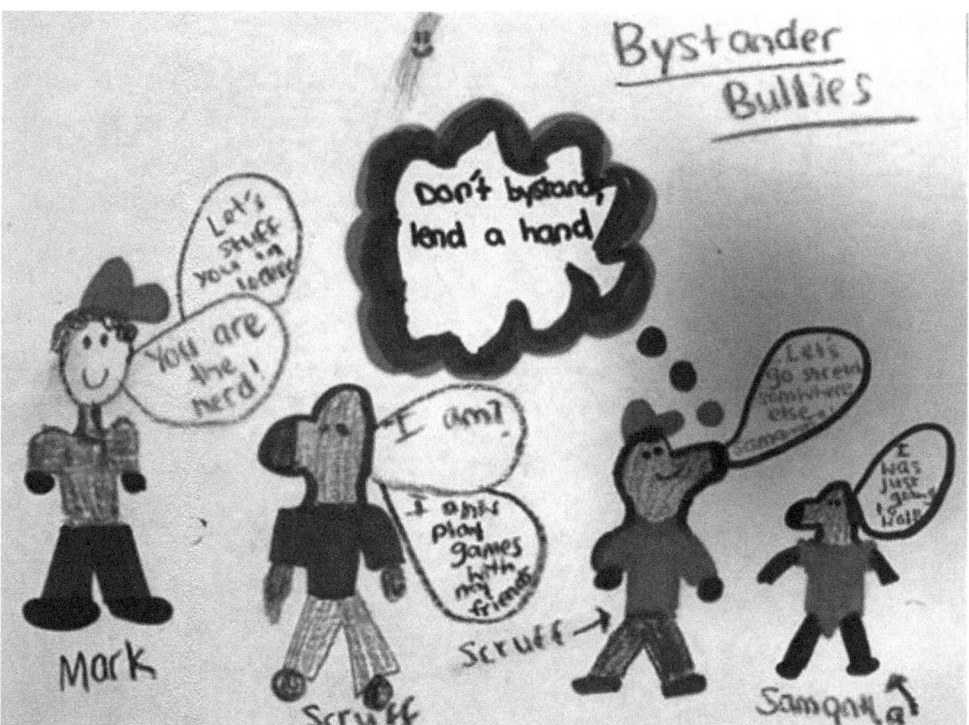

Figure 5.7 Drawing entitled "Bystander Bullies", which depicts the bullies and their words as well as antibullying strategies that were discussed in the video.

Frequency Comparison for Manifest and Latent Content

Manifest and Latent Content	Drawing	Nondrawing
Content (manifest) related to topic	63.2	36.8
Content (manifest) related to video	60	40
Content (latent) related to bullying	68.2	31.8

Participants self-directed with regard to the content of their drawings. As has been noted in various excerpts, children provided direct references to bullying as well as latent messages both through verbalizations and in drawings and through the use of imagery, whether pictorial or visual. The content of the drawings was at times overt, while at others it was symbolically contained within the context of the graphic depictions. Manifest content also was present in each interview, and latent messages were communicated verbally throughout the interviews in tandem with what children discussed and/or disclosed. As has been noted in various excerpts, children provided direct references to bullying as well as the video content. At times the covert or latent content was symbolically expressed.

Imagery was an overarching theme identified from the analysis of the data. Children in both cohorts utilized visual images, whether mental or graphic, that demonstrated an association with bullies or iconic figures either from pop culture or other sources such as movies or books, video games and other known sources. Imagery provided the context for disclosure of material associated with the topic. Categories that contributed to this theme included symbolism, metaphor and visualization. The concepts of manifest and latent, which were identified within fact-finding, emerged here as well. For purposes of this study, imagery included pictorial representation (a picture or a drawing in image form) as well as mental visualization (a mental image) or the representation of something in one's mind (such as a physical object). Images were used as representational devices for people, places, things, etc.

Overall, imagery and visualization factored into both the drawing and nondrawing interviews. Imagery was used as a means to convey and communicate information regardless of the study condition. Children who drew used imagery as a means of disclosing information, while those who were assigned to the nondrawing condition seemed to use mental imagery or visualization as a means of conveying information as well. Both cohorts seemed to rely upon imagery/visualization as a method for providing examples, whether metaphorically, symbolically or congruently, with regard to bullying. Children in the drawing condition were invited to use drawing as an open-ended prompt, meaning they could respond as they chose and depict images freely. Directives were not provided regarding the use of drawing. The media (art materials) served to foster expression regardless of whether it was representational, as demonstrated by P#1, P#5, P#7, P #9, P#11 or abstract, as with P#3.

Even though the children may not have initially been aware of what they were going to draw (as stated by P#7, P3# and even P#1), each had a story or a narrative to accompany their drawings. The use of drawing within the investigative interview process allowed for imaginal communication. The use of open-ended prompts seemed to support the procurement of narratives by the children. Imagery provided a means of gaining access to preverbal memory, which is correspondent to the encoding of traumatic memory (Hinz, 2009; Lusebrink, 1990). Memory is contingent upon sensory encoded knowledge, which is intrinsic to an art therapy–based interview process. Thus, children may have accessed or uncovered information through drawing because imagery taps into preverbal ways of knowing and allows for retelling in a manner that is developmentally congruent and consistent with the encoding of experience (Hinz, 2009; Lusebrink, 1990). As previously discussed, the risks associated with revealing event-specific information may be lessened through the use of drawing, especially when disclosing information relative to a sensory-based crime (such as sexual abuse).

Theme: Relationality

Relationality emerged as an overarching theme from the study. Learning and application, meaning making and self/other are the categories that contributed to the emergence of relationality. This theme resonated also with the dialogical relationship, which underlies the CIG. Each of the categories for relationality was dependent upon a relational component. It was through the exchange of information or conversational patterns between the interviewer and the children that meaning making took place as well as learning and application. The exchange of ideas led to application of learned information such as understanding of the strategies offered with regard to managing bullying. Problem solving and meaning making were contingent upon the dialogue or the transfer of information that occurred through a child's associations or narrative, as well as through graphic depiction, which was elaborated upon through descriptive measures. This was a factor with regard to self/other and awareness. Participants were able to relate what they experienced or what they learned from the videos with regard to the scenarios they witnessed and then transfer that knowledge or understanding through a relational process.

The children related personal narratives or stories that resonated with the video content, promoting awareness of interactive behaviors between self and other in response to bullying. Several of the children in both of the interview conditions were able to demonstrate awareness of self and other(s) with regard to how they had experienced bullying in their own lives in various settings: educational or other domains. The following table breaks out the categories and their respective definitions as well as the codes.

Relationality Matrix

Theme	Category	Definition	Codes
Relationality	Learning and Application	prevention/intervention (school-based message)	• bullying • definition • reference to self/others
		strategies	• stop, talk, walk • lend a hand • don't bystand
	Meaning Making	problem solving	• personal experience • narrative • application to self
	Self/Other	self-awareness	• relating video to self

Relationality: Meaning Making, Learning and Application, Self/Other

The categories that contributed to relationality are interrelated and will be explored together. Meaning making is a process that enables one to make sense of things. Examples of meaning making were demonstrated by children in both cohorts. Meaning making was a common denominator among the children. For example, P#4 offered that the videos were good because they teach a lot of life lessons like bullying "could happen at any time and if someone comes up to you and says something not very nice you have to defend yourself and use the skills from the video". As previously described under imagery, P#1's drawing helped him to problem-solve and make meaning through the use of metaphor (sharks as bullies).

Some of the children's statements are applicable to more than one category and theme. P#11 spoke about school-based prevention strategies and made connections to bullying in real life through the use of narrative, as well as imagery. She demonstrated problem solving by relating prevention strategies to her own life. P#5 was very engaged with drawing and demonstrated perfectionistic tendencies (which she also discussed verbally). She was very detail oriented. She spoke about a positive role model, her teacher. In her drawing she depicted her school mascot. The school mascot (owl) was emblematic of the virtues and strengths of her teacher. Although the manifest content may not directly relate to the videos, the latent content resonated with what she described as "the seven strengths to help prevent bullying". She described learning these ideologies at school and from her teacher as part of the curriculum, which was indicative of a school-based antibullying and prevention initiative. Fundamentally, the use of graphic depiction appeared to provide a way for her to make meaning from the videos or the experienced event, which is consistent with learning and application. Contextually, she drew an image that bridged what she knew (meaning making) as well as how she learned it (application and learning), and she related the school-based programming to the videos. Thus, there seemed to be a reciprocity and mutuality that emerged from talking and drawing for P #5 that extended beyond herself to the picture and included the interviewer and self. It was a cyclical process that necessitated interaction with another, given that interviews happen in a relationship that has a corresponding influence on the process.

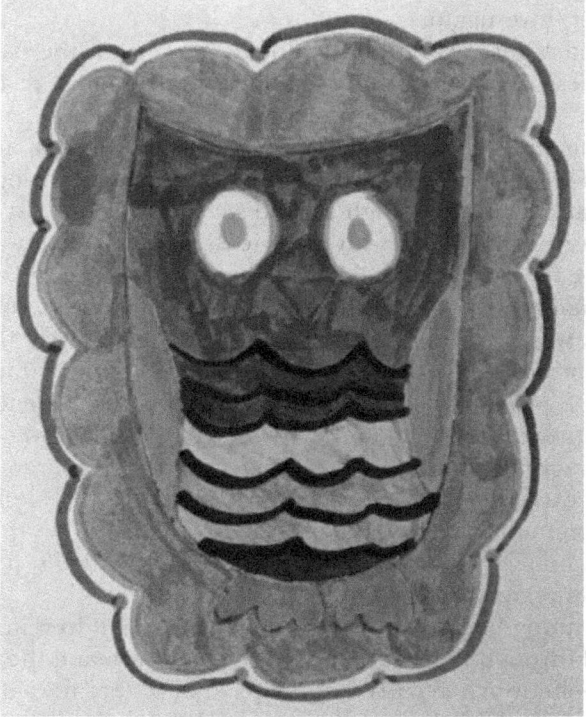

Figure 5.8 School mascot, owl is emblematic of the theme and categories as child's associations reflect meaning making, learning and application and self/other.

The interview relationship creates an intersubjective matrix, which is a relational milieu that encompasses the interviewer and the child. This concept refers to the conditions between two or more people, such as the level of consciousness existent between them (Skaife, 2001). Relationality was attributed to the interactive patterns and dialogue that was witnessed and observed regardless of the study condition. Pictorial description/depiction also fostered the dialogical or interactive piece of the process, which was ongoing throughout the interview process and is a hallmark of the CIG.

As children talked and drew, they depicted increased or perhaps enhanced details, which led to the disclosure of additional information indicating a relational element between drawing and talking. This was apparent in relation to the dialogical component of the interview process, which is related to self/other. This existed not only between the investigator and the children in a linear configuration (talk) but also in a circular relationship between drawing and talking. Drawing led to disclosure, and disclosure led to an increase in graphic details, which contributed to more information being recalled and disclosed. A symbiotic relationship between drawing and verbal associations was identified. A process of discovery emerged through the relational aspect that ensued between talking and drawing. There was a dependency one upon the other that motivated recall, which prompted uncovering and enhanced depiction or disclosure of information graphically and verbally.

Essentially, a pattern of movement between talking and drawing seemed to occur as graphic details gave rise to enhanced verbalization, and enhanced verbalization resulted in more elaborate pictorial details. Making meaning of art or images has been described as "a dynamic practice that can be described by three processes: cyclical, relational and personal" (Curtis, 2011, p. 9). These processes are congruent with the foundational principles of the CIG and were apparent in the interactions between the participants and the interviewer/investigator.

Relationality fosters interaction and dialogue, given that the CIG is an interactive and dynamic process. The categories were dependent upon a relational component. It was through the exchange of information or conversational patterns between the interviewer and the children that meaning making took place in addition to learning and application. These processes were contingent upon the dialogue or the transfer of information that occurred through a child's associations or narrative and with the drawing condition in conjunction with graphic depiction, which was elaborated upon through descriptive measures. This all factored into self/other and awareness as well.

Overall, relationality was correspondent with the dialogical component inherent in the CIG, which was apparent in both of the study conditions. One of the underlying foundational principles of the CIG is the idea of connectedness such that there is engagement in a process. The relationship piece is fundamental and intrinsic to the CIG, which is process oriented and contributes to facilitation of information. The relationship component within the CIG is critical to the procurement of fact-finding. Information is uncovered through imagery created in a dialogical process in which verbalization is concomitant (Cohen-Liebman, 2016). Disclosure in this context is identified as a "fundamentally dialogical process" (Jensen et al., 2005) in which fact-finding occurs within the interview relationship.

Examples of meaning making were demonstrated by children in both cohorts. This was acknowledged through the associations of the children and the patterns of interaction and engagement, which occurred in a myriad of different ways through emergent manifest and latent, symbolic and metaphoric and linear and nonlinear content. Prevention and intervention were concepts that were applied as a result of self-learning or through application via the interactive dimension of the process. Children disclosed information and discussed application of intervention and prevention strategies with regard to self and others as this pertained to the videos and with regard to the study context. This was not intended to be representative of sustainable change since this was not an intervention, but rather a component of this study. This information was communicated via engagement with the interviewer and was enhanced through the use of drawing with regard to verbalizations and associations.

Drawing as an open-ended prompt within a relational context is a means to enhanced disclosure in investigative interviews of children. The phenomenon of evidentiary disclosure within the CIG is predicated on the use of drawing as a primary resource as an open-ended prompt in investigative interviews. The interactive relationship or dialogical process is supported by drawing, which often precipitates verbalization and stimulates verbal elaboration by a child (Kelley, 1984; Cohen-Liebman, 1999, 2003). Interviews happen in a relationship that has a corresponding influence on the process. The interview relationship creates an intersubjective matrix, which is a relational milieu that encompasses the interviewer and the child. As has been noted previously, this concept refers to the conditions between two or more people, which contributes to meaning making and assimilation of information or learning and application. These processes do not happen in isolation, but emerge out of the interview or dialogical context.

Accuracy also factored into relationality, as was noted earlier in fact-finding. Accuracy is considered with regard to the information elicited and recalled by children in investigative interviews (Barlow et al., 2011; Macleod et al., 2013). As noted in the literature review, the interview is considered to be a type of conversation that is based upon an interactive process that engages both child and interviewer (Lamb & Brown, 2006). The interviewer encourages true accounts of experienced events at the onset of the process (Pipe et al., 2004). Interviewers have the responsibility to "help children function as informative conversational partners without compromising the accuracy of the information elicited" (Lamb & Brown, 2006, p. 217). In an investigative interview process, interviewers typically are advised to consider alternative explanations for core disclosures (central or main ideas) in an effort to establish relevancy and credibility (Cohen-Liebman, 1999). Regardless of the technique invoked to facilitate information gathering, accuracy should not be compromised (Patterson & Hayne, 2011). Accuracy is fundamental to fact-finding and is related to the theme of relationality, demonstrating the dynamic and interactive aspect of the CIG.

Although not a code or therefore a category in this study, empowerment is seemingly related to the theme of relationality and factors, as well with regard to clinical considerations. Empowerment is integral to the premise of the CIG, and it is fundamental to the different phases and factors prominently within the process (Cohen-Liebman, 1999). Empowerment is a construct that is advocated and maintained throughout the CIG interview. This concept is increasingly identified as contributory to promoting a positive experience for children in investigative interviews. It also conforms to the need for strategies that enhance testimony and promote accuracy, yet provide a sense of self-worth and positivity as a result of the process. The notion of supportive interviewing as having a correspondent impact on accuracy and rapport building is an area spurring research (Katz et al., 2014).

Underlying Mechanisms and the Drawing Effect

In an effort to understand how drawing enhances children's abilities to communicate about past experiences, research on the effect of drawing was reviewed (Gross & Hayne, 1998, 1999; Patterson & Hayne, 2011; Salmon et al., 2003). Researchers have agreed that the means through which drawing is an agent of facilitation is "unclear" (Patterson & Hayne, 2011; Thomas & Jolley, 1998) or "elusive" (Gross et al., 2009, p. 967). Reasons or mechanisms that may account for why drawing is effective as a tool or strategy to facilitate recall have been examined (Butler et al., 1995; Gross et al., 2009; Gross & Hayne, 1998, 1999; Pipe et al., 2004). Various explanations pertaining to the facilitation factor associated with drawing and the enhancement of recall and detail of material have been offered (Gross et al., 2009). Mechanisms have been identified and appear to be receiving support as possible explanations for the facilitative effect of drawing within investigative interviews of children (Jolley, 2010).

It has been speculated that drawing may be effective for keeping children focused for a longer amount of time as compared to a tell condition (Butler et al., 1995; Jolley, 2010). Other mechanisms that may contribute to the facilitative effect of drawing that were observed include reduction in the perception of demands or expectations associated with participation in investigative interviews, suggesting that drawing may provide social support. Additional mechanisms include organization of narratives by children and longer, more focused interviews when drawing is a component (Gross & Hayne, 1998; Gross et al., 2009). Some studies have suggested that children may draw to organize and detail a story (Butler et al., 1995; Salmon et al., 2003).

According to Davison and Thomas (2001), these "mechanisms either independently or in combination may offer an explanation regarding the recall facilitation from drawing" (Davison & Thomas, 2001, p. 157). Although various explanations have been offered as to why drawing might facilitate recall, little experimental work exists with regard to the study of the phenomenon according to some researchers (Jolley, 2010). In this study, the mechanisms that drive or contribute to the facilitative effect of drawing were considered secondary to the research question. Information gathered from the participants provided insight regarding the underlying mechanisms or variables identified in the literature that may account for the facilitative effect of drawing. The mechanisms and related studies that were identified from the literature and were correspondent to the study findings follow. Nine mechanisms were identified from the literature however, interviewer minimal responses or facilitative utterances and representational quality of drawings, were not explored as they exceeded the scope of the study and are not listed below. Facilitative utterances by interviewers versus participant response is directed at patterns of interaction between interviewer and child.

reduction in the perception of social demands	Cohen-Liebman, 1999; Driessnack, 2005; Patterson & Hayne, 2011; Pipe & Salmon, 2009; Thomas & Jolley, 1998
structured narratives	Butler et al., 1995; Gross et al., 2009; Macleod et al., 2013; Salmon et al., 2003; Wesson & Salmon, 2001
organization of narratives	Gross & Hayne, 1998; Gross et al., 2009
increased verbalization	Butler et al., 1995; Gross & Hayne, 1998, 1999; Gross et al., 2009; Patterson & Hayne, 2011; Salmon et al., 2003; Wesson & Salmon, 2001
prior knowledge of an event versus schematic knowledge	Gross et al., 2009; Davison & Thomas, 2001; Macleod et al., 2013; Salmon & Pipe, 2000
drawing as a function of recall	Butler et al., 1995; Davison & Thomas, 2001; Gross & Hayne, 1998, 1999; Gross et al., 2009; Jolley, 2010; Patterson & Hayne, 2011; Salmon & Pipe, 2000; Salmon et al., 2003; Wesson & Salmon, 2001
self-generated cues	Butler et al., 1995; Cohen-Liebman, 2017; Gross et al., 2009; Macleod et al., 2013

Participants were asked to explain what helps them to remember and what drawing affords regardless of the assigned study condition. The children's responses highlight how they recall and remember information and the role of drawing within memory processes. Drawing was acknowledged as contributing to recall and remembrance by children in both of the study conditions. The use of imagery was identified by participants in each condition as contributing to embedding (storing) and recall of information. The identified mechanisms that appeared to contribute to the facilitative factor of drawing were noted and identified within the study findings and reported through the children's own words.

Within both study conditions, the children's self-expression indicated resonance with several of the mechanisms ascribed to the facilitative effect of drawing from the identified in the literature. Excerpts from children in both study conditions offer explanation with regard to the use of drawing as a means to help recall and remember information. Each child at the conclusion of his or her interview was asked about the use of drawing, specifically with regard to how they use drawing and how it may impact their ability to recount information regardless of which condition they were assigned to. The children provided in their own words what drawing does for them. The responses were varied. Children explained the significance of drawing in such a way that was indicative or reflective of the individual mechanisms listed below. The mechanisms are numbered for purposes of aligning them with participant response (to follow) in no significant order. The number of children who identified the various mechanisms is noted in parentheses.

1. Reduction in the perception of social demands associated with the interview (7)
2. Self-generated cues (10)
3. Organization of narratives (7)
4. Increased verbalization (6)
5. Structured narratives (6)
6. Episodic versus schematic knowledge (6)
7. Drawing as a function of recall (7)

The children themselves were able to express or articulate through their graphic depictions and verbalizations how drawing promoted enhanced recall and disclosure of information. In addition, drawing was identified as a way to distill anxiety (P#1) or to relax (P#5), as a way of focusing (P#7), as a means of expression (P#3) and something to do to help manage underlying thoughts and feelings (P#1).

Self-generated cues seemed to be the most apparent mechanism identified from the children's associations, with mention or observation in 10 of the 12 interviews. Of the identified mechanisms that were deemed as contributory to the facilitative factor of drawing, four were identified or acknowledged almost equally by the children as contributing to the use of drawing as a means of retrieval and remembrance. Examples and excerpts from the children's narratives that reflect the underlying mechanisms follow. The associated mechanisms are listed in parentheses.

> P#1 – "I like to draw sharks. Drawing makes me happy. I draw mad things when I am sad. I filled up 4 or 5 sketch books already". P#1 provided that when he is bored and has nothing to do, he uses his sketch books. (Mechanisms 1, 2, 5.)
> P# 4 – "Well, I just think about what happened. I just really brain storm about what really happened and I speak what's on my mind". (Mechanisms 1, 2, 4, 5.)

P# 5 – "Like when I'm just talking it kind of puts more pressure on me because I have to think what happened. When I'm drawing, I can just relax and just draw and it just helps me. I can say what I'm thinking". With regard to drawing specifically she stated, "It helps you relax your mind and not be stressed and if the answer is good or bad you speak your mind". (Mechanisms 1, 2, 3, 4, 5, 7.)

P# 9 – "I normally do this every time I have like a theory like a scene in the movie or in the show or I just have a theory about it and a picture. There's like a camera in my brain something like that. And it's like I take pictures and stuff and I can memorize it and I can kind of remember stuff". When asked, what does drawing do for you? P#9 responded, "It helped me in the video. It helped me remember a few of the things like the main character was McGruff and he is a very helpful person". She also offered, "My teacher doesn't like it when we draw but she likes that we still use imagination and creativity. I think the drawing helped me to remember more stuff. Art is like something you can do to get your mind off of stuff. That's like you can go free or wild and whatever you want to draw". (Mechanisms 1, 2, 3, 4, 5, 7.)

P#10 – "I write things down. If I have a more descriptive picture of what I think or we were writing a narrative since we have like six parts of a story and you can draw it or write it. If I drew it, I wouldn't remember everything. If I wrote it, I won't remember everything but if since we were learning about sensory details, I would have a picture of what we were doing". When asked to explain sensory details and how she remembers them she said, "If you draw it and since most of the time I usually draw and since we usually note stuff, I usually write it down". (Mechanisms 2, 5, 7.)

P#12 – "I just think about why they're doing that. Like when I watch a video, I'm noticing like the main things happening not the minor events and I try to figure out when they're having a conversation. I try to figure out like the main not the minor events. I just like – like usually right after I watch the video I forget and then when I'm talking, I just keep on remembering. Like when things if I know I'm going to forget something I write it down immediately and like when I'm watching a video, I take notes. Obviously like when I'm watching a social studies video because we need to learn the information. But for drawing I don't draw to remember I always write to remember". (Mechanisms 1, 2, 3, 4, 5, 6, 7.)

The facilitative effect of drawing was addressed by the children through their associations and observed in their interactions, both with the media (drawing condition) and in their behavior. The children themselves were able to express or articulate through their graphic depictions (drawing condition) as well as verbalizations (both study conditions) how drawing and the use of imagery promoted enhanced recall and disclosure of information.

The children's responses offer information pertaining to why drawing facilitates communication about experienced events in investigative interviews from the perspective of the child and provide insight with regard to drawing as a facilitative agent for disclosure of information in relation to experienced events. The nondrawing children, like the drawing children, were able to offer explanations and describe what drawing in general affords for them personally with regard to memory and recall.

Although different underlying mechanisms have been explored as providing the impetus for the drawing effect, researchers have identified a constellation of variables as contributing to the facilitative effect of drawing. Researchers have determined that there is a "significant relation between children's drawings and the amount of information children reported during interviews" (Gross & Hayne, 1998, pp. 175–176). Some research indicates that children who draw disclose more information than children who do not draw within an investigative interview format which appears to correspond to the findings provided here although, as noted, the study findings cannot be generalized.

Self-generated cues appeared to be the mechanism most noted by children in both conditions. In addition, the reduction in the perception of social demands, organization of narratives and drawing as a function of recall were also noted by children in both study conditions as contributing to the facilitative effect of drawing when asked to explain what drawing does. The drawing condition appeared to derive advantages, as noted from consideration of the underlying mechanisms attributed to the drawing effect. From the small sample size (N = 6) that drew in this study, it was noted that drawing interviews seemed to share some related characteristics. The drawing cohort provided cogent narratives and details that were consistent with the information conveyed from witnessing the video clips. The children were more focused and they stayed on topic. They tended to provide logical and detailed narratives in relation to what they viewed/experienced with regard to the videos. The children demonstrated and conveyed episodic memory or information that was event specific.

Study Limitations

Several limitations were identified with regard to this study. Due to inherent difficulties, including legal, ethical and practical challenges to conducting a field study with the original target population, sexually abused children, an analogue or laboratory study was designed to address the research question. Impenetrable obstacles prohibited access to victims of sexual abuse at the initial stage of investigation, when investigative interviews are most likely to be conducted. In trying to simulate a real event, it was impossible to replicate and also unethical to implement an event that would mirror either the experience or the witnessing of an event that might promote trauma or a traumatic response.

For transparency purposes it is important to report that the interviewer was familiar or at least knew someone related to seven of the participants. This in and of itself had the potential to limit the study in a myriad of ways, although the participants did not seem to be impacted by circumstantial conditions, which might have been recognized if the children had been reluctant to engage or disclose information or been overly engaged. Attempts were made to minimize potential distractions. The researcher strived to maintain focus on the research study to mitigate potential conflicts and not allow external influences to infiltrate the process.

Another potential limitation encompasses the sample both in size and configuration. The sample is not reflective of a diverse population. The sample was somewhat homogenous in that the majority of the children came from the same socioeconomic demographic and had similar backgrounds with regard to lifestyle, culture and parental influence. The fact that there were four sibling groups is another factor to mention as possibly impacting the study. The results may have been skewed or impacted accordingly; however, most siblings were assigned to different cohorts with the exception of the triplet set given that two were assigned to the same due to the alternation of assignment. The findings as such are limited with regard to general assertions regarding a larger and more diverse or heterogeneous population. Also, the size of the study was as has been stated small, which restricts generalizability.

Whether or not the use of an animated video as the source of the analogue was a limitation merits mention. The idea of conducting an analogue study, let alone using a videotape scenario, rather than a staged or simulated interactive experience was a concern. The idea that children might be too far removed from the experience for it to be relative as an analogous situation was a concern that was postulated and examined. During the literature review, it was found that the use of video was described as a newer method of assessing the facilitative effect of drawing with regard to recall (Jolley, 2010). Video has been described as a form of analogous design that provides an opportunity to witness an event that is "interesting" but not "easily related to children's generic and script knowledge" (Jolley, 2010, p. 230). Jolley explained that this design integrates advantages while limiting disadvantages from other types of methodologies cited in the literature and studied specifically staged events and item recall. Jolley (2010), like other researchers, acknowledged that drawing promotes and functions as a self-generated cue that ultimately facilitates the retrieval of additional details about an event (Gross & Hayne, 1998, 1999). He offered that these studies "provide important support for the use of drawings as aids to children's recall" (Jolley, 2010, p. 233).

Another thought with regard to limitations revolves around the concepts of accuracy and inaccuracy. For coding purposes criteria must be specific to the study similarly to an investigative process. If a child did not specify a character in the video by name but provided a description, was that construed as accurate? In a forensic or investigative context, that could be problematic because in a forensic arena, fact-finding is intended to be accurate and credibility is at stake. In other words, false information or inaccurate material may contribute to a negative outcome in some fashion, whether investigatory or otherwise. Details are very important in the investigative/forensic realm.

From the perspective of the author/investigator, perhaps the concepts of accuracy and inaccuracy as they pertain to investigative interviewing merit examination. Given the nature of the findings and the emphasis on forensic relevancy, including episodic versus script memory, perhaps the way that accuracy and inaccuracy are defined and evaluated within these processes merit revisitation given that children may lack cognitive or verbal skills to articulate information formally but may be able to communicate salient and vital material in a nonlinear or descriptive manner. Given the nature of human interaction and engagement that underlies these processes, elements do not always correspond to simple and easy answers, necessitating a wider lens for understanding what a child may be communicating. In other words, it may be time to re-evaluate how terms are defined and evaluated in an effort to capture the nuances of how children relate information about experienced events, for example, how is accuracy determined, defined and addressed within these contexts? Such considerations may contribute to approach and method and offer understanding as well as appreciation of alternate modes of self-expression that are congruent with and maintain the objectives of fact-finding.

With regard to the study findings, a possible limitation may subsume subjectivity, which may have inadvertently contributed to coding. Moreover, juxtaposing forensic with social science can be a difficult divide to bridge given the respective purviews and cultural differences, as previously addressed in the literature review. Awareness of this dichotomy is justified and the potential impact upon the study is worthy of mention. Finally, it would be remiss for me not to state for transparency purposes that the results may be understood within the context of my work and my experience which emanate from my collective endeavors as a forensic art therapist, a child interview specialist, the clinical director at a multidisciplinary interviewing center, a psycho-legal evaluator and educator.

Implications for Future Study and Interdisciplinary Collaboration

Art therapy research is cultivating awareness of the practicality of the modality within nontraditional realms, forging interdisciplinary engagement. How information from the art therapy process is comprehended or understood is an ever-expanding area of exploration (Acosta, 2001; Lusebrink, 2014). Recognition of the use of drawing to assist children with disclosure that is accurate and detailed, criteria consistent with forensic application, merit continued study.

A number of implications contributed to the identification of areas for future research, specifically, in the realms of investigative interviewing, art therapy and the use of drawing as a facilitative agent for recall. The facilitative effect of drawing is related to the process, which merits examination in an effort to comprehend this phenomenon fully. Future study might expand upon the drawing effect and the underlying mechanisms ascribed to it by exploring how these processes work with regard to trauma and the brain. This may provide understanding with regard to the facilitative factor of drawing in a way that has not previously been considered or understood.

In essence, exploration that extends beyond the picture frame to include cognitive, neurological and biological underpinnings in tandem with the creative process may help to definitively establish the causal machinations of the facilitative effect of drawing. Research pertaining to the relationship between memory, imagery and recall from a neurobiological perspective may prove enlightening with regard to the impact of drawing as a facilitative agent within investigative interviews. Thus, research directed at understanding the processes that contribute to drawing as a means to enhance fact-finding and foster communication about experienced events from an interdisciplinary perspective including art therapy may be prudent.

Research from a physiological perspective to assess the impact of an investigative interview process on a child may provide useful information. This may provide another avenue for exploring how to enhance investigative interviewing practices including the use of drawing while safeguarding child victims and witnesses. This may offer an additional way to understand how processes related to recall, retrieval and memory are activated. By situating examination of the drawing effect within a multi-disciplinary context (study and research including trauma, psychology, neuroscience, biology, investigative interviewing, child maltreatment, art therapy and more), perhaps additional insight may be procured regarding drawing as a facilitative agent. A collaborative research initiative may foster innovative exploration leading to new ideas, alternate perspectives and enlightening discoveries that may inform practice and process.

Collaborative endeavors are needed to initiate a dialogue within the research community dedicated to understanding the role of drawing in facilitating information gathering or fact-finding. Understanding the effect of drawing in facilitating forensically relevant information with regard to encoding, storage and retrieval of information as well as the relationship between imagery and memory, including implicit and explicit, may be revealing. Ideas to explore include how imagery is linked to uncovering traumatic memory within the context of investigative interviewing. Art therapists and art therapy merit inclusion in the research efforts directed at exploring the facilitative effect of drawing within the context of investigative interviews of children.

> The tenets of art therapy are underscored with neurobiological principles. The art-making process and the artwork itself are integral components that help to understand and elicit verbal and nonverbal communication within an attuned . . . relationship. Explaining these tenets and their interventions in a neurobiological framework is especially relevant in the treatment of trauma (King, 2016b, p. 6).

It is hoped that study of the CIG will promote interdisciplinary opportunities in which art therapists are invited to be part of the conversation about investigative interviewing and the facilitative effect of drawing. An art therapy–based process contributes a different perspective.

Another thought for future studies is directed at videotaping the interview process. This may provide additional information with regard to the dynamic interplay between drawing and the dialogical relationship, including verbal and nonverbal interactions. For example, videotaping would permit observation of drawing in relation to verbalization. Correlation of such would be very helpful in determining exactly how and when a child responds pictorially within the interview process or in response to a verbal cue or prompt. Also, how or when verbalization is activated in response to a graphic depiction may be observed. This may be revealing for what stimulates or what triggers verbal and pictorial response and may highlight the nature of the dialogical or relational aspect of the process. How a child responds either visually or verbally may illuminate information that may be enlightening with regard to addressing the nature of the process. Similarly, to the study by Thyme et al. (2013), from an art therapy perspective, it would be helpful to be able to correlate associations with marks on paper. Also, videotaping would allow nonverbal behavior and nuances to be captured and understood with regard to the role they contribute within the process. This is important within the realm of investigative interviewing with regard to influential behaviors on the part of the interviewer, whether consciously or not such as nonverbal reinforcement behaviors, suggestibility, confirmatory bias, etc. Audiotapes and transcripts of textual data do not necessarily capture this type of behavior or interviewer influence (whether deliberate or not). Interviewers may be unaware of negative reinforcement behaviors during the interview process, as previously noted.

A mixed-methods design that explores the use of drawing within investigative interviewing using the CIG as both the instrument of study and the method is a recommendation for future study. The combination of quantitative and qualitative information might provide depth and understanding to the research question posed here that may encompass the recognition and identification of trends and patterns directed at assessing the facilitative effect of drawing. Codes and categories may provide variables to be explored quantitatively. Comingling these two approaches to research may provide an opportunity to obtain different perspectives with regard to the phenomenon under study. Findings may yield additional insight in an effort to enhance investigative interviewing practices. Mixed methods may also assist in understanding the findings, which may be generalizable depending upon the study variables, including sample size. Even though the data collated here were examined from a qualitative basis, frequency counts were a factor and constituted a quantitative element albeit the emphasis of the study design was not on frequency but rather the descriptive qualities.

Research initiatives exploring the linkage between bullying and child maltreatment with a nod to investigative interviewing practice is also an area that merits future study.

The literature review indicated the need for enhanced study regarding the relationship and impact between different forms of victimization. Several parallels associated with child sexual abuse and bullying were identified providing the impetus for continued examination given the identified gap in the literature surrounding the call for research in this area.

The CIG is an investigative interview process that in effect lends itself to other applications in which forensically relevant information or fact-finding is the goal. Exploring the use of the CIG as a means to interview and gather information from victims and/or witnesses of interpersonal violence or other traumatic experiences is recommended, including elder abuse. Further research to explore a verbal versus a verbal plus drawing interview process is also recommended with the use of another verbal interview format (not the CIG without drawing) for comparative purposes.

Contextual Findings

This qualitative comparative research study considered how drawing as an open-ended prompt in an investigative interview process enhanced memory recall and facilitated fact-finding or evidentiary disclosure when compared to an investigative interview without drawing. The purpose included the study of the CIG, a forensic art therapy investigative interview process. The underlying mechanisms associated with the drawing effect were also explored in an effort to address the problem, which was how to enhance children's abilities to communicate accurate information pertaining to experienced events in an investigative interview. Both verbal and pictorial data were collected to determine how evidentiary disclosure of an experienced or witnessed event was impacted when drawing was incorporated as a primary resource in an art therapy–based investigative interview process.

The data revealed the emergence of three overarching themes: fact-finding, imagery and relationality. The categories that contributed to the identification of the themes were considered as they evolved from the data analysis and with regard to forensic relevance. The themes that emerged were directly related to the CIG and as such indicate a correspondence with the process-oriented approach that underscores an art therapy–based investigative interview process. Fact-finding was aligned with an open invitational drawing process, while relationality appeared to be compatible with the dialogic and relational aspect of the process. The encoding, storage and recall of memory in image form was congruent with the theme of imagery that emerged from the study data and resultant findings. The use of imagery, whether mental visualization or graphic representation, appeared to be the facilitator or perhaps the factor that stimulated and triggered recall and memory.

Fact-finding encompassed the categories of memory and recall, accuracy and inaccuracy and details and information, which relate to forensic relevancy. These elements of investigative interviews contribute to understanding a child's experience. With regard to the CIG specifically, this theme was congruent with the encoding, storage and recall of memory in image form. The findings suggest that children in the drawing condition tended to provide episodic or forensically relevant information whereas the children in the nondrawing condition relied upon generalized or script knowledge.

The theme of imagery was reflective of the CIG in that an open invitational drawing process was the basis for elicitation of information. In essence, the study considered whether drawing as an open-ended prompt in an investigative interview facilitates communication and enhances elicitation of information regarding experienced events. The categories that were identified from the data were correspondent with the CIG. This theme resonated with an art therapy–based investigative interview and supported the juxtaposition of art therapy tenets, including the relationship between interviewer and child (dialogical/relational), art making and the creative process (drawing as an open-ended prompt) within the investigative format.

Finally, the third theme that was identified from the study was relationality, given the nature of the dynamic patterns of interaction that emerged verbally and non-verbally. The innate dynamism that pervades the investigative interview guideline, which functioned as the instrument as well as the object of study, exists on multiple levels. The CIG juxtaposes investigative (forensic) tenets with art therapy practices and principles. Although findings and data were examined in a seemingly linear pattern, in truth, the process itself is not linear. Rather, interactions are dynamic, with relationships occurring almost dialectically with overt/covert, manifest/latent, verbal/nonverbal configurations, as well as visualization that occurred mentally in addition to graphically or pictorially. The categories for this theme were learning and application, meaning making and self/other.

Finally, notable observations that emerged were identified and include; the drawing interviews were longer; the children were more focused; narratives were self-directed and cogent; and children were not easily distracted when drawing. Manifest content revealed themes related directly to the videos in at least half of the drawings, with latent identification discernible in almost all. Imagery and visualization factored into both the drawing and nondrawing interviews either pictorially or mentally. Metaphor and symbolism were utilized by children in both conditions. Imagery was identified as significant for encoding, storing and retrieving information.

The research question, which began with how rather than does, sought to uncover how an investigative interview predicated upon art therapy was responsive to facilitating fact-finding with school-aged children. Analysis of the data identified the use of imagery, whether mental visualization or pictorial depiction, as enhancing children's abilities to communicate accurate and relevant information. The use of imagery as indicated from the data analysis, which included frequencies (quantitative information) in conjunction with the qualitative descriptive information, revealed enhanced communication (fact-finding) or richer descriptions provided by the children in the drawing cohort with regard to the experienced event (video content). The themes that emerged were congruent with the fundamental foundational precepts associated with the CIG.

Forensic relevance was previously described for this study as relating to facts or details about experienced events. Script refers to general or previous knowledge about a topic, which is described through reference to content or context (Thoresen et al., 2009). In contrast, episodic memory fosters understanding of an episode or event that is rooted in personal experience. Overall, the study findings suggested that children in the drawing condition related information that was directly linked or event specific to the experienced event (the videos) rather than generalized information about the topic of bullying. The use of drawing as an open-ended prompt promoted disclosure of descriptive qualities that resonated with the facts or details children had observed in the videos prior to being interviewed. The descriptive qualities may not have manifested within the frequency counts, thus suggesting the discrepancies that were noted between some quantitative and qualitative findings. Qualitative material is often difficult to quantize.

Finally, seven of the nine underlying mechanisms that have been identified from the literature as possible associations with the facilitative effect of drawing were evident from the children's own words. These mechanisms were observed through the children's interactions and participation in the interview process, verbally and nonverbally. Promoting recall of experience through self-generated cues was the mechanism most identified by the children irrespective of study condition. This mechanism was acknowledged by the children as contributing to recall of information. Thus, the facilitative effect of drawing as a means of enhancing recall and providing richer narratives was acknowledged through the children's own statements. The children explained what drawing and the use of imagery afforded with regard to encoding, recall and retrieval of information. This in turn contributed to meaning making, learning and application in relation to the experienced event, which included observation of two animated videos that addressed strategies and techniques as well as prevention and intervention aimed at combating bullying.

The facilitative effect of drawing as a means of enhancing recall and providing richer narratives was acknowledged through the children's own statements.

Overall, imagery emerged as a key finding with regard to the research question and in understanding how an art therapy–based investigative interview process facilitated fact-finding as compared to a verbal investigative interview process. The findings revealed that imagery was a common denominator between the two study conditions. Foundational to the research question, the use of imagery, whether visual (mental) or graphic (pictorial), appeared to be the facilitator, or perhaps the factor that stimulated and triggered recall and memory. The dialogical component also was a key factor and was identified as contributing to the dynamic and interactive nature of the interview process, which emerged as multidimensional and multilayered.

A meshed model for qualitative content analysis was derived from an amalgamation of models from various researchers and their respective work, including Elo and Kyngäs (2008), Henning et al. (2004), Graneheim and Lundman (2004) and Thyme et al. (2013). The approach to blending qualitative content analysis with art psychotherapy as described by Thyme et al. (2013) provided a framework for data analysis. As such, a method for understanding the pictorial data within the context of the research question as well as the instrument of study, the CIG, emerged. It also enabled comparison with the information communicated (verbally, nonverbally and pictorially) by the participants in both study conditions.

According to Graneheim and Lundman (2004), "research findings should be as trustworthy as possible and every research study must be evaluated in relation to the procedures used to generate the findings" (p. 109). They advocate that the concepts that underlie trustworthiness with regard to qualitative research are "intertwined and interrelated" (Graneheim & Lundman, 2004). The concepts they put forth that are applicable for such studies are credibility, dependability and transferability. They state, however, that qualitative content analysis concepts are related to quantitative methods such as validity, reliability and generalizability. The evaluation criteria for the evaluation for qualitative content analysis is attributed to Lincoln and Guba (1985), who defined trustworthiness as important for an inductive approach to qualitative content analysis "because categories are created from the raw data without a theory-based categorization matrix" (Elo et al., 2014, p. 2). Lincoln and Guba (1985) posit that trustworthiness of a research study is important to evaluating its worth through consideration of the following criteria:

> **Credibility** – confidence in the "truth" of the findings
> **Dependability** – showing that the findings are consistent and could be repeated
> **Confirmability** – a degree of neutrality or the extent to which the findings of a study are shaped by the respondents and not researcher bias, motivation or interest
> **Transferability** – showing that the findings have applicability in other contexts

Elo et al. (2014) compiled a checklist for establishing trustworthiness that corresponds to Elo and Kyngäs's (2008) three phases of content analysis: preparation, organization and reporting. For preparation, they address data collection and sampling strategy; for organization, they consider categorization and interpretation; and in reporting, they address transferability, the use of excerpts, relevance to the data and description of the process. Credibility relates to the notion of confidence. In this regard it specifically refers to how well the data and the processes inherent to the method have addressed the study focus. This encompasses sampling (participants) and data gathering, as well as the amount of data collected. Determination of categories and themes contributes to credibility as well so that appropriate data have not been excluded and unnecessary material is not inadvertently included. Comparability is related to categories and themes such that similarities and differences may be determined and demonstrated through excerpts which highlight the data and findings. Another way to promote this is through dialogue and agreement with researchers or, in some cases, with member checking.

Also relevant to credibility is the role and the background as well as the experience of the researcher(s). With regard to this study, the investigator developed and implemented the CIG. The CIG has been in existence for more than 20 years and has been accepted within a judicial context as a viable resource for interviewing children. The investigator teaches a relevant course and has done so for almost 25 years. She is well versed in best practices and current trends pertaining to investigative interviewing of children and youth about experienced events, including traumatic encounters. As well, the qualitative researcher is "required to have the skill to build rapport with interviewees and the ability to respond insightfully within the context of an interview" (Sullivan & Sheehan, 2016, p. 77).

As noted by Denzin and Lincoln (2000), the researcher within the context of qualitative study is affiliated with the real world and addresses firsthand experiences, which contributes to elicitation and maximization of fact-finding or data gathering (Sullivan & Sheehan, 2016). Graneheim and Lundman (2004) note the importance of the researcher within qualitative content analysis; however, they indicate that it is a balancing act given that "it is impossible and undesirable for the researcher not to add a particular perspective to the phenomena under study. On the other hand, the researcher must 'let the text talk' and not impute meaning that is not there" (p. 111). Hopefully, this was achieved.

Dependability, as defined by Elo et al. (2014), refers to stability of data over time and under different conditions – in essence, meaning the study can be replicated. It is hoped that the study will be conducted at a later time with a larger and more diverse population. Conformity is identified as "objectivity or congruence with regard to the relevancy, accuracy and meaning of the data" (Elo et al., 2014, p. 2). Elo et al. (2014) note that this may be tricky when latent content is considered. The data were derived from the participants, and multiple excerpts from the data were reported to support the findings. It is noted that often data are analyzed by one researcher in this type of process, and thus it is incumbent upon the researcher to return again and again to the data with regard to interpretation, as well as corroboration through the data sources. The investigator invoked such a process for the study.

Transferability or generalization to other settings/populations and reporting findings is described by Graneheim and Lundman (2004) as transferring findings to another context. To achieve this principle, they advocate that context and process ascribed to the study components, including participants, data collection and the process of analysis, should be clear. This is fortified through the enumeration of the findings coupled with supportive excerpts from the data. According to De Wet (2010) rich and thick descriptions contribute to the determination of transferability. Lastly, some authors include transparency as well within the definition of trustworthiness (Thyme et al., 2013).

The author/investigator has attempted to be transparent with regard to sharing information and in an effort to establish trustworthiness given the identified variables including preparation, organization and analysis. Given the small sample size and other limitations, the inability to generalize the findings of this study has been duly acknowledged. It must be noted that what has been conveyed is rooted in the perspective of the researcher. Graneheim and Lundman (2004) state with regard to the trustworthiness of qualitative research, "There is no single correct meaning or universal application of research findings, but only the most probable meaning from a particular perspective" (Graneheim & Lundman, 2004, p. 110). Moreover, they state, "In qualitative research, trustworthiness of interpretations deals with establishing arguments for the most probable interpretations" (Graneheim & Lundman, 2004, p. 110).

Conclusion

Although research has been devoted to ascertaining how drawing works within investigative interview processes, drawing from an art therapy perspective within this milieu is a recent endeavor. The findings that emerged from this study situate the CIG as a dynamic and interactive process that is grounded in fact-finding, imagery and relationality. Drawing as an open-ended prompt within the CIG seemingly contributed to enhanced fact-finding or disclosure of event-specific (forensically relevant) information. The CIG is predicated upon eliciting information about a child's experience in a supportive and dialogical context. The premise is child centered, child focused and designed to empower a child. The CIG is based upon art therapy principles and practices juxtaposed with forensic tenets and judicial canons, ensuring that the process conforms with the demands of the legal system while safeguarding the emotional well-being of a child victim or witness (Cohen-Liebman, 2016).

The rationale for the study design was to explore how an art therapy–based investigative interview process compared to a verbal investigative interview process with regard to enhanced recall and elicitation of information pertaining to experienced events. The study explored the use of drawing as an open-ended prompt within a relational context to gather information about an experienced event. The study sought to retrieve data that were rich and descriptive between two study conditions: CIG with drawing and CIG without drawing.

Secondarily, the underlying mechanisms associated with the drawing effect were considered from an art therapy perspective. Content analysis provided a means for organizing, coding, aggregating and analyzing textual and imaginal data. Patterns and relationships between concepts emerged from analysis of the data (Shams et al., 2017) and were compared between the two study conditions. Dedoose, a qualitative data analysis software program, provided a means of managing and ordering data and enabled new levels of analysis (Gerbic & Stacey, 2005).

Three overarching themes emerged from the data: fact-finding, imagery and relationality. The themes were congruent with the three foundational principles of the CIG. The gaps that were addressed included 1) the inconclusive information and debatable acceptance that surrounds the use of drawing as an open-ended prompt in investigative interviews of school-aged children; 2) the identified need for research in forensic interviewing approaches for children; 3) the lack of systematic study of the CIG, an art therapy–based forensic interview process; 4) the need to explore the medium of drawing as a primary component in an investigative interview process, given the additional information that images provide; and 5) the elusiveness of the drawing effect and the underlying mechanisms attributed to it.

Children in the drawing condition appeared to self-generate retrieval cues, which seemed to trigger recall of information related to the videos and the strategies contributing to enhanced disclosure. Graphic elaboration stimulated recall of additional material, while verbalization contributed to enhanced recall both pictorially and verbally, demonstrating a cyclical process. Fact-finding was emergent as information was disclosed through imaginal and verbal means.

Underlying mechanisms attributed to the drawing effect were observed in the interactions of the children through the media (drawing condition) as well as in their associations and behavior. Children who drew disclosed information that was indicative of episodic or event-specific information, whereas script memory was demonstrated by the nondrawing study participants. The findings revealed that the drawing condition provided information that was forensically relevant.

Without the constraints of formal language, a child may depict his or her experience in a more tangible way (Cohen-Liebman, 2016, 2017). A child experiences and encodes a multiplicity of information. Drawing may encompass elements of an event and sensory details that may have occurred simultaneously and might be difficult to describe linearly. According to Wadeson (2010), "this form of expression more nearly duplicates experience" (p. 13). Drawing enables a child to depict the concurrence of temporal, spatial and sensory material (Cohen-Liebman, 2016).

The use of imagery facilitates expression due to the accessibility to unconscious material (Chapman, 2014). Verbal language may fail because there are no words to express what is encoded on a preverbal level. Drawing has been shown to overcome the inherent limitations of verbal interviews that require language (Steele & Kuban, 2013; Steele & Malchiodi, 2012). Drawing provides the means for disclosure of the various sensorial as well as logistical aspects associated with fact-finding. Traumatic experiences are considered to be stored implicitly, and implicit memory is sensory based. Trauma mitigates access to language and logic, making this sensorium or unconscious material unavailable (Steele & Kuban, 2013). Drawing provides the opportunity for children to externalize those "iconic meanings into a contextual format that makes it easier to then give them meaning" and "reorder . . . those memories in ways that can be managed" (Steele & Kuban, 2013, p. 70) and "experienced and remembered through images and sensations" (Steele & Malchiodi, 2012, p. 3).

In the absence of verbal language children need opportunities "to communicate what it is like without words" (Steele & Kuban, 2013, p. 7). Understanding how trauma and experienced events are encoded at the preverbal level underscores why imaginal expression resonates with uncovering or recall of memory in a fact-finding or investigative process suggesting continued exploration regarding the association of trauma, imagery and fact-finding.

Visualization, whether mental or graphic/pictorial, seemed to stimulate memory and recall, resulting in verbal elaboration in both study conditions. Recall and memory seemed to be reliant upon mental images, which were either communicated verbally (linearly) or through the use of graphic imagery (nonlinear disclosure). At times, confirmation of verbal statements was made through graphic depiction.

The use of drawing has garnered support as well as skepticism generating a spectrum of endorsement that ranges from avoidance and non-inclusion to recognition and praise. The literature review examined various ways drawing has been identified and studied within the realm of investigative interviewing. Study and focus have been directed at event drawing (Katz & Hershkowitz, 2010), memory trigger (Butler et al., 1995; Faller, 2005; Gross & Hayne, 1998, 1999) and as a means of providing comfort. The latter, comfort drawing, has been described "as a voluntary activity that children can start and stop at will" (Poole & Dickinson, 2014, p. 192). Other studies have explored the draw and tell technique (Katz & Hamama, 2013), which straddles event and comfort. Drawing has also been explored to determine if forensically relevant details increased in richness and abundance when incorporated within study designs (Katz et al., 2014; Katz & Hershkowitz, 2010). Additionally, whether drawing influences episodic or script memory and whether drawing hinders or helps retrieval of such information has been a matter of study with conflicting findings (Davison & Thomas, 2001; Gross et al., 2009; Jolley, 2010). The findings from study of the CIG appear to support that when children draw during the interview process, they recover or retrieve episodic or event-specific information, while children who did not draw tended to provide script or information predicated upon generalized or previous knowledge.

Several studies reviewed referenced drawing as a means to facilitate disclosure of personally meaningful or forensically relevant information (Butler et al., 1995; Gross & Hayne, 1998, 1999; Katz et al., 2014; Katz & Hershkowitz, 2010; Salmon et al., 2003; Wesson & Salmon, 2001). The "draw and talk" technique, primarily studied in analogue designs, was integrated into interviews to assess children's disclosures regarding personally experienced events. The results "under ideal circumstances" (nonsuggestive interventions) revealed an increase in the amount of information recalled, and accuracy was not tainted (Katz, & Hamama, 2013, p. 879). "The contribution of the drawings to the children's narratives was impressive", and according to the researchers, different children "produced richer testimonies when reporting more forensically relevant information with respect to the alleged abuse" (Katz & Hamama, 2013, p. 880).

The review of the literature also revealed that studies (Butler et al., 1995; Gross & Hayne, 1998, 1999; Gross et al., 2009; Patterson & Hayne, 2007; Salmon et al., 2003; Wesson and Salmon, 2001) have determined that "under some circumstances, drawing facilitated children's reports about a wide range of experiences" (Gross et al., 2009, p. 966). Research has focused on recall of factual information rather than on children's narrative reporting of events or autobiographical material and the effect of drawing on these scenarios (Gross et al., 2009). Some research indicated that drawing facilitated subjects' ability to recall and report both narrative information and factual (or educational) information (Gross et al., 2009). In addition, drawing has been demonstrated to enhance reporting of material (Macleod et al., 2013). The findings from the study addressed here contribute to these areas of exploration although the findings cannot be generalized.

The literature review considered the polarity implicit with regard to the role of drawing within the interview context. It has been suggested that young children are unable to produce their own internal retrieval cues that support the recall of information (Gentle et al., 2014; Katz & Hershkowitz, 2012; Lamb & Brown, 2006). According to Lamb et al. (2008), aids, props, cues and media do not necessarily help children retrieve information, and as such "their effects depend on the way they were used" (p. 164). They identified that the facilitative effects of "allowing" children to draw while talking are thought to derive from a number of possible mechanisms which they define as including the generation of self-retrieval cues that remind children of additional details as they draw or "construct" the drawing. Essentially, they consider drawing to be a self-report measure.

Although some researchers have identified that drawing contributes to the elicitation of forensically relevant information, the content of the drawing is still not evaluated within the process (Katz & Hamama, 2013). As such, studies that consider the use of drawing in interviews are not focused on the content or interpretation of the material drawn (Patterson & Hayne, 2011).

Some studies that address the role of drawing within investigative interviews relegate drawing to a strategy (tool or technique) rather than a method (process or an approach). Graphic content and context are not considered in relation to what and even how children report information in investigative interviews given that children are not typically engaged in a manner that affords the opportunity to explain their drawing content in depth. Manifest (overt graphic content) and latent (underlying or symbolic content) material are not considered or explored.

Drawing and the imaginal or pictorial content, as well as the relationship between what a child says as they draw (within the interview context), have not been topics of focus in empirical work with regard to investigative interviewing. These topics are central to the practice and the processes inherent in art therapy and speak to the viability of this study (at least in the author's opinion). Within an art therapy–based process such as the CIG, a child's associations regarding marks on paper (drawing/imagery) are a fundamental component of the process and contribute to understanding a child's experience.

The research conducted by Driessnack (2006) concluded that "too often, clinicians and researchers disregard children's words used to explain or accompany their drawings and instead substitute their own explanations" (p. 1416). In the studies examined by Driessnack (2005, 2006), when children were asked to draw in interviews, the content of their drawings was not evaluated; rather, drawing was used functionally as a means to stimulate recall. The child's associations, at least within the context of an art therapy process, are vital to understanding the meaning of a child's graphic productions. The goal is not to interpret for the child, but rather to have the child explain what the imagery depicts or represents. This meaning making component emerges within the dialogical relationship that encompasses fact-finding.

The need to balance strategies to enhance fact-finding as well as safeguard the emotional well-being of children are areas of interest. As such, measures that "ensure that the investigation is an empowering experience that generates feelings of trust, self-worth and justice" are advocated and are areas of current study (Katz et al., 2014, p. 858). Emphasis has been focused on maximizing testimonial capability in an effort to help children retrieve and report information that is not only rich but also reliable, with attention directed at "interviewing tactics" that not only enhance testimony but also "modify" interviews to attend to children's emotional needs (Katz et al., 2014, p. 859). As such, more sensitive interviews or interviewing is advocated (Katz et al., 2014). Accordingly, "[n]o studies have attempted to assess the way children comprehend their experience in investigative interviews, including how drawing can shape the children's interview experience" (Katz et al., 2014, p. 860). Katz and colleagues provide that information from a clinical context may provide insight with regard to the "potential of drawing to lead to a more positive perception of the interview by children" (Katz et al., 2014, p. 860). Drawing has been evaluated as a means for providing social support in both clinical and legal contexts (Gross & Hayne, 1998). From a clinical perspective, researchers are identifying the need for interviews to have built-in safeguards or support for children with emphasis directed at a child-centered approach rather than an interviewer-led process in which the expectation is a question-and-answer format. As such, a call for investigative interviews to integrate parallel lines (Katz et al., 2014) is advocated in an effort to maintain the well-being of those engaged in the (fact-finding) process and as a means to prevent secondary traumatization.

The CIG offers a forum that meets this challenge, given the intrinsic psycho-legal orientation. The blend of forensic and psychological epistemologies has been described as foundational to the CIG (Cohen-Liebman, 2016), which emanated from the investigator's (author's) practice of FAT (Cohen-Liebman, 2016). Social science and forensic tenets are melded and contribute to a process that meets the demands of the legal system while preserving the emotional well-being of children and youth (Cohen-Liebman, 2016). Thus, the CIG offers an investigative approach or a fact-finding method that is informative yet supportive, legally compliant yet clinically responsive (Cohen-Liebman, 2016).

Beyond the Picture Frame

The use of drawing offers much for investigating, interviewing and testifying within the realm of child sexual abuse. Drawing is much more that a picture. It entails what a child says within the construct of a dialogical process in relation to graphic depiction. Exploring memory processes, and the relationship of imagery and trauma as well as the drawing effect within an interdisciplinary context will hopefully promote understanding and appreciation for the use of drawing as a means to elicit and enhance communication, foster self expression and facilitate personal narratives about experienced events.

It is hoped that the findings contribute to the dialogue on investigative interviewing. Additionally, it is hoped that through the systematic exploration of the CIG, the study contributes to the debate regarding the advantages and disadvantages of the use of drawing within investigative interviewing and the utility of an art therapy–based process.

The use of drawing within an investigative or fact-finding endeavor that juxtaposes art therapy and forensic tenets affords a different perspective not previously explored. The impact of the study potentially will be a contribution to the discussion surrounding interviewing best practices for school-aged children. When drawing is integrated in a primary capacity as an open-ended prompt, children may disclose what they cannot or are afraid to say. *Drawing to disclose* may in effect provide investigators with forensically relevant information by appealing to the sensorial nature of a child's experience via graphic or imaginal expression which may stimulate recall leading to (enhanced) verbal expression.

The study discussed a novel application of art therapy for investigative purposes using a specific fact-finding, imagery-based and relational format: the CIG. The findings revealed that children who drew provided more forensically relevant (episodic) or qualitatively descriptive information than children who did not draw. Coupled with investigation of the theoretical principles and foundational constructs of the CIG, it is hoped that this study will contribute to the call for evaluative research on the effect of drawing on the content of children's reports in forensic interviews (Patterson & Hayne, 2011). It is hoped as well that the study and the resultant findings provide a response to the call for "how, when, and whether drawing should be introduced in forensic contexts" (Pipe et al., 2004, p. 451) in addition to insight regarding the relevance and appropriateness of the use of drawing in forensic interviews (Driessnack, 2005).

Furthermore, the findings from this study hopefully demonstrate the use of drawing and its effectiveness in assisting children to communicate and recall information in various contexts. Giving children the opportunity to draw may moderate the retrieval process. This is achieved through the generation of retrieval cues that are sensory and internally created, helping children organize their narratives, which in turn, allows them to "share their voice" (Driessnack, 2006, pp. 420–421).

Understanding the process is central to appreciating drawing as a facilitative agent within an art therapy–based investigative interview. I hope that an art therapy–based investigative interview process predicated upon fact-finding, imagery and relationality will be understood as a plausible means for eliciting information from child victims and witnesses (and potentially other populations) about experienced events within a fact-finding milieu. The use of an open-ended prompt in the form of drawing may provide a resource to communicate accurate and reliable information that extends beyond the picture frame.

References

Acosta, I. (2001). Rediscovering the dynamic properties inherent in art. *American Journal of Art Therapy, 39*(3), 93.

Aldridge, J., Lamb, M. E., Sternberg, K. J., Orbach, Y., Esplin, P. W., & Bowler, L. (2004). Using a human figure drawing to elicit information from alleged victims of child sexual abuse. *Journal of Consulting and Clinical Psychology, 72*(2), 304.

Allen, B., & Tussey, C. (2012). Can projective drawings detect if a child experienced sexual or physical abuse? A systematic review of the controlled research. *Trauma, Violence, & Abuse, 13*(2), 97–111.

American Academy of Child and Adolescent Psychiatry. (1990). *Guidelines for the evaluation of child and adolescent sexual abuse.* Author.

American Art Therapy Association (AATA). (2013). *Fact sheet.* www.arttherapy.org/upload/aata factsheet.pdf

American Art Therapy Association (AATA). (2015). www.arttherapy.org

American Professional Society on the Abuse of Children. (1990). *Guidelines for psychosocial evaluation of suspected sexual abuse in young children.* Author.

American Professional Society on the Abuse of Children. (2002). *Practical guidelines: Investigative interviewing in cases of alleged child abuse.* Author.

American Prosecutors Research Institute and National Center for the Prosecution of Child Abuse. (2004). *Investigation and prosecution of child abuse.* Sage.

Anderson, J., Ellefson, J., Lashley, J., Miller, A. L., Olinger, S., Russell, A., & Weigman, J. (2010). CornerHouse forensic interviewing protocol: RATAC. *Thomas M. Cooley Journal of Practical and Clinical Law, 12*(2), 193–331.

Arieti, S. (1976). *Creativity: The magic synthesis.* Basic Books.

Arnheim, R. (1994). The thoughts that made me move. *The Arts in Psychotherapy, 21*(4), 245–246.

Barlow, C. M., Jolley, R. P., & Hallam, J. L. (2011). Drawings as memory aids: Optimising the drawing method to facilitate young children's recall. *Applied Cognitive Psychology, 25*, 480–487.

Betensky, M. (1987). Phenomenology of therapeutic art expression and art therapy. In J.A. Rubin (Ed.), *Approaches to art therapy: Theory and technique* (pp. 149–166). New York, NY: Brunner/Mazel.

Betensky, M. (1995). *What do you see: Phenomenology of therapeutic art expression.* Jessica Kingsley.

Bird, J. (2012). Towards Babel: Language and translation in art therapy. In H. Burt (Ed.), *Art therapy and postmodernism: Creative healing through a prism.* Jessica Kingsley.

Bolger, K. E., & Patterson, C. J. (2001). Developmental pathways from child maltreatment to peer rejection. *Child Development, 72*(2), 549–568.

Bourg, W., Broderick, R., Flagor, R. Kelly, D., Ervin, D., & Butler, J. (1999). *A child interviewer's guidebook.* Sage Publications, Inc.

Brooks, C. M., & Milchman, M. S. (1991). Child sexual abuse allegations during custody litigation: Conflicts between mental health expert witnesses and the law. *Behavioral Sciences and the Law, 9*(1), 21–32. https://doi.org/10.1002/bsl.2370090104

Brown, D. A. (2011). The use of supplementary techniques in forensic interviews with children. In M. E. Lamb, D. J. LaRooy, L. C. Malloy, & C. Katz (Eds.), *Children's testimony: A handbook of psychological research and forensic practice* (pp. 217–250). Wiley-Blackwell.

Brown, D. A., Lamb, M. E., Lewis, C., Pipe, M. E., Orbach, Y., & Wolfman, M. (2013). The NICHD investigative interview protocol: An analogue study. *Journal of Experimental Psychology: Applied, 19*(4), 367–382.

Brown, D. A., & Lamb, M. E. (2009). Forensic interviews with children: A two-way street: Supporting interviewers in adhering to best practice recommendations and enhancing children's capabilities in forensic interviews. In K. Kuehnle & M. Connell (Eds.), *The evaluation of child sexual abuse allegations: A comprehensive guide to assessment and testimony* (pp. 299–325). John Wiley & Sons.

Brown, D. A., Pipe, M. E., Lewis, C., Lamb, M. E., & Orbach, Y. (2007). Supportive or suggestive: Do human figure drawings help 5-to 7-year-old children to report touch? *Journal of Consulting and Clinical Psychology, 75*(1), 33.

Browne, A., & Finkelhor, D. (1986). Impact of child sexual abuse: A review or research. *Psychological Bulletin, 99*, 66–77.

Bruck, M., & Ceci, S. J. (1999). The suggestibility of children's memory. *Annual Review of Psychology, 50*(1), 419–439.

Bruck, M., Melnyk, L., & Ceci, S. J. (2000). Draw it again Sam: The effect of drawing on children's suggestibility and source monitoring ability. *Journal of Experimental Child Psychology, 77*, 169–196.

Buck, J. (1970). *House-tree-person technique manual* (Rev. ed.). Western Psychological Services.

Burgess, A. W., & Hartman, C. R. (1993). Children's drawings. *Child Abuse & Neglect, 17*, 161–168.

Burgess, A. W., Hartman, C. R., Wolbert, W. A., & Grant, C. A. (1987). Child molestation: Assessing impact in multiple victims (Part I). *Archives of Psychiatric Nursing, 1*(1), 33.

Burgess, A. W., McCausland, M. P., & Wolbert, W. A. (1981). Children's drawings as indicators of sexual trauma. *Perspectives in Psychiatric Care, 19*(2), 50–57.

Burt, H. (Ed.). (2012). *Art therapy and postmodernism: Creative healing through a prism.* Jessica Kingsley.

Butler, S., Gross, J., & Hayne, H. (1995). The effect of drawing on memory performance in young children. *Developmental Psychology, 31*, 597–608.

Carnes, C. (2000). *Forensic evaluation of children when sexual abuse is suspected.* National Children's Advocacy Center.

Case, C., & Dalley, T. (2014). *The handbook of art therapy.* Routledge.

Ceci, S. J., & Bruck, M. (1993). Suggestibility of the child witness: A historical review and synthesis. *Psychological Bulletin, 113*, 403–439.

Ceci, S. J., & Bruck, M. (1995). *Jeopardy in the courtroom: A scientific analysis of children's testimony.* American Psychological Association.

Cerf, C., Hespe, D., Gantwerk, B., Martz, S., & Vermeire, G., (2011). *New Jersey bullying parent guide: Guidance for parents on the anti-bullying bill of rights act (P.L.2010, c.122).* New Jersey Department of Education.

Chan, H. C. O., & Wong, D. S. (2015). The overlap between school bullying perpetration and victimization: Assessing the psychological, familial, and school factors of Chinese adolescents in Hong Kong. *Journal of Child and Family Studies, 24*(11), 3224–3234.

Chapman, L. (2014). *Neurobiologically informed trauma therapy with children and adolescents: Understanding mechanisms of change.* WW Norton & Company.

Cheit, R. (2014). *The witch hunt narratives: Politics, psychology and the sexual abuse of children.* Oxford University Press.

Clements, P. T., Benasutti, K. M., & Henry, G. C. (2001). Drawing from experience: Using drawings to facilitate communication and understanding with children exposed to sudden traumatic deaths. *Journal of Psychosocial Nursing and Mental Health Services, 39*(12), 12–20.

Cohen-Liebman, M. S. (1995). Drawings as judiciary aids in child sexual abuse litigation: A composite list of indicators. *The Arts in Psychotherapy,* special issue on sexual abuse, *22*(5), 475–483.

Cohen-Liebman, M. S. (1999). Draw and tell: Drawings within the context of child sexual abuse investigations. *The Arts in Psychotherapy, 26*(3), 185–194.

Cohen-Liebman, M. S. (2002). Intro to art therapy. In A. P. Giardino & E. R. Giardino (Eds.), *Recognition of child abuse for the mandated reporter* (3rd ed., pp. 227–257). G.W. Medical Publishing.

Cohen-Liebman, M. S. (2003). Drawings in forensic investigations of child sexual abuse. In C. Malchiodi (Ed.), *Handbook of art therapy* (pp. 167–179). Guilford Press.

Cohen-Liebman, M. S. (2016). Forensic art therapy. In D. Gussak & M. Rosal (Eds.), *The Wiley Blackwell handbook of art therapy* (pp. 469–477). Wiley-Blackwell.

Cohen-Liebman, M. S. (2017). *Drawing and disclosure of experienced events in an art therapy investigative interview process with school aged children: A qualitative comparative analogue study* (Doctoral dissertation). Retrieved from ProQuest Dissertations and Theses database.

Cohen-Liebman, M. S. (2020). Drawing to disclose: Empowering child victims and witnesses in investigative interviews. In M. Berberian & B. Davis (Eds.), *Art therapy practices for resilient youth.* Routledge.

Cohen-Liebman, M. S. (2021). Drawing to disclose: Findings from an art therapy-based investigative interview process. In V. Huet & L. Kapitan (Eds.), *The art of practice & research: Art therapy international practice research conference proceedings.* Cambridge Scholars Publishing.

Conte, J. R., Sorenson, E., Fogarty, L., & Rosa, J. D. (1991). Evaluating children's reports of sexual abuse: Results from a survey of professionals. *American Journal of Orthopsychiatry, 61*(3), 428.

Conte, J. R., & Vaughan-Eden, V. (2018). Child sexual abuse. In B. Klika & J. Conte (Eds.), *The APSAC handbook on child maltreatment* (4th ed., pp. 95–110). Sage Publications, Inc.

Cook, C. R., Williams, K. R., Guerra, N. G., & Kim, T. (2009). Variability in the prevalence of bullying and victimization. In *Handbook of bullying in schools: An international perspective* (pp. 347–362). Routledge.

Cox, S. (2005). Intention and meaning in young children's drawing. *International Journal of Art & Design Education, 24*(2), 115–125.

Curtis, E. K. (2011). Understanding client imagery in art therapy. *Journal of Clinical Art Therapy, 1*(1), 9–15.

Davison, L. E., & Thomas, G. V. (2001). Effects of drawing on children's item recall. *Journal of Experimental Child Psychology, 78,* 155–177.

Davies, D., Cole, J., Albertella, G., McCulloch, L., Allen, K., & Kekevian, H. (1996). A model for conducting forensic interviews with child victims of abuse. *Child Maltreatment, 1*(3), 189–199.

De Wet, C. (2010). Victims of educator-targeted bullying: A qualitative study. *South African Journal of Education, 30*(2).

Dedoose (2017). http://www.dedoose.com

Denzin, N. K., & Lincoln, Y. S. (2000). Introduction: The discipline and practice of qualitative research. In N. K. Denzin & Y. S. Lincoln (Eds.), *Handbook of qualitative research* (2nd ed., pp. 1–28). Sage Publications, Inc.

DiLeo, J. H. (1973). *Children's drawings as diagnostic aids.* Brunner/Mazel.

Drennan, J., Brown, M. R., & Sullivan Mort, G. (2011). Phone bullying: Impact on self-esteem and well-being. *Young Consumers, 12*(4), 295–309.

Driessnack, M. (2005). Children's drawings as facilitators of communication: A meta-analysis. *Journal of Pediatric Nursing, 20,* 415–423.

Driessnack, M. (2006). Draw-and-tell conversations with children about fear. *Qualitative Health Research, 16*(10), 1414–1435.

Dunn-Snow, P. (2015). Art therapy: Definitions and dimensions. *Delta Kappa Gamma Bulletin, 81*(4), 79–80.

Edwards, D. (2004). *Art therapy.* Sage.

Egberg-Thyme, K., Wiberg, B., & Sundin, E. (2008). *The entangled butterfly and the blue cactus: Two case studies on time-limited psychodynamic art psychotherapy.* Retrieved from http://urn.kb.se/resolve?urn=urn:nbn:se:umu:diva-3286

Ehring, T., Kleim, B., & Ehlers, A. (2011). Combining clinical studies and analogue experiments to investigate cognitive mechanisms in posttraumatic stress disorder. *International Journal of Cognitive Therapy, 4*(2), 165–177.

Elo, S., Kääriäinen, M., Kanste, O., Pölkki, T., Utriainen, K., & Kyngäs, H. (2014). Qualitative content analysis: A focus on trustworthiness. *Sage Open, 4*(1), 1–10.

Elo, S., & Kyngäs, H. (2008). The qualitative content analysis process. *Journal of Advanced Nursing, 62*(1), 107–115.

Espelage, D. L., Bosworth, K., & Simon, T. R. (2000). Examining the social context of bullying behaviors in early adolescence. *Journal of Counseling & Development, 78*(3), 326–333.

Espelage, D. L., Holt, M. K., & Poteat, V. P. (2010). Individual and contextual influences on bullying. In J. L. Meece & J. S. Eccles (Eds.), *Handbook of research on schools, schooling, and human development* (pp. 146–159). Routledge.

Espelage, D. L., Mebane, S. E., & Swearer, S. M. (2004). Gender differences in bullying: Moving beyond mean level differences. In *Bullying in American schools: A social-ecological perspective on prevention and intervention* (pp. 15–35). Routledge.

Espelage, D. L., & Swearer, S. (2003). Research on school bullying and victimization: What have we learned and where do we go from here? *School Psychology Review, 32,* 365–383.

Everson, M. D., & Boat, B. W. (2002). The utility of anatomical dolls and drawings in child forensic interviews. In M. L. Eisen, J. A. Quas, & G. S. Goodman (Eds.), *Memory and suggestibility in the forensic interview* (pp. 383–408). Lawrence Erlbaum Associates.

Faller, K. C. (1993). *Child sexual abuse: Assessment and intervention issues.* U.S. Department of Health and Human Services, National Center on Child Abuse and Neglect.

Faller, K. C. (2003). *Understanding and assessing child sexual maltreatment.* Sage.

Faller, K. C. (2005). Anatomical dolls: Their use in assessment of children who may have been sexually abused. *Journal of Child Sexual Abuse, 14*(3), 1–21.

Faller, K. C. (2007). *Interviewing children about sexual abuse: Controversies and best practice.* Oxford University Press.

Faller, K. C. (2014). Forty years of forensic interviewing of children suspected of sexual abuse, 1974–2014: Historical benchmarks. *Social Sciences, 4*(1), 34–65.

Finkelhor, D., Ormrod, R. K., & Turner, H. A. (2007). Poly-victimization: A neglected component in child victimization. *Child Abuse & Neglect, 31*(1), 7–26.

Finkelhor, D., Ormrod, R. K., & Turner, H. A. (2009). The developmental epidemiology of childhood victimization. *Journal of Interpersonal Violence, 24*(5), 711–731.

Franklin, M. (1994). A feeling for words: Arnheim on language. *The Arts in Psychotherapy, 21*(4), 261–267.

Gantt, L., & Tripp, T. (2016). Treating preverbal trauma with art therapy. In J. L. King (Ed.), *Art therapy, trauma, and neuroscience: Theoretical and practical perspectives* (pp. 67–99). Routledge.

Gee, S., & Pipe, M. E. (1995). Helping children to remember: The influence of object cues on children's accounts of real events. *Developmental Psychology, 31,* 746–758.

Gentle, M., Powell, M. B., & Sharman, S. J. (2014). Mental context reinstatement or drawing: Which better enhances children's recall of witnessed events and protects against suggestive questions? *Australian Journal of Psychology, 66*(3), 158–167.

Gerbic, P., & Stacey, E. (2005). A purposive approach to content analysis: Designing analytical frameworks. *The Internet and Higher Education, 8*(1), 45–59.

Gilroy, A., & McNeilly, G. (2000). *The changing shape of art therapy: New developments in theory and practice.* Jessica Kingsley Publishers.

Goodenough, F. (1926). *Measurement of intelligence by drawings.* World Book.

Goodman-Brown, T. B., Edelstein, R. S., Goodman, G. S., Jones, D. P., & Gordon, D. S. (2003). Why children tell: A model of children's disclosure of sexual abuse. *Child Abuse & Neglect, 27*(5), 525–540.

Gould, J. W. (1998). *Conducting scientifically crafted child custody evaluations.* Sage.

Gould, J. W., & Stahl, P. M. (2009). The art and science of child custody evaluations. *Family and Conciliation Courts Review, 38*(3), 392–414.

Graham, S. (2010). What educators need to know about bullying behaviors. *Phi Delta Kappan, 92*(1), 66-69.

Graham, S., Bellmore, A. D., & Mize, J. (2006). Peer victimization, aggression, and their co-occurrence in middle school: Pathways to adjustment problems. *Journal of Abnormal Child Psychology, 34*(3), 349–364.

Graneheim, U. H., & Lundman, B. (2004). Qualitative content analysis in nursing research: Concepts, procedures and measures to achieve trustworthiness. *Nurse Education Today, 24*, 105–112. http://dx.doi.org/10.1016/j.nedt.2003.10.001

Gross, J., & Hayne, H. (1998). Drawing facilitates children's verbal reports of emotionally laden events. *Journal of Experimental Psychology: Applied, 14*, 163–179.

Gross, J., & Hayne, H. (1999). Drawing facilitates children's verbal reports after long delays. *Journal of Experimental Psychology: Applied, 5*, 265–283.

Gross, J., Hayne, H., & Drury, T. (2009). Drawing facilitates children's reports of factual and narrative information: Implications for educational contexts. *Applied Cognitive Psychology, 23*, 953–971.

Gross, J., Hayne, H., & Poole, A. (2006). The use of drawing in interviews with children: A potential pitfall. In J. R. Marrow (Ed.), *Focus on child psychology research* (pp. 119–144). Nova.

Gussak, D. (2013). *Art on trial: Art therapy in capital murder cases.* Columbia University Press.

Gussak, D., & Cohen-Liebman, M. S. (2001). Investigation vs. intervention: Forensic art therapy and art therapy in forensic settings. *American Journal of Art Therapy, 40*, 123–135.

Gussak, D., & Rosal, M. L. (2016). An introduction. In D. Gussak & M. Rosal (Eds.), *The Wiley Blackwell handbook of art therapy.* Wiley-Blackwell.

Harachi, T., Catalano, R., & Hawkins, J. D. (1999). United States. In P. K. Smith, Y. Morita, J. Junger-Tas, D. Olweus, R. Catalano, & P. Slee (Eds.), *The nature of school bullying: A cross-national perspective* (pp. 279–295). Routledge.

Harris, S. (2010). Toward a better way to interview child victims of sexual abuse. *National Institute of Justice Journal, 267*, 12–15. www.ncjrs.gov/pdffiles1/nij/233282.pdf.

Harris-Williams, M. H. (2010). *The aesthetic development: The poetic spirit of psychoanalysis: Essays on Bion, Meltzer, Keats.* Karnac Books.

Hawker, D. S., & Boulton, M. J. (2000). Twenty years' research on peer victimization and psychosocial maladjustment: A meta-analytic review of cross-sectional studies. *The Journal of Child Psychology and Psychiatry and Allied Disciplines, 41*(4), 441–455.

Haynie, D. L., Nansel, T., Eitel, P., Crump, A. D., Saylor, K., Yu, K., & Simons-Morton, B. (2001). Bullies, victims, and bully/victims: Distinct groups of at-risk youth. *The Journal of Early Adolescence, 21*(1), 29–49.

Hebert, M., Cenat, J., Blais, M., Lavoie, F., & Guerrier, M. (2016). Child Sexual abuse, bullying, cyberbullying, and mental health problems among high school students: A moderated mediated model. *Depression and Anxiety, 33*, 623–629.

Henning, E., van Rensburg, W., & Smit, B. (2004). *Finding your way in qualitative research.* Van Schaik.

Hershkowitz, I., Lamb, M. E., Orbach, Y., Katz, C., & Horowitz, D. (2012). The development of communicative and narrative skills among preschoolers: Lessons from forensic interviews about child abuse. *Child Development, 83*, 611–622.

Hiltz, B., & Bauer, G. (2003). Drawings in forensic interviews of children. *APRI Update, 16*(3), 1–2.

Hinz, L. D. (2009). *Expressive therapies continuum: A framework for using art in therapy*. Routledge.

Hoffman, C. D. (2005). Investigative interviewing: Strategies and techniques. *The International Foundation for Protection Officers*. https://www.ifpo.org/wp-content/uploads/2013/08/inter viewing.pdf

Holt, M. K., Finkelhor, D., & Kantor, G. K. (2007a). Hidden forms of victimization in elementary students involved in bullying. *School Psychology Review, 36*, 345–360.

Holt, M. K., Finkelhor, D., & Kantor, G. K. (2007b). Multiple victimization experiences of urban elementary school students: Associations with psychosocial functioning and academic performance. *Child Abuse & Neglect, 31*(5), 503–515.

Home Office. (2007). *Achieving best evidence in criminal proceedings: Guidance on interviewing victims and witnesses, and using special measures*. Home Office.

Hong, J. S., Espelage, D. L., Grogan-Kaylor, A., & Allen-Meares, P. (2012). Identifying potential mediators and moderators of the association between child maltreatment and bullying perpetration and victimization in school. *Educational Psychology Review, 24*(2), 167–186.

Hopperstad, M. H. (2008). How children make meaning through drawing and play. *Visual Communication, 7*(1), 77–96.

Howells, V., & Zelnik, T. (2009). Making art: A qualitative study of personal and group transformation in a community arts studio. *Psychiatric Rehabilitation Journal, 32*(3), 215.

Hritz, A. C., Royer, C. E., Helm, R. K., Burd, K. A., Ojeda, K., & Ceci, S. J. (2015). Children's suggestibility research: Things to know before interviewing a child. *Anuario de Psicología Jurídica, 25*(1), 3–12.

Huss, E. (2009). "A coat of many colors": Towards an integrative multilayered model of art therapy. *The Arts in Psychotherapy, 36*(3), 154–160.

Jensen, T. K., Gulbrandsen, W., Mossige, S., Reichelt, S., & Tjersland, O. A. (2005). Reporting possible sexual abuse: A qualitative study on children's perspectives and the context for disclosure. *Child Abuse & Neglect, 29*(12), 1395–1413.

Jolley, R. P. (2010). *Children and pictures: Drawing and understanding*. Wiley-Blackwell.

Junge, M., & Asawa, P. (1994). *A history of art therapy in the United States*. The American Art Therapy Association, Inc.

Junge, M., & Linesch, D. (1993). Our own voices: New paradigms for art therapy research. *The Arts in Psychotherapy, 20*, 61–67.

Juvonen, J., Graham, S., & Schuster, M. A. (2003). Bullying among young adolescents: The strong, the weak, and the troubled. *Pediatrics, 112*(6), 1231–1237.

Kanetsuna, T., & Smith, P. K. (2002). Pupil insights into bullying, and coping with bullying: A binational study in Japan and England. *Journal of School Violence, 1*(3), 5–29.

Karlholm, D. (2009). Action drawing: Notes on the (dis) revelatory nature of drawing. *Konsthistorisk Tidskrift, 78*(2), 92–103.

Katz, C. (2014). The dead end of domestic violence: Spotlight on children's narratives during forensic investigations following domestic homicide. *Child Abuse & Neglect, 38*, 1976–1984.

Katz, C., Barnetz, Z., & Hershkowitz, I. (2014). The effect of drawing on children's experiences of investigations following alleged child abuse. *Child Abuse & Neglect, 38*(5), 858–867.

Katz, C., & Hamama, L. (2013). "Draw me everything that happened to you": Exploring children's drawings of sexual abuse. *Children and Youth Services Review, 35*(5), 877–882.

Katz, C., & Hershkowitz, I. (2010). The effects of drawing on children's accounts of sexual abuse. *Child Maltreatment, 15*(2), 171–179.

Katz, C., & Hershkowitz, I. (2012). The effect of multipart prompts on children's testimonies in sexual abuse investigations. *Child Abuse & Neglect, 36*(11), 753–759.

Katz, C., & Hershkowitz, I. (2013). Repeated interviews with children who are the alleged victims of sexual abuse. *Research on Social Work Practice, 23*(2), 210–218.

Kelley, S. J. (1984). The use of art therapy with sexually abused children. *Journal of Psychosocial Nursing and Mental Health Services, 22*(12), 12–18.

Kellogg, R. (1969). *Analyzing children's art*. Mayfield Publishing Company.

Kemp, A. R. (2017). *Abuse in society: An introduction*. Waveland Press, Inc.

Kempe, A. (2007). *A good knight for children: C. Henry Kempe's quest to protect the abused child.* Book-locker.com, Inc.

Kendall-Tackett, K. A. (1992). Beyond anatomical dolls: Professionals' use of other play therapy techniques. *Child Abuse & Neglect, 16*(1), 139–142.

King, J. (2016a). Art therapy a brain based profession. In D. Gussak & M. Rosal (Eds.), *The Wiley Blackwell handbook of art therapy* (pp. 77–90). Wiley-Blackwell.

King, J. (Ed.). (2016b). *Art therapy, trauma, and neuroscience: Theoretical and practical perspectives.* Routledge/Taylor & Francis Group, LLC.

Knutson, J. F., & Schartz, H. A. (1997). Evidence pertaining to physical abuse and neglect of children as parent-child relational diagnoses. *DSM-IV Sourcebook, 3,* 713–804.

Kohlbacher, F. (2006). The use of qualitative content analysis in case study research. *Forum Qualitative Sozialforschung/Forum: Qualitative Social Research, 7*(1). www.qualitative-research.net/index.php/fqs/article/view/75/153

Koppitz, E. M. (1968). *Psychological evaluation of children's human figure drawings.* Grune & Stratton.

Koppitz, E. M. (1984). *Psychological evaluation of human figure drawings by middle school pupils.* Grune & Stratton.

Kramer, E. (1993). *Art as therapy with children.* Magnolia Street Publishers.

Krippendorff, K. (2013). *Content analysis. An introduction to its methodology* (3rd ed.). Sage Publications.

Lamb, M. E., & Brown, D. A. (2006). Conversational apprentices: Helping children become competent informants about their own experiences. *British Journal of Developmental Psychology, 24*(1), 215–234.

Lamb, M. E., & Thierry, K. L. (2005). Understanding children's testimony regarding their alleged abuse: Contributions of field and laboratory analog research. In D. M. Teti (Ed.), *Handbook of research methods in developmental psychology* (pp. 489–508). Blackwell Publishers.

Lamb, M. E., Brown, D. A., Hershkowitz, I., Orbach, Y., & Esplin, P. W. (2018). *Tell me what happened: Questioning children about abuse.* John Wiley & Sons.

Lamb, M. E., Hershkowitz, I., Orbach, Y., & Esplin, P. W. (2008). *Tell me what happened: Structured investigative interviews of child victims and witnesses* (Vol. 36). Wiley-Blackwell.

Lamb, M. E., La Rooy, D., Malloy, L. C., & Katz, C. (2011). *Children's testimony: A handbook of psychological research and forensic practice.* Wiley Publications.

Lamb, M. E., Orbach, Y., Hershkowitz, I., Esplin, P. W., & Horowitz, D. (2007). A structured forensic interview protocol improves the quality and informativeness of investigative interviews with children: A review of research using the NICHD investigative interview protocol. *Child Abuse & Neglect, 31*(11), 1201–1231.

Leclerc, J. (2006). The unconscious as paradox: Impact on the epistemological stance of the art psychotherapist. *The Arts in Psychotherapy, 33,* 130–134.

Leclerc, J. (2012). When the image strikes: Postmodern thinking and epistemology in art therapy. In H. Burt (Ed.), *Art therapy and postmodernism: Creative healing through a prism* (pp. 367–378). Jessica Kingsley.

Liang, H., Flisher, A. J., & Lombard, C. J. (2007). Bullying, violence, and risk behavior in South African school students. *Child Abuse & Neglect, 31*(2), 161–171.

Limber, S., & Small, M. (2003). State laws and policies to address bullying in schools. *School Psychology Review, 32,* 445–455.

Lincoln, Y. S., & Guba, E. G. (1985). *Naturalistic inquiry.* Sage.

Lindberg, M. A., Chapman, M. T., Samsock, D., Thomas, S. W., & Lindberg, A. W. (2003). Comparisons of three different investigative interview techniques with young children. *The Journal of Genetic Psychology, 164*(1), 5–28.

Lippert, T., Cross, T. P., Jones, L., & Walsh, W. (2009). Telling interviewers about sexual abuse: Predictors of child disclosure at forensic interviews. *Child Maltreatment, 14*(1), 100–113.

Lippert, T., Cross, T. P., Jones, L., & Walsh, W. (2010). Suspect confession of child sexual abuse to investigators. *Child Maltreatment, 15*(2), 161–170.

Lusebrink, V. B. (1990). *Imagery and visual expression in therapy.* Plenum Press.

Lusebrink, V. B. (2014). Art therapy and neural basis of imagery: Another possible view. *Art Therapy: Journal of the American Art Therapy Association, 31*(2), 87–90.

Lyon, T. D., Ahern, E. C., & Scurich, N. (2012). Interviewing children versus tossing coins: Accurately assessing the diagnosticity of children's disclosures of abuse. *Journal of Child Sexual Abuse, 21*(1), 19–44.

Lyon, T. D., Lamb, M. E., & Myers, J. (2009). Legal and psychological support for the NICHD interviewing protocol. *Child Abuse & Neglect, 33,* 71–74.

Machover, K. (1980). *Personality projection in the drawing of the human figure: A method of personality investigation.* Charles C. Thomas.

Macleod, E., Gross, J., & Hayne, H. (2013). The clinical and forensic value of information that children report while drawing. *Applied Cognitive Psychology, 27*(5), 564–573.

Malloy, L. C., Brubacher, S. P., & Lamb, M. E. (2011). Expected consequences of disclosure revealed in investigative interviews with suspected victims of child sexual abuse. *Applied Developmental Science, 15*(1), 8–19.

Mayring, P. (2000). Qualitative content analysis. [28 paragraphs]. *Forum Qualitative Sozialforschung/ Forum: Qualitative Social Research [On-line Journal], 1*(2). http://qualitative-research.net/fqs/ fqs-e/2-00inhalt-e.htm

McConeghey, H. (1994). Arnheim and art therapy. *The Arts in Psychotherapy, 21*(4), 287–293.

McNamee, C. M. (2004). Using both sides of the brain: Experiences that integrate art and talk therapy through scribble drawings. *Art Therapy, Journal of the American Art Therapy Association, 21*(3), 136–142.

McNiff, S. (1994). Rudolf Arnheim: A clinician of images. *The Arts in Psychotherapy, 21*(4), 249–259.

Melinder, A., Alexander, K., Cho, Y. I., Goodman, G., Thoresen, C., Lonnum, K., & Magnussen, S. (2010). Children's eyewitness memory: A comparison of two interviewing strategies as realized by forensic professionals. *Journal of Experimental Child Psychology, 105,* 156–177.

Merriam, S. B. (2009). *Qualitative research in practice: Examples for discussion and analysis.* Jossey-Bass.

Miller, T. W., Veltkamp, L. J., & Janson, D. (1987). Projective measures in the clinical evaluation of sexually abused children. *Child Psychiatry and Human Development, 18*(1), 47–57.

Miller-Perrin, C. L., & Perrin, R. D. (2013). *Child maltreatment: An introduction* (3rd ed.). Sage Publications.

Moon, C. H. (2001). *Studio art therapy: Cultivating the artist identity in the art therapist.* Jessica Kingsley.

Morrell, M. (2011). Signs and Symbols: Art and language in art therapy. *Journal of Clinical Art Therapy, 1*(10, 25–32.

Myers, J. E. (1998). *Legal issues in child abuse and neglect practice* (Vol. 1). Sage Publications, Inc.

Nansel, T. R., Overpeck, M., Pilla, R. S., Ruan, W. J., Simons-Morton, B., & Scheidt, P. (2001). Bullying behaviors among US youth: Prevalence and association with psychosocial adjustment. *Jama, 285*(16), 2094–2100.

National Center for Education Statistics. U.S. Department of Education, NCES. www.https//nces.ed.gov

National Crime Prevention Council. www.ncpc.org/

National Sexual Violence Resource Center, NSVRC. (2012). www.nsvrc.org

Naumburg, M. (1987). *Dynamically oriented art therapy: Its principles and practices.* Magnolia Street Publishers.

O'Donohue, W. T., & Fanetti, M. (2016). *Forensic interviews regarding child sexual abuse. A guide to evidence-based practice.* Springer.

Olafson, E. (2012). A call for field-relevant research about child forensic interviewing for child protection. *Journal of Child Sexual Abuse, 21*(1), 109–129.

Olweus, D. (1993). Bully/victim problems among schoolchildren: Long-term consequences and an effective intervention program. In S. Hodgins (Ed.), *Mental disorder and crime* (pp. 317–349). Sage Publications.

Olweus, D. (1994). Bullying at school: Basic facts and effects of a school-based intervention program. *Journal of Child Psychology and Psychiatry, 35*(7), 1171–1190.

Olweus, D. (2013). School bullying: Development and some important challenges. *Annual Review of Clinical Psychology, 9,* 751–780.

Orbach, Y., Hershkowitz, I., Lamb, M. E., Sternberg, K. J., Esplin, P. W., & Horowitz, D. (2000). Assessing the value of structured protocols for forensic interviews of alleged child abuse victims. *Child Abuse & Neglect, 24,* 733–752.

Patterson, T., & Hayne, H. (2011). Does drawing facilitate older children's reports of emotionally laden events? *Applied Cognitive Psychology, 25,* 119–126.

Pepler, D., Jiang, D., Craig, W., & Connolly, J. (2008). Developmental trajectories of bullying and associated factors. *Child Development, 79*(2), 325–338.

Pipe, M. E., Lamb, M. E., Orbach, Y., & Esplin, P. W. (2004). Recent research on children's testimony about experienced and witnessed events. *Developmental Review, 24*(4), 440–468.

Pipe, M. E., & Salmon, K. (2009). Dolls, drawings, body diagrams, and other props: Role of props in investigative interviews. In K. Kuehnle & M. Connell (Eds.), *The evaluation of child sexual abuse allegations: A comprehensive guide to assessment and testimony* (pp. 365–395). Wiley-Blackwell.

Pipe, M. E., & Wilson, J. C. (1994). Cues and secrets: Influences on children's event reports. *Developmental Psychology, 30*(4), 515.

Poole, D. A., & Bruck, M. (2012). Divining testimony? The impact of interviewing props on children's reports of touching. *Developmental Review, 32*(3), 165–180.

Poole, D. A., & Dickinson, J. J. (2014). Comfort drawing during investigative interview: Evidence of the safety of a popular practice. *Child Abuse & Neglect, 38,* 192–201.

Poole, D. A., & Lamb, M. E. (1998). *Investigative interviews of children: A guide for helping professionals.* American Psychological Association.

Poole, D. A., & Lamb, M. E. (2009). *Investigative interviews of Children: A guide for helping professions.* American Psychological Association.

Poole, D. A., & Lindsay, D. S. (1996). Effects of parents. suggestions, interviewing techniques, and age on young children's event reports. In *Recollections of trauma: Scientific research and clinical practice.* Plenum Press.

Poole, D. A., & Lindsay, D. S. (2001). Children's eyewitness reports after exposure to misinformation from parents. *Journal of Experimental Psychology: Applied, 7*(1), 27.

Poole, D. A., & Lindsay, D. S. (2002). Reducing child witnesses' false reports of misinformation from parents. *Journal of Experimental Child Psychology, 81*(2), 117–140.

Robbins, A. (2000). *The artist as therapist.* Jessica Kingsley.

Robbins, A., & Sibley, L. B. (1976). *Creative art therapy.* Brunner/Mazel.

Rowlands, A. L. (2003). *The use of drawing to facilitate children's event memory recall* (Doctoral dissertation). University of York, England.

Rubin, J. A. (1999). *Art therapy: An introduction.* Psychology Press.

Rubin, J. A. (2001). *Approaches to art therapy: Theory and technique.* Taylor & Francis Group, LLC.

Salmon, K. (2001). Remembering and reporting by children: The influence of cues and props. *Clinical Psychology Review, 21,* 267–300.

Salmon, K. (2006). Toys in clinical interviews with children: Review and implications for practice. *Clinical Psychologist, 10*(2), 54–59.

Salmon, K., & Pipe, M. E. (1997). Props and children's event reports: The impact of a 1-year delay. *Journal of Experimental Child Psychology, 65*(3), 261–292.

Salmon, K., & Pipe, M. E. (2000). Recalling an event one year later: The impact of props, drawing and a prior interview. *Applied Cognitive Psychology, 14,* 261–292.

Salmon, K., Bidrose, S., & Pipe, M. E. (1995). Providing props to facilitate children's event reports: A comparison of toys and real items. *Journal of Experimental Child Psychology, 60,* 174–194.

Salmon, K., Roncolato, W., & Gleitzman, M. (2003). Children's report of emotionally laden events: Adapting the interview to the child. *Applied Cognitive Psychology, 17*(1), 65–79.

Saywitz, K., Lyon, T., & Goodman, G. (2018). When interviewing children: A review and update. In B. Klika & J. Conte (Eds.), *The APSAC handbook on child maltreatment* (pp. 310–329). Sage Publications, Inc.

Schreier, M. (2012). *Qualitative content analysis in practice.* Sage Publications.

Shams, H., Garmaroudi, G., & Nedjat, S. (2017). Factors related to bullying: A qualitative study of early adolescent students. *Iranian Red Crescent Medical Journal, 19*(5), 1–11.

Sheppard, D. I., & Zangrillo, P. A. (1996, March–April). Coordinating investigations of child abuse. *Voices,* 21–25.

Shetgiri, R. (2013). Bullying and victimization among children. *Advances in Pediatrics, 60*(1), 33.

Shields, A., & Cicchetti, D. (2001). Parental maltreatment and emotion dysregulation as risk factors for bullying and victimization in middle childhood. *Journal of Clinical Child Psychology, 30*(3).

Skaife, S. (2001). Making visible: Art therapy and intersubjectivity. *International Journal of Art Therapy: Inscape, 6*(2), 40–50.

Smith, P. K., Cowie, H., Olafsson, R. F., & Liefooghe, A. P. (2002). Definitions of bullying: A comparison of terms used, and age and gender differences, in a Fourteen – Country international comparison. *Child Development, 73*(4), 1119–1133.

Sorenson, E., Bottoms, B., & Perona, A. (1997). *Handbook on intake and forensic interviewing in the children's advocacy center setting.* Office of Juvenile Justice and Delinquency Prevention.

Soundy, C. S. (2012). Searching for deeper meaning in children's drawings. *Childhood Education, 88*(1), 45–51.

Steele, W. (2003). Using drawing in short-term trauma resolution. In C. Malchiodi (Ed.), *Handbook of art therapy* (pp. 139–151). Guilford Press.

Steele, W., & Kuban, C. (2013). *Working with grieving and traumatized children and adolescents: Discovering what matters most through evidence-based sensory interventions.* John Wiley & Sons, Inc.

Steele, W., & Malchiodi, C. (2012). *Trauma-informed practices with children and adolescents.* Taylor & Francis.

Steinmetz, M. (1997). *Interviewing for child sexual abuse: Strategies for balancing forensic and therapeutic factors.* Jalice.

Stemler, S. (2001). An overview of content analysis. *Practical Assessment, Research & Evaluation, 7*(17), 137–146.

Sternberg, K. J., Lamb, M. E., Davies, G. M., & Westcott, H. L. (2001). The memorandum of good practice: Theory versus application. *Child Abuse & Neglect, 25*(5), 669–681.

Sternberg, K. J., Lamb, M. E., Hershkowitz, I., Yudilevitch, L., Orbach, Y., Esplin, P. W., & Hovav, M. (1997). Effects of introductory style on children's abilities to describe experiences of sexual abuse. *Child Abuse & Neglect, 21*(11), 1133–1146.

Stopbullying.gov. (n.d.). A federal government website managed by the U.S. Department of Health & Human Services 200 Independence Avenue, S.W. – Washington, D.C. 20201.

Strange, D., Garry, M., & Sutherland, R. (2003). Drawing out children's false memories. *Applied Cognitive Psychology, 17*(5), 607–619.

Sullivan, J., & Sheehan, V. (2016). What motivates sexual abusers of children? A qualitative examination of the spiral of sexual abuse. *Aggression and Violent Behavior, 30,* 76–87.

Thomas, G. V., & Jolley, R. P. (1998). Drawing conclusions: A re-examination of empirical and conceptual bases for psychological evaluation of children from their drawings. *British Journal of Clinical Psychology, 37,* 127–139.

Thoresen, C., Lønnum, K., Melinder, A., & Magnussen, S. (2009). Forensic interviews with children in CSA cases: A large sample study of Norwegian police interviews. *Applied Cognitive Psychology, 23*(7), 999–1011.

Thyme, K. E., Wiberg, B., Lundman, B., & Graneheim, U. H. (2013). Qualitative content analysis in art psychotherapy research: Concepts, procedures, and measures to reveal the latent meaning in pictures and the words attached to the pictures. *The Arts in Psychotherapy, 40*(1), 101–107.

Tinnin, L. (1990). Biological processes in nonverbal communication and their role in the making and interpretation of art. *American Journal of Art Therapy, 29*(1), 9–13.

Tobey, A. E., & Goodman, G. S. (1992). Children's eyewitness memory: Effects of participation and forensic context. *Child Abuse & Neglect, 16*(6), 779–796.

Tsaousis, I. (2016). The relationship of self-esteem to bullying perpetration and peer victimization among schoolchildren and adolescents: A meta-analytic review. *Aggression and Violent Behavior, 31,* 186–199.

Ulman, E. (1992). Art therapy: Problems of definition. *American Journal of Art Therapy, 30*(3), 78–88.

Van der Kolk, B. A. (2014). *The body keeps the score: Brain, mind, and body in the healing of trauma.* Viking.

Vick, R. M. (2003). A brief history of art therapy. In C. Malchiodi (Ed.), *Handbook of art therapy* (pp. 5–15). Guilford Press.

Vieth, V. (2008). Letter to the editor. *Child Abuse & Neglect, 32*, 1003–1006.

Wadeson, H. (2010). *Art psychotherapy* (2nd ed.). John Wiley & Sons, Inc.

Wadeson, H. (2016). An eclectic approach to art therapy revisited. In D. Gussak & M. Rosal (Eds.), *The Wiley Blackwell handbook of art therapy*. Wiley-Blackwell.

Wakefield, H., & Underwager, R. (1998). The application of images in child abuse investigations. In J. Prosser (Ed.), *Image-based research: A sourcebook for qualitative researchers* (pp. 176–194). Falmer Press.

Wesson, M., & Salmon, K. (2001). Drawing and showing: Helping children to report emotionally laden events. *Applied Cognitive Psychology, 15*, 301–320.

Wheelock, A., Bebell, D., & Haney, W. (2000). What can student drawings tell us about high-stakes testing in Massachusetts. *Teachers College Record*.

Willcock, E., Morgan, K., & Hayne, H. (2006). Body maps do not facilitate children's reports of touch. *Applied Cognitive Psychology, 20*, 607–615.

Williams, S. J. (2001). *Can the child witness provide accurate testimony?* (Doctoral dissertation). University of Bristol.

Williams, S. J., Wright, D. B., & Freeman, N. H. (2002). Inhibiting children's memory of an interactive event: The effectiveness of a cover-up. *Applied Cognitive Psychology, 16*(6), 651–664.

Yates, A., Beutler, L. E., & Crago, M. (1985). Drawings by child victims of incest. *Child Abuse & Neglect, 9*(2), 183–189.

Afterword

Forensic Art Therapy was intended to introduce and acquaint the reader with this nontraditional application of the modality and investigative method. I envisioned the text as a compendium of resourceful material for individuals including the novice as well as the seasoned professional engaged in investigating, interviewing and testifying on behalf of victims and witnesses. These stratums interrelate and underlie Forensic Art Therapy. Legal proceedings, testimonial capability and practical tips and strategies for effective witnessing and compelling testimony were shared. Ethical issues inherent in the forensic arena were identified. Understanding how drawing functions in investigative interviews and what drawing affords the child, the team and the process was considered. Finally, a forensic art therapy investigative interview process, the CIG, was explained, and recent research and associated findings were discussed.

I hope the material is helpful and useful as well as applicable for students and professionals dedicated and devoted to assisting vulnerable populations. Disclosure of experienced events that may be traumatic in nature is a process that invokes support, empowerment and acceptance. Within the context of an art therapy-based investigative interview process, a victim or witness may be able to express what one is unable to say or perhaps give voice to the unspeakable due to the facilitative effect of drawing. Acceptance and understanding of a forensic art therapy investigative interview process may provide an alternative to traditional verbal techniques and contribute another dimension to the realm of investigative interviewing.

Finally, I conclude this labour of love with a few reflections pertaining to an integral and essential staple associated with my work.

How we perceive a box of crayons and what we choose to do with the crayons provokes innumerable potentialities . . .

A Box of Crayons

A box of crayons is neither simple nor concrete
A box of crayons is replete with subtle offerings that speak
Scribbled marks on paper organized or maybe not very neat
Self-expression via imagery is hardly incomplete
A new box of crayons with colors so bright yet the intensity is not in plain sight
A box of crayons holds the key perhaps to one's identity
For sure you must know that inside each box is a treasure trove
Each color each stick is so significant
For one color is not merely a singular entity

If two or more merge they become blended beyond singularity

Remove the paper wrapping and you shall see a new way of emoting

Eliciting a lack of uniformity and cultivating individuality, originality and creativity

Mentality is conveyed through expression that manifests through graphic synergism

Thoughts and feelings expressed underscored with symbolism and metaphors

The crayons and colors whether static or swirl give rise to critical analysis that will reveal

Just what we are thinking but have tried to conceal

Unaware of our thought processes too latent to prevail

The crayons cultivate and implore exploration galore

Through color and shape, kinesthetic or more we uncover what once was too aberrant to ignore

Just who we are and what we have hidden may be revealed without bidding

Thus, a box of crayons provides a new way of seeing and believing

We record our thoughts and what we have learned through visual record in which introspection is born

My teaching philosophy is predicated upon keeping people engaged and informed

About real-world application of the things, we self-discover, apply and learn

Marcia Sue Cohen-Liebman, PhD

Glossary of Terms

Adversary System of Justice

The most effective way to arrive at just results. It is predicated upon opposing sides presenting evidence or knowledge and facts by witnesses to an impartial trier of fact. The goal is the acquisition of the truth. This practice necessitated that the trier of fact was provided with informed and unbiased material, including opinions proffered by experts.

Analogue Studies

Frequently employed in research pertaining to investigative interviewing. An analogue study simulates a real and objective experience. An analogue design means that variables are known.

Beyond a Reasonable Doubt

This is the standard or legal burden of proof that the prosecution must meet in a criminal proceeding, meaning that no other explanation logically can be determined from the facts.

Burden of Proof

This is what must be met in court to prove someone's guilt. It is the responsibility of the prosecution to meet the burden in order to prove that a crime was committed. The standard or amount of proof varies depending upon the nature of the case. There are three standards: preponderance of evidence, clear and convincing evidence and beyond reasonable doubt. In a civil matter, the burden of proof is "a preponderance of evidence", which is considered the least demanding of the burdens of proof, meaning it is the easiest to meet with 51% certainty (Myers, 2011) whereas if the matter is a criminal case, then the accused must be found guilty or not guilty.

Charge Enhancements

Contextual information that can contribute to the determination of charges (as per law enforcement, who decides whether to present evidence to the prosecution, who will make a determination), as well as the identification of additional arenas to explore within an investigative interview. Examples for child sexual abuse include use of force, bribes, threats, coercion, pornography, etc.

Child Advocacy

This is an overarching term that refers to individuals, professionals and organizations that advocate for children's rights.

Child Maltreatment

Child maltreatment is a general term that encompasses various forms of child abuse and neglect, including physical abuse, sexual abuse, emotional abuse and psychological abuse (Miller-Perrin & Perrin, 2012).

Civil Proceedings

Civil proceedings encompass many types of litigation, including cases that may be associated with family court or juvenile court where child welfare is a primary focus. The aim is typically centered around protection and resolution. Civil proceedings are distinct from criminal proceedings. In a civil case, the burden to be met to establish guilt is a "preponderance of evidence".

Closing Statements/Arguments

Summation of the evidence presented during a legal proceeding such as a trial.

Common Interview Guideline (CIG)

An art therapy-based investigative interview guideline for facilitating fact-finding that is predicated upon the juxtaposition of art therapy principles and practices with legal or judicial tenets. The CIG blends these diametric elements resulting in a forensically oriented but emotionally supportive process. It advocates fluidity and flexibility with regard to the five phases that comprise it: rapport building, developmental screening/skills assessment, anatomy identification, fact-finding and closure. The CIG is not a standardized and scripted process. It incorporates the use of free or nondirected drawing in the capacity of an open-ended prompt.

Competency

Ascertainment of a child's ability to comprehend truth, as well as understanding the need to tell the truth. Assessment of competency (within a legal or forensic context including an investigative interview) in conjunction with a child's cognitive capabilities and communication skills will impact child's perceived ability to provide testimony and be examined on direct and cross examination.

Content Analysis

Content analysis is a systematic, replicable technique for textual analysis in which content categories are identified through coding (Stemler, 2001). The technique of content analysis is not restricted to the domain of textual analysis. Originally intended as a quantitative methodology for communication or textual data, qualitative content analysis was expanded interdisciplinarily in the mid-20th century and broadened to encompass other forms of media. Through this differentiation, qualitative content analysis expanded into different models of communication, including nonverbal (Wheelock et al., 2000).

Core Details

Primary or significant material in a fact-finding process that typically remains constant.

Credibility Assessment

Contributes to establishing or determining believability. With regard to a child, concern is directed at whether a child's testimony (or disclosure in an investigative interview) is sound (perhaps reliable) and will be believed on the witness stand. Types of memory are considered with regard to how a child stores and recalls information. Whether or not information is episodic (referring to a personal experienced event) or scripted (generalized knowledge about a topic or previous knowledge about something) may factor into consideration and contribute to evaluation with regard to determination of credibility.

Criminal Proceedings

The defendant (offender) must be found to have committed a crime with unlawful intent. The focus is directed at offender accountability. The defendant must be found to be guilty or not guilty beyond a reasonable doubt. Strict adherence to rules of evidence pervades criminal proceedings which are directed toward punitive measures, restitution and even rehabilitation.

Cross Examination

Objectives and strategies associated with this judicial process are designed to impeach the testimony and ultimately credibility of a witness. Cross is known as an antibiased device (Myers, 1992).

Curriculum Vitae (CV) for Court

Summary or expanded outline showcasing an individual's qualifications. Qualifications are highlighted, including education, background, training and experience, as well as areas related to expertise such as publications, awards, affiliations, academic positions, professional presentations, prior court involvement as a witness, areas of specialization and other criteria.

Daubert

A test to determine reliability. Referred to as relevance analysis. Adopted in 1993 for federal courts, it is a two-step process. When enacted, a judge conducts an inquiry to assess the reliability of scientific principles supporting an expert's testimony. In assessing reliability, the judge considers whether the principle can be and has been tested to determine its reliability and validity and how often accurate results are yielded (Myers, 1992, 2019).

Dedoose

An electronic data management and cross-platform application for analyzing qualitative and mixed-methods research (Gerbic & Stacey, 2005). It is considered an alternative to qualitative data analysis software and has been used for social science research. It is described as "[a] cross-platform application for analyzing qualitative and mixed methods research with text, photos, audio, videos, spreadsheet data and more" (www.dedoose.com, 2017).

Defendant

The defendant is the accused and is the person or perhaps a body such as an institution that is being brought up on charges or a legal action.

Deposition

A deposition is a proceeding that is used by attorneys to ascertain the content of the testimony of an opposing witness. Depositions consist of sworn testimony taken in the presence of a recorder and are certified by the witness as correct. No trier of fact is present. Normally the attorney who requested the deposition asks the questions, but the witness has counsel present to object or advise not to answer.

Dialogical

Dialogue or communication with another to explore a subject or topic.

Direct Testimony

Designed to elicit the facts in the most effective manner from a witness.

Discovery Process

The collection or exchange of information or evidence conducted prior to a legal proceeding (pretrial).

Drawing Effect

The drawing effect pertains to the use of drawing in relation to the recall of memory and its effectiveness in assisting children to communicate about experience(s). Underlying mechanisms attributed to the drawing effect have been identified (postulated) and continue to be studied. The role of imagery with regard to the encoding, storage, retrieval and recall of information in various contexts is also considered with regard to the drawing effect.

Episodic Memory

Episodic memory fosters understanding of an episode or event that is rooted in personal experience. Episodic details contribute to the assessment and understanding of a particular experience. Episodic memory (event-specific) versus script memory (generalized knowledge) is considered with regard to assessing whether information communicated is forensically relevant.

Epistemology

Knowledge or the theory of knowledge.

Evidence

Encompasses a wealth of forms. Evidence can include testimony by witnesses, and it is also defined as written documents or objects. Evidence is admissible unless some rule exists to exclude it. Evidence is defined as "any matter, verbal or physical that can be used to support the existence of a factual proposition (Lilly, 1996, p. 2). It is considered anything "which tends to provide or disprove" a matter in question and is directly related to the case.

Expert Witness

An individual testifying as an expert witness garners special privileges in court. The person must demonstrate and meet certain qualifications to be considered and presented in the guise of an expert witness including knowledge, skill, education, training and experience (Rule 702). An expert may testify in the form of an opinion and may answer hypothetical questions.

Fact-Finder

The fact-finder is an impartial individual (judge) or body (jury) tasked with determining the facts of a matter (case) based upon the evidence presented.

Forensic Art Therapy

The juxtaposition of art therapy principles and practices with standard forensic procedure and protocol. This application extended the modality beyond evaluation/diagnoses and intervention/treatment into the realm of investigation, a novel application.

Forensic Relevance

Forensic relevance refers to information and the manner in which it is disclosed relative to an experienced event. Episodic details contribute to the assessment and understanding of a particular experience. Forensic relevance increases and is enhanced with the quantity as well as the quality of the information disclosed by a child within an investigative process. Moreover, consideration of this information (as it relates to a forensic or legal matter) distinguishes a fact-finding process (investigative) from a clinical process.

Forensic Science

The application of scientific methods, principles and techniques to evaluate evidence related to judicial inquiry.

Frye Rule

Also known as the general acceptance rule – a test to determine reliability when expert testimony is based on scientific principles or techniques of questionable reliability. It means that the trier of fact must be convinced that the principle is generally accepted as reliable in the relevant professional community. Such evidence may garner a special admissibility hearing to thwart the presentation of unreliable scientific principles or techniques in court. The Frye rule was the standard for many years before Daubert was recognized. Four sources of evidence can be used to establish general acceptance in accordance with the Frye rule: informed testimony (testify to general acceptance), relevant literature, guidelines from professional organizations and prior court decisions.

Hearsay

Hearsay is a statement made to a witness by someone not in the court. It is offered by a witness to prove the truth of the fact and may be admissible in certain circumstances.

Hired Gun

This is an expert hired by one side to present an opinion favorable to that side. Compensation is customary, and as such the expert is typically brought into court to support a position or an agenda.

Interviewing Tool

Media such as aids, tools and props including dolls, puppets and body templates used in a supportive capacity in an investigative (interview) process.

Judiciary Aid

Provides evidentiary material that may be admissible in a judicial proceeding.

Jury

A group composed of individuals from the community. To serve as a juror, one must be a U.S. citizen, 18 years old and live in the jurisdiction of the court.

Jury Instructions

The judge will instruct the jury about rules of law relative to the case following closing arguments and prior to deliberations.

Juvenile Court

Juvenile court handles civil or family law matters. A range of cases that pertain to protection of children are addressed, including abuse, neglect and delinquency.

Latent

Symbolic or underlying meaning related to the manifest content of something such as an image.

Lay Witness

A fact witness or an individual who testifies about facts pertaining to a topic or a subject that the witness has experience with or personal knowledge. Direct observations may be provided. A lay witness may not offer an opinion on the matter before the court.

Leading Question

The answer is contained within the question.

Legal Proceedings

In the United States there are two types of legal proceedings: civil and criminal. Each has a respective burden of proof that is distinct and distinguishes the type of proceeding.

Line of Questioning

A line of questioning refers to a single question or a series of related questions asked by the examining attorney.

Litigation

Action directed at resolution of a legal matter in dispute.

Mandated Reporting

Legal obligation by certain professionals to report suspicions of abuse or suspected abuse to designated authorities or agencies.

Manifest

That which is visible, such as in a drawing the collection of lines, shapes and colors. Overt or obvious content.

Media

For purposes of this manuscript and as designated, art or drawing materials.

Mock Court

Mock court is based on the simulation and enactment of a trial (judicial proceeding). Mock court is relevant to understanding and interacting in a court of law and offers an experiential component to acquire knowledge about courtroom participation. Litigation tactics are practiced to prepare participants with an understanding of courtroom strategy to enhance performance on the witness stand.

Multidisciplinary Team

Representatives from a host of disciplines combine their respective skills, strengths, backgrounds and expertise to foster a collaborative and cooperative affiliation in a coordinated effort to address an issue such as child abuse investigations.

Novel Scientific Evidence

Novel scientific evidence is subjected to a special admissibility test if proffered expert testimony is believed to be based upon novel scientific principles. A hearing may be conducted to evaluate the admissibility of the evidence. The special admissibility test is applicable when expert testimony is judged by the court to be less accessible to lay analysis than other types of evidence. The special admissibility test is applicable when expert testimony is based on scientific principles of questionable reliability (Myers et al., 1989).

Objections

In a trial, rules exist that pertain to procedure, conduct of participants and the submission of evidence. To ensure a fair process, objections may be raised in response to the areas where rules are applied. There are three broad types of objections: procedure and rules, admission and use of testimony and evidence and conduct of a participant with regard to procedure or evidence.

Ontology

Reality or existence.

Open-Ended Prompts

Open-ended or invitational prompts are used to elicit free recall.

Opening Statements

The prosecutor will introduce and present the allegations or the charges against the defendant. As such, the prosecution presents and sets the stage or the groundwork of the case in court. The prosecutor will explain to the trier of fact what will be proved and how that will happen through presentation of witnesses and evidence. The prosecutor will explain in a conversational manner who the client is and why the client and, by extension the trier of fact, is in the courtroom. This individual will explain the circumstances that gave rise to the proceeding. The prosecutor will inform the judge or jury what will be presented (the evidence) and who will be providing information (the witnesses to be called) to help the trier of fact understand the facts of the case.

Opinion Testimony

Opinion testimony is offered based upon reliable certainty. Only an expert may provide an opinion. Experts are not supposed to speculate or guess as to an opinion.

Overruled

When an objection is overruled by the judge, the witness is allowed to answer the question because the judge disagrees with the reason offered by the objecting attorney.

Peer Review

Process whereby feedback and/or commentary is offered. Ideally, this material is provided in a constructive and helpful manner by peers or team members.

Peripheral

Minor or secondary material that is supportive information related to core or central material. Peripheral details may change; however, core material should remain constant and consistent.

Plaintiff

The plaintiff (civil court) may also be referred to as the complainant or in a criminal case, the prosecution. It is the job of the prosecution, meaning the attorney who represents the state or the entity pursuing justice (so to speak), to meet the burden of proof. As such, the prosecution is responsible for bringing legal action (on behalf of an individual or entity).

Preliminary Hearing

A judge determines if enough evidence has been rendered by the prosecution to justify a defendant standing trial.

Preponderance of Evidence

According to Myers (2011), this is the least demanding of the burdens of proof, meaning it is the easiest to meet with 51% certainty. This standard is associated with civil proceedings.

Prosecution

The person or entity responsible for bringing an action on behalf of an individual (or entity) in criminal court.

Redirect Testimony

This type of testimony allows for rehabilitation of a witness and follows cross.

Rehabilitative Evidence

This type of evidence is designed to inform or assist the judge and/or jury to understand a fact or matter. Rehabilitative evidence does not necessarily rise to the same level of expertise as substantive evidence, meaning that the information presented by an expert is offered to dispel misconceptions and to educate the judge or jury about a topic.

Relationality

Emerged as a theme in the research presented in Part V and encompassed categories that foster interaction and dialogue, given that the CIG is an interactive and dynamic process.

Relevance Analysis (Daubert)

A test to determine reliability. It is a two-step process. When enacted, a judge conducts an inquiry to assess the reliability of scientific principles supporting an expert's testimony. In assessing reliability, the judge considers whether a principle can be and has been tested to determine its reliability and validity and how often accurate results are yielded.

Reporting Mandates

These require certain professionals to report suspected child abuse cases and/or neglect to designated authorities.

Rule 702

The federal rule that is the basic principle governing admission of expert testimony in a court of law.

Script Memory

This is considered generalized knowledge about a topic or previous knowledge/understanding about something rather than episodic or event specific memory.

Scripting

This is an exercise designed to understand the expectations as a witness, primarily in terms of direct testimony and to prepare accordingly. Questions and answers are written out and areas of weakness are identified in advance and in anticipation of cross examination. This exercise is a tool used for preparation for witnesses and prosecutors so that expectations are known and to avert surprises on the witness stand.

Self-Generated Cues

Prompts produced by a person that facilitate retrieval of information or memory recall. Self-generated cues have been determined to promote recall of experience (Butler et al., 1995; Gross et al., 2009; Macleod et al., 2013). They may reduce reliance on external retrieval cues (Butler et al., 1995; Jolley, 2010; Wesson & Salmon, 2001; Williams, 2001). Self-generated cues such as drawing have been identified as contributing to increased verbalization and pictorial details as well as disclosure of forensically relevant information (Cohen-Liebman, 2017, 2020, 2021).

Social Science

Refers to human behavior and society. In court, expert witnesses provide information to assist the trier of fact to understand the behavior of individuals and groups of people.

Subpoena

A command by the court and merits a response. A subpoena has an official court seal and is signed by a court clerk, judge or attorney.

Substantive Evidence

Substantive evidence is offered to prove a matter or an issue. This type of evidence is associated with a high level of expertise and may be directed at an opinion by an expert.

Sustained

Response to an objection made in a court of law. If sustained, the witness may not answer the question because the judge agrees with the objecting attorney that the question is improper under the rules of evidence.

Testimony

Testimony is admitted into evidence via a procedure in which the witness is identified, testifies under oath and is subjected to questioning by both plaintiff and defense attorneys.

Theme

A theme is given to identify each particular line of questioning (on direct examination).

Trial

This is a judicial procedure conducted to determine if the rights of a person or entity have been violated. Rules govern how a trial is to be conducted, whether in real life or in a mock scenario.

Trier of Fact

A trier of fact, meaning a judge or jury, is the person or body responsible for determining the fact at issue in a court of law. The trier of fact is tasked with concluding from the evidence the facts of the case. The trier of fact is provided with informed and unbiased material, including opinions proffered by experts to determine the truth (Myers, 1992). The trier of fact has sole province on deciding the issue before the court.

Verdict

Decision or judgement about a legal matter in dispute.

Voir Dire

Foundation for expertise and may be conducted as a separate hearing (hearing within a hearing) to establish qualification of an expert. Intended to establish an individual's credentials for testimonial capability. Means "to speak the truth" and is a preliminary examination of a potential witness's qualifications. The proceeding is directed at establishing the qualifications of the witness in order for the witness to present testimony.

Wilkerson v. Pearson (1985)

This was a landmark case that established the credibility of art therapists as expert witnesses and the validity of drawings as judiciary aids.

Witness

Witnesses are integral to the trial system and provide various roles within the court. They educate, inform, disabuse commonly held misperceptions and provide expert opinions. They present evidence in various forms, including information and knowledge.

References

Butler, S., Gross, J., & Hayne, H. (1995). The effect of drawing on memory performance in young children. *Developmental Psychology, 31*, 597–608.

Cohen-Liebman, M. S. (2017). *Drawing and disclosure of experienced events in an art therapy investigative interview process with school aged children: A qualitative comparative analogue study* (Doctoral dissertation). Retrieved from ProQuest Dissertations and Theses database.

Cohen-Liebman, M. S. (2020). Drawing to disclose: Empowering child victims and witnesses in investigative interviews. In M. Berberian & B. Davis (Eds.), *Art therapy practices for resilient youth* (pp. 285–312). Routledge.

Cohen-Liebman, M. S. (2021). Drawing to disclose: Findings from an art therapy-based investigative interview process. In V. Huet & L. Kapitan (Eds.), *The art of practice & research: Art therapy international practice research conference proceedings* (pp. 77–85). Cambridge Scholars Publishing.

Dedoose (2017). http://www.dedoose.com

Gerbic, P., & Stacey, E. (2005). A purposive approach to content analysis: Designing analytical frameworks. *The Internet and Higher Education, 8*(1), 45–59.

Gross, J., Hayne, H., & Drury, T. (2009). Drawing facilitates children's reports of factual and narrative information: Implications for educational contexts. *Applied Cognitive Psychology, 23*, 953–971.

Jolley, R. P. (2010). *Children and pictures: Drawing and understanding.* Wiley-Blackwell.

Lilly, G. C. (1996). *An introduction to the law of evidence* (3rd ed.). West Publishing Co.

Macleod, E., Gross, J., & Hayne, H. (2013). The clinical and forensic value of information that children report while drawing. *Applied Cognitive Psychology, 27*(5), 564–573.

Miller-Perrin, C. L., & Perrin, R. D. (2012). *Child maltreatment: An introduction* (3rd ed.). Sage Publications, Inc.

Myers, J. E. B. (1992). *Legal issues in child abuse and neglect.* Sage Publications Inc.

Myers, J. E. B. (2011). Juvenile court. In J. E. B. Myers (Ed.), *The APSAC handbook on child maltreatment* (3rd ed., pp. 53–66). Sage Publications, Inc.

Myers, J. E. B. (2019). *Mental health law in a nutshell.* West Academic Publishing.

Myers, J. E. B., Bays, J., Becker, J., Berliner, L., Corwin, D. L., & Saywitz, K. J. (1989). Expert testimony in child sexual abuse litigation. *Nebraska Law Review, 68*(1–2), 1–145.

Stemler, S. (2001). An overview of content analysis. *Practical Assessment, Research & Evaluation, 7*(17), 137–146.

Wesson, M., & Salmon, K. (2001). Drawing and showing: Helping children to report emotionally laden events. *Applied Cognitive Psychology, 15*, 301–320.

Wheelock, A., Bebell, D., & Haney, W. (2000). What can student drawings tell us about high-stakes testing in Massachusetts. *Teachers College Record.*

Wilkerson v. Pearson, 210 New Jersey, Super. 333, 335. Chancery Division. (1985).

Williams, S. J. (2001). *Can the child witness provide accurate testimony?* (Doctoral dissertation). University of Bristol.

Index

Note: numbers in *italics* indicate a figure.

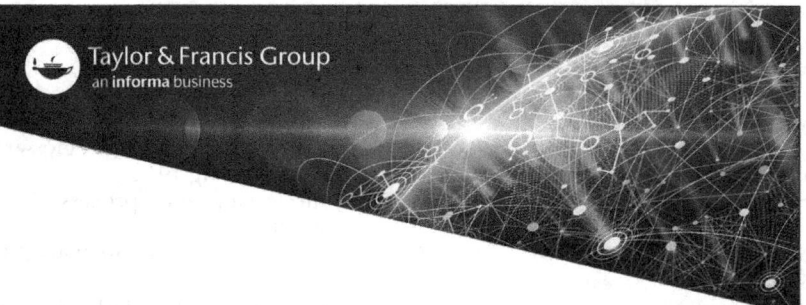
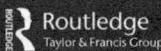
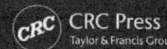

9781032125343